A Manual of Neonatal Intensive Care

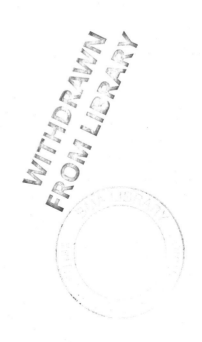

A Manual of Neonatal Intensive Care

FIFTH EDITION

Janet M Rennie MA MD FRCP FRCPCH FRCOG DCH
Consultant and Senior Lecturer in Neonatal Medicine, Elizabeth Garrett Anderson
Obstetric Wing, University College London Hospitals, London, UK

Giles S Kendall BSc(Hons) MB BS MRCPCH PhD
Consultant in Neonatal Medicine, Elizabeth Garrett Anderson Wing, University
College London Hospitals, London, UK
Honorary Senior Lecturer in Neonatal Neuroimaging and Neuroprotection, Institute
for Women's Health, University College London, London, UK

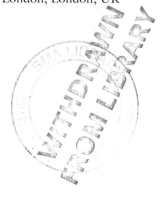

CRC Press
Taylor & Francis Group
Boca Raton   London   New York

CRC Press is an imprint of the
Taylor & Francis Group, an **informa** business

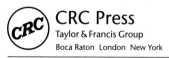

CRC Press
Taylor & Francis Group
6000 Broken Sound Parkway NW, Suite 300
Boca Raton, FL 33487-2742

© 2013 by Taylor & Francis Group, LLC
CRC Press is an imprint of Taylor & Francis Group, an Informa business

No claim to original U.S. Government works

Printed by CPI on sustainably sourced paper
Version Date: 20130426

International Standard Book Number-13: 978-0-340-92771-7 (Paperback)

Visit the Taylor & Francis Web site at
http://www.taylorandfrancis.com

and the CRC Press Web site at
http://www.crcpress.com

Contents

Abbreviations

ACTH	adrenocorticotrophic hormone
ACV	assist control ventilation
ADH	antidiuretic hormone
AED	antiepileptic drug
AFP	alpha-fetoprotein
ANP	atrial natriuretic peptide
APTT	activated partial thromboplastin time
ARF	acute renal failure
ASD	atrial septal defect
BAPM	British Association of Perinatal Medicine
BP	blood pressure
BPD	bronchopulmonary dysplasia
CAH	congenital adrenal hyperplasia
CCAM	congenital cystic adenomatoid malformation
CDH	congenital diaphragmatic hernia
CHD	congenital heart disease
CLD	chronic lung disease
CMV	cytomegalovirus
CNS	central nervous system
CNST	Clinical Negligence Scheme for Trusts
CONS	coagulase-negative staphylococci
CP	cerebral palsy
CPAP	continuous positive airways pressure
CRP	C-reactive protein
CSF	cerebrospinal fluid
CSVT	cerebral sinovenous thrombosis
CTG	cardiotocogram (cardiotocography)
CVC	central venous catheter
CVP	central venous pressure
CVS	chorionic villus sampling
CXR	chest X-ray
DAT	direct antiglobulin
DDH	developmental dysplasia of the hip
DEHSI	diffuse excessive high signal intensity
DIC	disseminated intravascular coagulation
DMSA	dimercaptosuccinic acid
DPG	diphosphatidylglycerol
DPL	dipalmitoyl lecithin
DZ	dizygotic
EBM	expressed breast milk
ECF	extracellular fluid
ECG	electrocardiogram
ECMO	extracorporeal membrane oxygenation
EDD	expected date of delivery

EDF	end-diastolic flow
EEG	electroencephalogram
ELBW	extremely low birth weight
EPO	erythropoietin
ETT	endotracheal tube
FBC	full blood count
FDP	fibrin degradation product
FFP	fresh frozen plasma
FHR	fetal heart rate
FISH	fluorescent in-situ hybridization
FRC	functional residual capacity
GBS	group B beta haemolytic streptococcus
GFR	glomerular filtration rate
GMH-IVH	germinal matrix–intraventricular haemorrhage
hCG	human chorionic gonadotrophin
HCV	hepatitis C virus
HDN	haemolytic disease of the newborn
HELLP	hypertension, elevated liver enzymes and low platelets
HFNC	high-flow nasal cannula
HFOV	high frequency oscillatory ventilation
HIE	hypoxic ischaemic encephalopathy
HIV	human immunodeficiency virus
HPA	human platelet antigen
HMD	hyaline membrane disease
HTLV	human T-cell lymphotropic virus
HVS	high vaginal swab
IAP	intrapartum antibiotic prophylaxis
ICH	intracranial haemorrhage
ICP	intracranial pressure
IEM	inborn error of metabolism
IMV	intermittent mandatory ventilation
IPL	intraparenchymal lesion
IPPV	intermittent positive pressure ventilation
IUGR	intra-uterine growth restriction
IV	intravenous
IVC	inferior vena cava
IVH	intraventricular haemorrhage
IVIG	intravenous immunoglobulin
LBW	low birth weight
LP	lumbar puncture
MAP	mean airway pressure
MAPCA	major aortopulmonary collateral arteries
MAS	meconium aspiration syndrome
MCAD	medium chain acyl-CoA dehydrogenase
MCT	medium chain triglyceride
MCUG	micturating cysto-urogram
MRI	magnetic resonance imaging
MRSA	meticillin-resistant *Staphylococcus aureus*
MZ	monozygotic
NCEPOD	National Confidential Enquiry into Patient Outcome and Death
NCPAP	nasal continuous positive airway pressure

NEC	necrotizing enterocolitis
NG	nasogastric
NHSLA	NHS Litigation Authority
NICE	National Institute for Health and Clinical Excellence
NICU	neonatal intensive care unit
NIPE	Newborn and Infant Physical Examination
NNAP	National Neonatal Audit Programme
NNU	neonatal unit
NO	nitric oxide
NPSA	National Patient Safety Agency
NSC	national screening committee
NT	nuchal translucency
PAPP-A	pregnancy-associated plasma protein A
PCR	polymerase chain reaction
PCV	packed cell volume
PDA	patent ductus arteriosus
PEEP	positive end expiratory pressure
PHVD	post-haemorrhagic ventricular dilatation
PIE	pulmonary interstitial emphysema
PIH	pregnancy-induced hypertension
PIP	peak inspiratory pressure
PKU	phenylketonuria
PN	parenteral nutrition
PPHN	persistent pulmonary hypertension of the newborn
PPROM	preterm premature rupture of the membranes
PSV	pressure support ventilation
PT	prothrombin time
PTV	patient trigger ventilation
PUJ	pelvi-ureteric junction
PUV	posterior urethral valve
PVH	periventricular haemorrhage
PVL	periventricular leukomalacia
RBC	red blood cell
RCOG	Royol College of Obstetricians and Gynaecologists
RCPCH	Royal College of Paediatrics and Child Health
RDS	respiratory distress syndrome
ROP	retinopathy of prematurity
RSV	respiratory syncytial virus
RV	right ventricle
RVT	renal vein thrombosis
SGA	small for gestational age
SIMV	synchronized intermittent mandatory ventilation
SIPPV	synchronized intermittent positive pressure ventilation
SNRI	serotonin–norepinephrine reuptake inhibitors
SSRI	selective serotonin reuptake inhibitors
SVC	superior vena cava
SVT	supraventricular tachycardia
T_e	expiratory time
TGV	thoracic gas volume
T_i	inspiratory time
TPN	total parenteral nutrition

TRAb	thyrotrophin receptor stimulating antibody
TRH	thyrotrophin releasing hormone
TSH	thyroid–stimulating hormone
TST	tuberculin skin test
TTN	transient tachypnoea of the newborn
TTTS	twin–twin transfusion syndrome
UAC	umbilical artery catheter
USS	ultrasound scan
UTI	urinary tract infection
UVC	umbilical venous catheter
VEGF	vascular endothelial growth factor
VG	volume guarantee
VKDB	vitamin K deficiency bleeding
VLBW	very low birth weight
VSD	ventricular septal defect
VTV	volume targeted ventilation
VUJ	vesico-ureteric junction
WBC	white blood cell (count)
WPW	Wolff–Parkinson–White syndrome

Preface

Preface to the 5th edition

Unbelievably, it is now over 30 years since the publication of the first edition of *A Manual of Neonatal Intensive Care* (1981). In that time, generations of residents and neonatal nurses have come to rely on the book as a source of sound practical advice with an explanation of the reasons behind the recommended course of action. As before, we have aimed to distill the wisdom acquired from long experience into a readable text supplemented with lists and tables. In a rapidly advancing field such as this, some management strategies are controversial and lack an evidence base, and in this situation we have suggested the course of action which we have found most helpful while briefly outlining the alternatives. We hope that all who read and use the book will find it helpful, and that it will stimulate their enthusiasm for neonatology, a specialty which is challenging, varied and exciting. No working day on a neonatal unit is ever the same; but an understanding of normal neonatal physiology and the common response of the newborn to illness can help everyone who works in this pressurized environment to respond and plan treatment appropriately. That has been our aim in writing the book. We have referred to the baby as he and the mother as she for simplicity, and hope that this does not offend the reader.

Acknowledgements

There were times during the period between the publication of the fourth edition and delivery of the material for this fifth edition when the team at Hodder Arnold, and more recently CRC Press, must have despaired of ever seeing the book published. Thanks are due to Gavin Jamieson for his unending patience and encouragement and to Francesca Naish for finally setting us deadlines which we managed to meet. Our colleagues at UCLH have remained as supportive as ever. We would like to thank Fiona Maguire and Elizabeth Erasmus for input into the chapters on parenteral and enteral nutrition, respectively. We gratefully acknowledge the work of Cliff Robertson, sole author of the first three editions. Particular thanks are due to our spouses, Ian Watts and Kin Yee Shiu, and to the younger generation of Kendalls, Han Se and Lin Mei, who have seen their father less than ever over the last year or so.

Janet Rennie, Giles Kendall
London
June 2012

PART 1
Organization and delivery of care

1

Epidemiology and neonatal outcomes

Key points
- Around 7% of all births are of low birth weight (<2500 g) or preterm (<37 completed weeks of pregnancy).
- About 15 per 1000 pregnancies are twin pregnancies, but 25% of all babies with very low birth weight (<1500 g) are twins or higher multiples.
- The outcome for babies born at 25 weeks of gestation or less has improved, but there is still a high risk of death, with motor and/or learning difficulty in a high percentage of the survivors.

Epidemiology: definitions in perinatal medicine

Neonatologists need knowledge and understanding of current international, national and local statistics in order to provide adequate information during the counselling of parents when there is the expectation of a preterm or complicated birth. To make sense of the published statistics it is first essential to define the terms that are commonly used in perinatal medicine (Fig. 1.1).

- **Preterm:** any baby born below 37 weeks' completed gestation, i.e. less than 259 completed days of gestation, measured from the first day of the last normal menstrual period. **Extreme preterm** is often used to describe delivery below 26 weeks' completed gestation.
- **Low birth weight:** a baby with a birth weight of less than 2500 g (up to and including 2499 g).
- **Very low birth weight:** birth weight of less than 1500 g.
- **Extremely low birth weight (ELBW):** birth weight of less than 1000 g.
- **Stillbirth:** a stillborn baby is defined as a baby born after the 24th week of pregnancy who did not show any signs of life at any time after being born. If there are no signs of life at birth, a baby born before 24 weeks' gestation is classed as a miscarriage. The stillbirth rate (see below) is the number of stillbirths expressed per 1000 live births and stillbirths.
- **Live birth:** a birth at any gestation (including below 24 weeks) where the baby shows signs of life after delivery.
- **Neonatal death:** the death of a neonate born with signs of life (see above) within the first 28 days after delivery. It is often subdivided into **early neonatal death** within the first 7 days of life and **late neonatal death** occurring after the 7th day but before the completed 28th day of life.

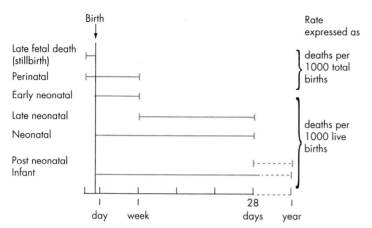

Fig. 1.1 Definition of stillbirth and infant mortality rates

- **Infant mortality rate:** the number of infants dying within the first year of life per 1000 live births.
- **Perinatal mortality rate:** the number of stillbirths and neonatal deaths in the first week of life per 1000 total births (live and stillborn).

The Millennium Development Goal is to achieve a two-thirds reduction in mortality in children younger than 5 years by 2015; there was a worldwide reduction of 3.1 million neonatal deaths between 1990 and 2010. Most of the deaths still occur in sub-Saharan Africa or south Asia, with less than 1% of the deaths in high-income countries.

The value of understanding the outcomes of babies born prematurely extends beyond the counselling of parents and families. Such studies allow the guidance of health and social care provision, both in the perinatal period and extending into childhood.

Around 7% of all births in the UK are of babies with birth weight <2500 g, and about 1.2% of all births are of babies <1500 g. The percentage of ELBW babies has risen considerably from 0.27% in 1983 to around 0.5% in 2009. Unfortunately national data in England and Wales did not record gestational age until 2005, when the linkage with the NHS numbers for babies was established. Data are available for Scotland from the early 1970s and show a steadily rising trend with an increase in the number of multiple preterm births.

The availability of gestational age-specific mortality data for England and Wales shows that there is, as expected, a steadily declining mortality as gestational age increases, with the exception of post-dates babies of 42 weeks (Fig. 1.2). Note the logarithmic scale on the *y*-axis.

Within the UK, the mortality figures vary considerably by the ethnic origin of the mother, and international comparisons of perinatal mortality data are often performed. The World Health Organization has recommended that babies of gestational age below 22 weeks and birth weight below 500 g should be excluded from comparisons between countries because of differences in incidence and reporting of births of such babies.

Valuable information about the outcome of extremely preterm babies born in England and Wales is available from the two EPICure studies. These were prospective, geographical studies which included all deliveries below 26 weeks, for 1995 and 2006. The survival figures for babies admitted to the neonatal intensive care unit (NICU) born below 26 weeks are shown in Fig. 1.3; improvement in survival is seen between the 1995 and 2006 cohort, which is significant at 24 and 25 weeks' gestation.

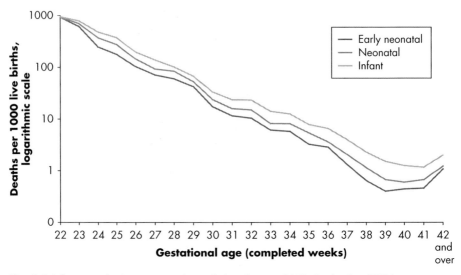

Fig. 1.2 Infant mortality by gestational age, babies born in 2008, England and Wales. *Source:* ONS childhood mortality statistics, unpublished data. Data from Office of National Statistics, compiled by Allison Mc Farlane; from Rennie and Robertson (2012) with permission

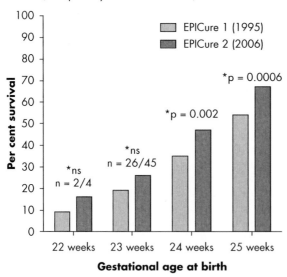

Fig. 1.3 Outcome of babies born below 26 weeks' gestation

There are, however, limitations in the applicability of national geographical outcomes due to small numbers of the most extreme preterm infants and changing patterns of neonatal care with time (use of surfactant, antenatal steroids, temperature control, increased use of non-invasive ventilation, centralization of care, minimal handling, etc.).

Neonatal outcomes

In surviving infants born extremely preterm, a number of significant medical morbidities are seen which appear largely unchanged across the 10 years between EPICure 1 and 2 (Fig. 1.4). Although cerebral palsy (CP) has long been monitored as

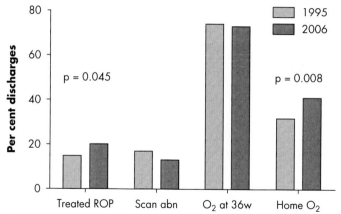

Fig. 1.4 Major neonatal morbidities at discharge in infants born <26 weeks. abn, abnormal; ROP, retinopathy of prematurity; w, weeks

an adverse outcome of preterm birth, and there is no doubt that there is an increased risk of CP in extremely preterm babies, far more survivors of preterm birth are disabled by their learning problems.

Severe motor outcomes such as CP are relatively rare, affecting approximately 10% of very low birth weight babies. In EPICure 1, in infants born at less than 26 weeks, 14% of surviving babies showed moderate motor disability and 4% severe motor disability. Cognitive outcomes appear to be a continuum of disability, with a very significant fall away in cognitive outcomes in babies born at less than 32 weeks of gestation (Fig. 1.5). However, when assessed by the requirement for special educational needs provision in school, the effects of even mild degrees of prematurity can be detected (Fig. 1.6).

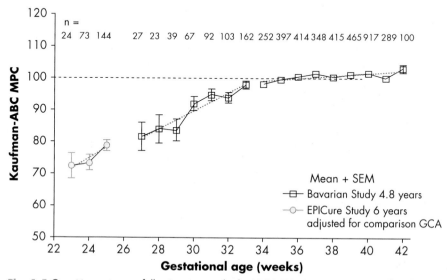

Fig. 1.5 Cognitive outcomes following preterm birth. ABC MPC, Assessment Battery for Children Mental Processing Composite; GCA, general conceptual ability; SEM, standard error of the mean. With permission from Marlow *et al.* (2005)

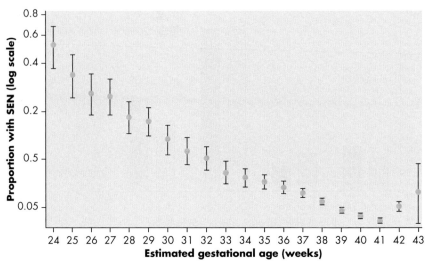

Fig. 1.6 Percentage of children with special educational needs (SEN) by gestation at delivery (note the logarithmic scale). Redrawn from Mackay *et al.* (2010). From Rennie and Robertson (2012) with permission

It should also be recognized that the assessment of neurodisability following extreme preterm birth varies dependent on the age of assessment. Although severe disability is readily detectable early, some of the milder forms of disability are not detectable until later childhood. In addition to adverse motor and cognitive outcomes, more detailed follow-up has demonstrated significantly increased behavioural symptoms (especially social, thought and attention difficulties), emotional disorders such as anxiety and depression, and autistic-like disorders. Our understanding of how prematurity affects individuals into adult life is currently very limited.

When discussing outcomes with families it is important to recognize that it takes knowledge and experience to pitch the information at the right level, to include enough detail to explain but not confuse; overall we aim to be 'honest but not cruel'. Trainee paediatricians are often asked about a baby's prognosis, partly because they are present on the neonatal unit at all hours of the day and night and partly because parents like to canvass a second opinion. It cannot be stressed too often that much damage can be done by inaccurate and ill-timed advice. As in any other area of neonatology, if in doubt, ask! Encourage your consultants to document what they have already told the parents and to let you sit in on the counselling sessions. Always remember that there is a huge spectrum of disability, that there are always exceptions, and that quality of life is a value judgement. Conflicting advice gives rise to anger and bitter resentment in parents.

In discussing the outcome after preterm birth, survival rates depend where you start, e.g. survival of all/live born/admitted to NICU. As a rule of thumb, in surviving infants the rates of serious impairments are currently:

- 23 weeks – 60% (mean IQ 72)
- 24 weeks – 60% (mean IQ 76)
- 25 weeks – 40% (mean IQ 80).

However, recognize that outcomes are:

1. individual and therefore quoting a mass of statistics is of limited value
2. different for boys and girls
3. related to birth weight, and birth weight for gestation as well as gestation alone.

References

Mackay, DF, Smith, GC, Dobbie, R, *et al.* (2010) Gestational age at delivery and special educational need: retrospective cohort study of 407,503 schoolchildren. *PLoS Medicine*, 7: e1000289.

Marlow, N, Wolke, D, Bracken, MB, Samara, M (2005) Neurologic and developmental disability at six years of age after preterm birth. *New England Journal of Medicine*, **352**: 9–19.

Further reading

Johnson, S (2007) Cognitive and behavioural outcomes following very preterm birth. *Seminars in Fetal and Neonatal Medicine*, **12**: 363–73.

Marlow, N, Johnson, S (2012) Outcome following preterm birth. In Rennie, JM (ed.) *Rennie & Roberton's Textbook of Neonatology*, 5th edition. Edinburgh: Elsevier, pp. 71–88.

Nosarti, C, Murray, RM, Hack, M (2010) *Neurodevelopmental Outcomes of Preterm Birth: From Childhood to Adult Life.* Cambridge University Press.

Web links

www.statistics.gov.uk

www.nichd.nih.gov/about/org/cdbpm/pp/prog_epbo/epbo_case.cfm (NICHD Neonatal Research Network (NRN): Extremely Preterm Birth Outcome Data)

2

Organization of neonatal care

Key points
- Do not admit babies to neonatal units without a good reason; unnecessary routine admissions include babies of diabetic mothers and babies delivered by instrumental means.
- *In-utero* transfer of a baby expected to require intensive or specialist care is preferable to *ex-utero* transfer, but safe transport *ex utero* is better than leaving a sick baby in a unit which is not staffed or equipped to manage him.
- The current structure of neonatal services in the UK is via 'networks' with nationally agreed quality standards, defined by the National Institute for Health and Clinical Excellence.

Definition of levels of care

More than half a million babies are born every year in the UK; less than 1% of these babies will die. At least half the deaths occur in very premature babies with a birth weight less than 1.5 kg. About 10% of all babies are admitted to UK neonatal units, with a wide range between hospitals from 4% to 35% (Audit Commission 1992). Most of these admissions are for 'special care', for example jaundice requiring phototherapy or blood glucose monitoring. Maternity units which provide 'transitional care', usually on postnatal wards staffed with midwives with experience and expertise in the care of the well small baby, have reduced admissions to their special care nurseries to 5%. About 2% of babies need full intensive care, mainly because they are born very prematurely and need ventilatory support for respiratory distress syndrome. The definitions of levels of care are given in Table 2.1.

For the purpose of this book we will refer to all units as neonatal units (NNUs) rather than intensive care or special care units, and readers will no doubt have a clear – if not altogether unbiased – opinion of what level of care their own units provide. Neonatal units in the UK are now organized into 23 networks. The NHS has published a framework for Neonatal Intensive Care, found at www.dh.gov. uk/en/Publicationsandstatistics/Publications/PublicationsPolicyAndGuidance/ DH_107845. This comprehensive document identifies important regional organization to support NNUs and includes a set of quality standards for the audit of neonatal practice. NNUs within a network usually operate with common protocols and take part in benchmarking and audit, often via contributions to national minimum datasets. The National Institute for Health and Clinical Excellence (NICE) has set quality standards for specialist neonatal care (Table 2.2).

Table 2.1 Categories of babies requiring neonatal care (BAPM 1992, 2001, 2010)

Intensive care

Owing to the complex needs of both the baby and his/her family the ratio of neonatal nurses to baby should be 1 nurse: 1 baby. This nurse should have no other managerial responsibilities during the time of clinical care but may be involved in the support of a less experienced nurse working alongside her in caring for the same baby. Babies in this category include those:

1. receiving any respiratory support via a tracheal tube and in the first 24 hours after its withdrawal;
2. receiving nasal continuous positive airway pressure (NCPAP) for any part of the day and less than 5 days old;
3. below 1000 g current weight and receiving NCPAP for any part of the day and for 24 hours after withdrawal;
4. less than 29 weeks gestational age and less than 48 hours old;
5. requiring major emergency surgery, for the pre-operative period and post-operatively for 24 hours;
6. requiring complex clinical procedures:
   - full exchange transfusion;
   - peritoneal dialysis;
   - infusion of an inotrope, pulmonary vasodilator or prostaglandin and for 24 hours afterwards;
7. any other very unstable baby considered by the nurse-in-charge to need 1:1 nursing;
8. a baby on the day of death.

High-dependency intensive care

The ratio of neonatal nurses qualified in specialty responsible for the care of babies requiring high-dependency care should be 1 nurse: 2 babies. Babies in this category include those:

1. receiving NCPAP for any part of the day and not fulfilling any of the criteria for intensive care;
2. below 1000 g current weight and not fulfilling any of the criteria for intensive care;
3. receiving parenteral nutrition;
4. having convulsions;
5. receiving oxygen therapy and below 1500 g current weight;
6. requiring treatment for neonatal abstinence syndrome;
7. requiring specified procedures that do not fulfil any criteria for intensive care:
   - care of an intra-arterial catheter or chest drain;
   - partial exchange transfusion;
   - tracheostomy care until supervised by a parent;
8. requiring frequent stimulation for severe apnoea.

Special care

A nurse should not be responsible for the care of more than four babies receiving special or normal care.

Special care is provided for all other babies who could not reasonably be expected to be looked after at home by their mother.

Table 2.2 Specialist neonatal care quality standard (NICE 2010)

In-utero and postnatal transfers for neonatal special, high-dependency, intensive and surgical care follow perinatal network guidelines and care pathways that are integrated with other maternity and newborn network guidelines and pathways.
Networks, commissioners and providers of specialist neonatal care undertake an annual needs assessment and ensure each network has adequate capacity.
Specialist neonatal services have a sufficient, skilled and competent multidisciplinary workforce.
Neonatal transfer services provide babies with safe and efficient transfers to and from specialist neonatal care.
Parents of babies receiving specialist neonatal care are encouraged and supported to be involved in planning and providing care for their baby and regular communication with clinical staff occurs throughout the care pathway.
Mothers of babies receiving specialist neonatal care are supported to start and continue breast feeding, including being supported to express milk.
Babies receiving specialist neonatal care have their health and social care plans coordinated to help ensure a safe and effective transition from hospital to community care.
Providers of specialist neonatal services maintain accurate and complete data, and actively participate in national clinical audits and applicable research programmes.
Babies receiving specialist neonatal care have their health outcomes monitored.

■ Provision of intensive care facilities

UK neonatal units have evolved into a three-tier structure (Department of Health 2008), similar to the structure in the USA and Australia:

Level 1: Special care units provide special care for their own local population. Depending on arrangements within their neonatal network, they may also provide some high-dependency services.

Level 2: Local neonatal units provide neonatal care for their own catchment population, except for the sickest babies. They provide all categories of neonatal care, but they transfer babies who require complex or longer-term intensive care to a neonatal intensive care unit, as they are not staffed to provide longer-term intensive care. The majority of babies over 27 weeks of gestation will usually receive their full care, including short periods of intensive care, within their local neonatal unit.

Level 3: Neonatal intensive care units are sited alongside specialist obstetric and feto-maternal medicine services. They provide the whole range of medical (and sometimes surgical) neonatal care for their local population, along with additional care for babies and their families referred from the neonatal network.

The British Association of Perinatal Medicine (BAPM) (1996, 2010) recommends 1–1.9 intensive care cots per 1000 births and suggests that prolonged intensive care (level 1 care) should be undertaken only by those units providing more than 500 days of intensive care per year. While a three-tier system has much to commend it, and similar systems have evolved in other specialties which are 'high-cost low-volume', it does require an organized transport structure. There are disadvantages in transferring small, sick babies long distances after delivery, although careful management during transfer (see p. 62) can reduce the risks. Peaks in demand, unanticipated preterm birth and unexpected severe neonatal illness such as meconium aspiration syndrome or overwhelming group B beta-haemolytic *Streptococcus* sepsis mean that postnatal transport will never be entirely avoided. The alternative is *in-utero* transport, which has its own drawbacks. One is that mothers may remain, undelivered, in the accepting institution for some weeks.

■ References

Audit Commission (1992) *Children First: A Study of Hospital Services.* Audit Commission Services report no. 7. London: HMSO.

BAPM (1992) Categories of babies requiring neonatal care. *Archives of Disease in Childhood,* **67**: 868–9.

BAPM (1996) *Standards for Hospitals Providing Neonatal Care.* London: BAPM, RCPCH.

BAPM (2001) *Standards for Hospitals Providing Neonatal Intensive and High Dependency Care,* 2nd edition. London: BAPM, RCPCH.

BAPM (2010) *Service Standards for Hospitals Providing Neonatal Care,* 3rd edition. London: BAPM, RCPCH.

Department of Health (2008) *Toolkit for High Quality Neonatal Services.* London: DH.

National Institute for Health and Clinical Excellence (2010) *Quality Standards Programme: Specialist Neonatal Care.* Available from www.nice.org.uk and www.ic.nhs.uk.

3

Clinical governance, risk management and legal aspects of neonatal practice

Key points

▪ All neonatologists should strive to produce excellence in care of babies and support for families.

▪ The processes of benchmarking, clinical governance and risk management can help ensure excellence in health care provision.

▪ In England, medical negligence claims are administered through the Clinical Negligence Scheme for Trusts. Individual Trusts can reduce their financial contribution to the scheme by adhering to a series of standards of care.

▪ Deaths of babies in neonatal units often occur as a result of redirection of care from 'preservation of life at all costs' to a package of 'comfort care'. This should not be considered as 'withdrawal of care'.

At the centre of all neonatal practice is the desire to deliver excellence in the care of newborn infants and appropriate support for their families. The Department of Health published a framework for Neonatal Intensive Care in 2009 (www.dh.gov.uk/en/Publicationsandstatistics/Publications/PublicationsPolicyAndGuidance/DH_107845). This 'toolkit' includes a set of quality standards for neonatal care and sets standards for staffing and family-centred care, including advice on network clinical governance. The British Association of Perinatal Medicine and the Royal College of Obstetricians and Gynaecologists also have useful publications which set standards. All neonatal units should collect basic data, including the number of cot days, together with information about critical incidents and serious untoward events, infection rates, complaints, transfers refused, and details of staff compliance with training requirements such as neonatal life support. Units in England contribute data to the National Neonatal Audit Programme (NNAP) (hosted by the Royal College of Paediatrics and Child Health (RCPCH), www.rcpch.ac.uk). Units can benchmark their standards using the NNAP or internationally via the Vermont Oxford Network (www.vtoxford.org) or EuroNeoNet (www.euroneostat.org). All NHS providers are registered with the Care Quality Commission (which replaced the Healthcare Commission in April 2009), which has powers to enforce standards, such as standards of documentation and hygiene.

Clinical governance

Clinical governance is a quality assurance process designed to ensure that standards of care are maintained and improved and that any specific Trust (and the entire NHS) is accountable to patients. Clinical governance is traditionally based on seven key pillars:

1. Clinical effectiveness and research.
   a. Evidence-based medicine; changing practice where appropriate.
   b. Implementing relevant guidelines, e.g. National Institute for Health and Clinical Excellence guidelines.
2. Audit.
3. Risk management.
   a. Complying with protocols.
   b. Learning from incidents and near misses (After Action Review, Critical Incident Reports).
4. Education and training.
5. Patient and public involvement.
6. Using information and IT.
7. Staff management.

Serious untoward incident reporting and investigation

All Trusts have a system in place for reporting untoward incidents and it is the duty of all clinicians to use these systems. Any incident which is deemed to be serious enough triggers a serious untoward incident investigation, which involves collecting statements from all those involved and writing a report with a 'root cause analysis', which is shared with the parents and is a disclosable document in any civil litigation which may ensue. If you are involved in such an investigation it is your duty to cooperate with any request to write a statement. Any such statement should be limited to fact and is not the place for opinion. If the matter goes to litigation, the only people who are allowed the luxury of expressing an opinion are any expert witnesses called by the court.

The National Patient Safety Agency (NPSA, www.nrls.npsa.nhs.uk) published important alerts so that the wider community could learn from mistakes occurring elsewhere in the NHS. The NPSA declared 'never events', some of which are particularly relevant to neonatal cases, such as misplaced nasogastric tubes and failure to respond to oxygen desaturation. The NPSA was formed in 2001 and was closed in 2012, although many of its functions (such as training in root cause analysis) will apparently continue in other forums.

Medical negligence

The NHS funds clinical negligence claims at a national level via the NHS Litigation Authority (NHSLA, an organization established in 1995). The NHSLA administers the Clinical Negligence Scheme for Trusts (CNST). Trusts which meet particular standards are granted a discount (10%, 20% or 30%) from their contributions to the national costs. This system provides a strong financial incentive for Trusts to comply with CNST quality standards and gives these standards more impact.

Medical negligence claims have increased considerably since 1990, and in April 1999 new civil procedure rules were established, following Lord Woolf's report into civil justice published in 1996 (www.dca.gov.uk). The total cost of funding claims via the NHSLA is around £800 million a year, although the NHSLA is liable for at least £16.9 billion in 'forward claims'. Claims involving maternity services form the largest single portion of the NHSLA's budget. This is because the average successful cerebral palsy claim currently costs around £8 million. Claims specifically aimed at neonatal care are less common, but the maternity/neonatal service generally is a high-risk area for any Trust. Common 'high-risk' situations leading to litigation in neonatal medicine are:

■ early neonatal encephalopathy associated with intrapartum hypoxic ischaemia;
■ complications of procedures;
■ hypocarbia associated with periventricular leukomalacia;
■ extreme hyperbilirubinaemia;
■ hypoglycaemia;
■ meningitis.

■ Consent

Consent has to be given by someone with parental responsibility. Parents have the right to decide what treatment their children should receive, and doctors should act in partnership with parents wherever possible. Consent does not have to be in writing to be valid, but it is common practice to use a consent form for major procedures in order to document what the procedure entails, and that the risks and benefits have been explained.

A mother automatically has parental responsibility for her child from birth. A father has parental responsibility only if he is married to the mother when the child is born or has acquired legal responsibility for his child through one of these routes:

■ by jointly registering the birth of the child with the mother;
■ by a parental responsibility agreement with the mother;
■ by a parental responsibility order, made by a court;
■ by marrying the mother of the child.

Living with the mother (even for a long time) does not give a father parental responsibility. In an acute emergency or when the parents refuse to consent to treatment that is immediately necessary for the preservation of the life or long-term health of the child, doctors are empowered to act and should carry out such immediate treatment as they deem necessary.

Very young mothers

Women under the legal age of consent (16) can give consent for procedures on themselves and their baby if they are deemed 'Gillick competent'; that is, able to understand and make decisions. The term arose from a case in which the mother of young teenage girls campaigned against a circular which stated that contraception could be prescribed to young girls without their parent's consent (*Gillick v West Norfolk and Wisbech Area Health Authority* [1985] 3 All ER 402 (HL)).

Very ill mothers

Occasionally an unmarried mother becomes so ill at the time of birth that she requires admission to intensive care herself (examples we have encountered include stroke, serious infection, and hypertension, elevated liver enzymes and low platelets (HELLP) syndrome). In this situation it is good practice to involve her partner and parents, if they are available.

Psychiatrically ill mothers

The starting point in seeking consent in such cases is the mother's consultant psychiatrist. Occasionally, as with mothers who are themselves too ill to give consent, it is necessary to involve social services in order to obtain valid consent for operative procedures.

■ Death

From April 2008 all child deaths in England have been reported to Child Death Overview Panels, as part of child safeguarding. These panels have a statutory responsibility to review and investigate child deaths. Neonatal deaths form the largest group of cases – almost 1800 deaths in the year ending March 2011. Only a small number were deemed to have had potentially modifiable factors. National data can be obtained from the Office for National Statistics. National statistical information on perinatal deaths was formerly reported and analysed by CESDI (Confidential Enquiry into Stillbirth and Death in Infancy), which was established in 1992 and superseded by CEMACH (Confidential Enquiry into Maternal and Child Health) in 2003. The future of CEMACH is under review, with a new service provider promised from April 2012.

When to inform the coroner

Neonatal deaths that should be referred to the coroner include cases in which:

- ■ cause of death is unknown, or sudden and unexpected;
- ■ death occurred during an operation or before recovery from the effects of an anaesthetic;
- ■ the deceased infant was not seen by the certifying medical practitioner, either after death or within 14 days of death;
- ■ death may have been caused by violence or neglect;
- ■ death may have been due to an accident;
- ■ death may have been in any other way unnatural or there are suspicious circumstances.

Once the coroner has completed the investigation, samples taken as part of the autopsy fall under the Human Tissue Act (see below) and should be handled according to parents' wishes. If there is a potential issue of litigation due to neglect by hospital staff, the case should always be discussed with HM Coroner.

All tissue samples taken during a coroner's autopsy are done so under the authority of HM Coroner. According to the Coroners (Amendment) Rules (2005), only samples that have a bearing on the cause of death, or help to establish the identity of the deceased, may be taken during a coronial autopsy. These samples remain under the coroner's jurisdiction until the investigation has been concluded, after which the tissue samples are subject to the Human Tissue Act and require parental consent for further handling. Parents then have the same options as if the autopsy had been conducted by the hospital (i.e. retention and use for research or other purposes, disposal by the hospital, or return to the family), but it is noteworthy that if no communication has been received by the family within 3 months of the coroner's function having ceased, the tissue samples, including all blocks and slides, must be disposed of by the hospital according to current legislation in the UK (HTA Code of Practice 5, 2009).

Scaling down intensive care to 'comfort care'

Many deaths on a neonatal unit are the result of withdrawing full intensive care support, which is not the same as withdrawing all care. In our view, babies should always receive a package of care which involves warmth, hygiene, analgesia (if required), love and nutrition. This package of care is often termed 'comfort care', and if full intensive care appears futile, or the outlook for the baby's quality of life is considered by all those involved to be grim, it is appropriate to re-orientate the goals of care towards comfort care. Sometimes babies who have appeared desperately ill do not in fact die when care is redirected in this way, and parents should be warned that death is not always inevitable in this situation.

Redirecting care towards comfort care should be done only after full consultation with staff and the baby's family. It is unrealistic to expect to achieve complete consensus and the aim is to achieve as much common ground as possible. The RCPCH document 'Witholding or withdrawing life sustaining treatment in children' (2nd edition, 2004, www.rcpch.ac.uk) is a useful resource, as is the 2006 Nuffield Council report (www.nuffieldbioethics.org). When discussing redirection of care it is essential to document that appropriate discussions have been held, and it is always wise to involve a senior colleague. It goes without saying that these discussions should be initiated and chaired by a consultant.

RCPCH framework

The RCPCH put forward five situations in which it may be ethical and legal to consider withholding or withdrawing life-sustaining medical treatment in children. These have been tested in the courts on a number of occasions and are widely accepted. They are:

1. The 'brain dead' child.
2. The 'permanent vegetative state'.
3. The 'no chance' situation where disease is so severe that life-sustaining treatment simply delays death without significant alleviation of suffering, rendering medical treatment inappropriate.
4. The 'no purpose' situation where there may be survival with treatment but the degree of impairment will be so great that it is unreasonable to expect the patient to bear it.
5. The 'unbearable' situation where, in the face of progressive or irreversible illness, the child or family feel that further treatment is more than can be borne.

In neonatal practice most decisions regarding redirection of care relate to criteria 3 and 4.

Dealing with conflict

On rare occasions there is no unanimity of view about treatment (or withdrawal of intensive care) among the team, or between the parents, or between the team and the parents. Reports of 'miracle survivors' do not help, and the usual situation is that parents 'want everything to be done' when the treating team feel that continuing intensive care is futile, painful and likely to result in death or survival of a seriously disabled individual. Some parents want a guarantee of success before agreeing to treatment for their child, and this, too, can cause conflict if the team perceive the prospects of treatment (for example, resuscitation and intensive care at 26 weeks of gestation) to be reasonably good. In this situation, seeking an independent second opinion can be extremely helpful, but on occasion there will have to be recourse to the law.

Landmark legal cases

Tracing cases which have reached litigation provides an interesting perspective on the way that attitudes have changed. In 1981 the court was faced with the case of a baby with Down syndrome; neither the parents nor the baby's consultant paediatrician wanted him to live. In 2012 this attitude towards such a baby appears arcane. Other legal cases show similar shifts, with the courts supporting the view that it is not always appropriate to offer full cardiopulmonary resuscitation to a baby with irrevocable and serious brain injury. In general courts have supported the medical view, with occasional findings in favour of the parents.

■ Further reading

Forman, V (2009) *This Lovely Life: A Memoir of Premature Motherhood*. New York: Mariner Books.

Leigh, MAMS, Rennie JM (2012) Ethical and legal aspects of neonatology. In Rennie, JM (ed.) *Rennie & Roberton's Textbook of Neonatology*, 5th edition. Edinburgh: Elsevier, pp. 102–114.

McHaffie, HE (2001) *Crucial Decisions at the Beginning of Life*. Oxford: Radcliffe Medical Press.

Miller, GD (2007) *Extreme Prematurity: Practices, Bioethics and the Law*. New York: Cambridge University Press.

Nuffield Council on Bioethics (2006) Critical care decisions in fetal and neonatal medicine: ethical issues. Available from www.nuffieldbioethics.org.

Rennie JM, Leigh, B (2008) The legal framework for end-of-life decisions in the UK. *Seminars in Fetal and Neonatal Medicine*, **13**(5): 296–300.

PART 2
Pregnancy and early neonatal life

4

Maternal–fetal medicine for the neonatologist

Key points
- Babies whose mothers were hypothyroid as a result of auto-antibody disease should be reviewed at around 2 weeks of age, with thyroid function tests, because they are at risk of thyrotoxicosis.
- Twin–twin transfusion syndrome diagnosed before 26 weeks carries a significant risk of demise of one twin and brain damage in the survivor.
- Women with preterm membrane rupture should be treated with oral erythromycin and there is an approximately 50% chance that they will deliver within a week, so preparation for preterm delivery should be made.

Prenatal diagnosis of fetal disease

Screening

In the UK the National Screening Committee (NSC) (www.nsc.nhs.uk and www.screening.nhs.uk) manages the programme, evaluating new tests and ensuring that screening tests do more good than harm at reasonable cost. Antenatal screening is optional and the tests which are offered are under constant review. Informed consent is vital and the NSC has a range of information available.

The current recommendations for pregnancy screening in the UK are shown in Fig 4.1. A 'fetal anomaly' ultrasound scan is performed at 18–20 weeks of pregnancy and this is supplemented by an earlier fetal nuchal translucency scan and/or estimation of serum markers. Tests are aimed at the detection of Down syndrome and other fetal abnormalities which can be diagnosed with ultrasound imaging. Tests for syphilis, HIV, hepatitis B, maternal blood group, sickle cell and thalassaemia are offered. Testing for rubella susceptibility is offered in order that women with low antibody levels can seek vaccination; this test does not detect congenital rubella.

Laboratory tests on maternal serum used in screening

High levels of alpha-fetoprotein (AFP) (above 2.5 multiples of the median) are present in maternal serum at 15–22 weeks of pregnancy when the fetus has an open neural tube defect. Once fetal abnormality is excluded, a high AFP level is linked to adverse outcomes of pregnancy, including low birth weight and placental abruption. Interpretation is dependent on gestational age and the presence of a single fetus.

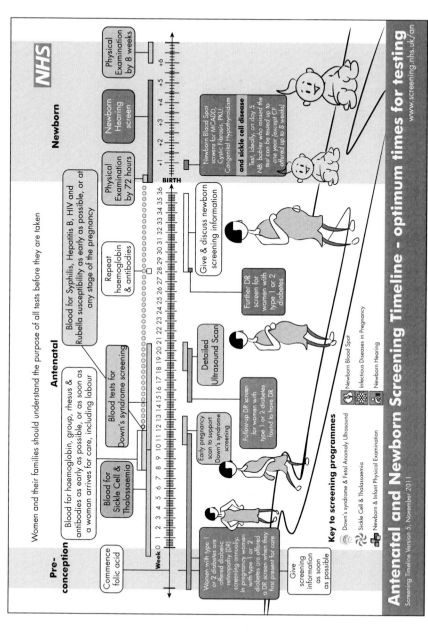

Fig. 4.1 Current 'timeline' of the UK antenatal screening programme. MCADD, medium chain acyl dehydrogenase deficiency; PKu, phenylketonuria © 2013, UK National Screening Committee (www.screening.nhs.uk), used with permission

In the first trimester the currently recommended screening test for Down syndrome includes tests of free beta-human chorionic gonadotrophin (beta-hCG) and pregnancy-associated plasma protein A (PAPP-A), measured between 11 weeks 0 days and 13 weeks 6 days of pregnancy, combined with nuchal translucency (see below). In the second trimester (15–20 weeks) AFP and free beta-hCG is used to screen for Down syndrome. An integrated test combines the results of PAPP-A in the first trimester and beta-hCG, unconjugated oestriol and AFP between 15 and 20 weeks. This test requires two visits and the results can be combined with nuchal translucency measurement.

Ultrasound tests used in screening

Nuchal translucency (NT) describes the measurement of the depth of fluid at the back of the fetal neck (Fig. 4.2). The measurement is made between 11 and 14 weeks of pregnancy, and is increased in fetuses with Down syndrome and other conditions. NT can be combined with results from first-trimester serum screening and maternal age to produce a composite risk for Down syndrome.

Nuchal translucency tests are conducted between 11 and 14 weeks of pregnancy.

Diagnostic tests used in the diagnosis of fetal abnormality

Chorionic villus sampling

Chorionic villus sampling (CVS) is a test which can be used to sample placental tissue between 11 and 13 weeks of pregnancy. CVS earlier in pregnancy was found to increase the risk of limb abnormalities and has been abandoned. This test is usually estimated to have a 1% risk of miscarriage, which makes it unacceptable for some women.

Amniocentesis

Amniocentesis is used to obtain amniotic fluid, which contains fetal skin cells that can be analysed for their chromosome make-up. Amniocentesis can be performed via either the trans-abdominal or the vaginal route. When the procedure is used for diagnostic testing it is usually carried out at around 15–20 weeks of pregnancy, although it can be performed from 10 weeks. The test has a 1% risk of miscarriage.

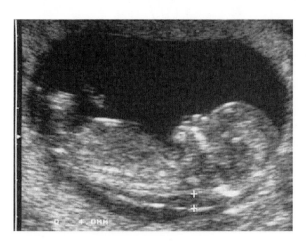

Fig. 4.2 Ultrasound estimation of nuchal translucency (callipers shown by ++)

Percutaneous umbilical blood sampling of fetal blood

Fetal blood can be obtained from the umbilical cord, with the needle guided by ultrasound, from the second trimester onwards. Direct sampling of fetal blood allows special cytogenetic, immunological and other tests to be performed, and blood can be assessed for viral load in cases of maternal HIV and possible cytomegalovirus infection. Percutaneous umbilical blood sampling has a 1–2% risk of fetal loss, with a 5% risk of preterm delivery.

Free fetal DNA in the maternal circulation

This test is not yet routine clinical practice, but in future extraction of the small amounts of fetal material present in the maternal circulation should allow genetic studies to be carried out without invasive testing.

Diagnostic imaging of the fetus with ultrasound and MRI

The quality of fetal ultrasound imaging has improved considerably over the last decade. Ultrasound is used to estimate fetal growth and can reveal a vast range of abnormalities, from congenital cardiac disease to exomphalos. Fetal magnetic resonance imaging (MRI) has also advanced, owing to faster data-acquisition times. The indications for fetal MRI are not yet agreed or standardized, but many centres offer MRI of the fetal brain if there is significant ventriculomegaly or a posterior fossa abnormality. Agenesis of the corpus callosum is the most common additional finding in cases of ventriculomegaly diagnosed with ultrasound imaging.

■ Maternal conditions affecting the fetus

Maternal health can have a major impact on fetal wellbeing. Maternal problems which can affect the fetus include infectious disease, chronic maternal illnesses and occasionally trauma. A summary is given in Table 4.1. For the management of perinatal infections affecting both mother and baby, see Chapter 16.

Table 4.1 Important maternal conditions affecting the fetus (excluding infectious disease, see Chapter 16)

Maternal condition	Effect on fetus and neonate
Asthma	Usually little, but occasionally mothers with severe asthma can deteriorate significantly during pregnancy, requiring intensive care and consideration of delivery
Cardiac disease	Usually little effect on the fetus, but mothers can require close monitoring, sometimes leading to a preterm delivery, and anticoagulation can be a problem for some. Increased risk of CHD in fetuses of mother with CHD
Diabetes mellitus	Increased risk of congenital abnormality and macrosomia, neonatal hypoglycaemia (see Chapter 18). Outlook for the fetus is poor if the mother develops ketoacidosis
Drug/alcohol dependency	Risk of fetal alcohol syndrome. Possible link between crack cocaine and fetal stroke; for management of neonatal abstinence syndrome see Chapter 28
Epilepsy	Need for additional folate in mothers taking antiepileptic drugs which are folate antagonists. Risk of fetal valproate and other syndromes

(continued)

Table 4.1 (Continued)

Maternal condition	Effect on fetus and neonate
Hypertension	Risk of placental insufficiency, labetalol can cause neonatal hypotension and hypoglycaemia
Liver disease	Risk of stillbirth in cholestasis, acute fatty liver of pregnancy. Hepatitis B carriage requires appropriate vaccination of the baby (Chapter 16)
Myasthenia gravis	Anticholinesterase antibodies can cause transient neonatal myasthenia
Psychiatric disease	Maternal selective serotonin reuptake inhibitors can cause a neonatal withdrawal syndrome, and antipsychotics can cause extrapyramidal reactions in babies. Lithium can be teratogenic and cause neonatal toxicity
Rheumatoid arthritis	Aspirin can cause neonatal bleeding, and possibility of high levels of morphine acquired via breast milk in babies whose mothers are slow metabolizers of codeine
Systemic lupus erythematosus	High miscarriage rate, and anti-Ro antibodies can cause fetal heart block
Thrombocytopenia – idiopathic thrombocytopenic purpura	Usually no serious effect on the fetus, which may have a low platelet count (for neonatal alloimmune thrombocytopenic purpura see Chapter 23)
Thrombophilia and thromboembolic disease	Common cause of maternal death and morbidity. Warfarin is contraindicated in pregnancy, especially in the first trimester, because it is teratogenic and can cause fetal intracranial bleeding. Genetic thrombophilic tendencies, e.g. factor V Leiden, can be associated with stroke in affected fetuses
Thyroid disease	Risk of neonatal thyrotoxicosis if mother has thyrotrophin receptor stimulating antibodies, which can cross the placenta (see Chapter 19)

CHD, congenital heart disease.

Epilepsy

Most women with a seizure disorder are already receiving treatment before they become pregnant and many will have attended pre-pregnancy counselling. From the fetal point of view, the problems centre around the teratogenic effect of several commonly used antiepileptic drugs, and both fetal phenytoin and valproate syndromes are described. High-dose folic acid (5 mg/day) is indicated from before conception to reduce the risk of neural tube defects and cleft palate, and vitamin K (10 mg/day) from 36 weeks. The latter is indicated to prevent early-onset vitamin K deficiency bleeding (Chapter 23). Occasional maternal seizures are not usually a problem for the fetus, but status epilepticus presents a high risk of fetal hypoxia with a 50% risk of fetal loss.

Diabetes

Screening for diabetes in pregnancy is currently recommended in women who have a body mass index more than 30 kg/m^2 at booking, who have delivered a baby weighing more than 4.5 kg, who come from an ethnic group with a high prevalence, who have had diabetes in a previous pregnancy or who have a first-degree relative with diabetes.

Women with diabetes remain at high risk of having a fetus with a congenital malformation. The aim of treatment, maintaining tight control with a haemoglobin A1c of below 6.1% before conception and in the first trimester, is to achieve a perinatal mortality close to the norm. Babies of diabetic mothers (whether gestational or not) require screening for neonatal hypoglycaemia (see Chapter 18).

Thyroid disease

Thyroid disease may be diagnosed for the first time during pregnancy, and there is a condition of transient gestational hyperthyroidism.

Graves' disease is the most common cause of hyperthyroidism in young women in the UK, being responsible for about 85% of cases. However, not all women with thyrotoxicosis have Graves' disease, defined as hyperthyroidism caused by thyrotrophin receptor stimulating antibodies (TRAbs). Pregnancy outcome is worse in the presence of maternal thyroid disease, and 1–5% of neonates whose mothers have Graves' disease develop hyperthyroidism as a result of transplacental passage of TRAbs. TRAb concentrations should be measured in early pregnancy in women with a history of Graves' disease even if they have been effectively treated with surgery or radioiodine, and fetuses whose mothers have high levels should be monitored carefully, with particular reference to growth and fetal heart rate (FHR) estimation. Drugs are the mainstay of management in symptomatic mothers, aiming to use the lowest dose possible to achieve a euthyroid state. 'Block and replace' regimens are not recommended in pregnancy because of the risk of fetal hypothyroidism.

Maternal hypothyroidism is usually secondary to Hashimoto's thyroiditis, when the mother is usually producing thyroid-inhibiting antibodies. Thyroid-stimulating hormone (TSH) receptor antibody titres do not distinguish between the stimulating and blocking types of antibody; babies are at risk of hypothyroidism but rarely can become thyrotoxic. In mothers with hypothyroidism in whom the TSH receptor antibody status is elevated or unknown, it is advisable to review the baby around 2 weeks after birth, measuring TSH and free thyroxine. In mothers who are hypothyroid as a result of hypoplasia of the gland, the routine Guthrie card screen of TSH should suffice because the risk of disease in the baby is low (about 5%).

See Chapter 19 for further information about the management of neonatal thyrotoxicosis and hypothyroidism.

Liver disease

Cholestasis of pregnancy presents with itching and jaundice, with an elevation of bile acids. There is a risk of sudden fetal death and induction of labour is usually recommended at 37 weeks, although the itching can be controlled for a time with ursodeoxycholic acid. Acute fatty liver of pregnancy is a much more serious disease with a high mortality and the woman requires urgent delivery whatever the gestation. HELLP (hypertension, elevated liver enzymes and low platelets) syndrome is an aggressive form of pre-eclampsia and may be part of the spectrum of acute fatty liver of pregnancy. HELLP syndrome is a very serious obstetric emergency, with a high perinatal mortality.

Screening bloods taken at booking sometimes reveal previously unsuspected chronic hepatitis B carriage, in which case the woman's partner should be offered an evaluation and vaccination of the newborn baby is indicated, with immunoglobulin where appropriate (Chapter 16).

Hypertension in pregnancy

Between 10% and 15% of all pregnant women are hypertensive. Some have pre-existing hypertension and some (7%) become hypertensive during pregnancy as a result of either pregnancy-induced hypertension (PIH) or pre-eclampsia. PIH is defined as new hypertension appearing after 20 weeks and resolving after delivery, with a diastolic blood pressure of at least 90 mmHg on two occasions, whereas pre-eclampsia is new hypertension with significant (>300 mg/24 h) proteinuria. Pre-eclampsia is an important cause of prematurity; the most effective (sometimes life-saving) treatment is delivery. Magnesium sulphate is the drug of choice for severe pre-eclampsia, HELLP syndrome and eclampsia, and can produce neonatal hypotonia.

Multiple pregnancy

The spontaneous twinning rate varies considerably between populations, being very low in Japan and high in some African populations. The prevalence of multiple pregnancies has risen steadily since the early 1980s, although there has been a recent decline in triplets and higher-order multiples. Currently, about 15 per 1000 babies born in the UK are one of twins. Dizygotic (DZ) twins are formed when two ova are released and fertilized, whereas monozygotic (MZ) twins form from division of a single zygote. About two-thirds of twins in the UK are dizygotic, and the diagnosis is obvious when the twins are of different sex. Determination of the pattern of placentation is important, but MZ twins whose zygote division occurs early can have two chorions. Like-sex DZ twins can only be distinguished from the one-third of MZ twins with dichorionic placentas by DNA analysis. For practical purposes, demonstration of a monochorionic placenta means that the twins are MZ, although there are rare exceptions. About 1% of MZ twins are monoamniotic and this carries the special and serious risk of fetal death from cord entanglement, leading to debates about the timing of elective preterm delivery.

Twin pregnancies are at high risk and require special monitoring; discordant growth is common whether or not there is twin–twin transfusion syndrome (TTTS). Following demise of one twin, the risk of preterm delivery before 34 weeks is 65%, and there is an incidence of neurological abnormality in survivors of 9% (higher if the pregnancy is monochorionic).

Twin–twin transfusion syndrome

Monochorionic placentas have vascular anastomoses allowing inter-twin transfusion, and when this exchange becomes unbalanced TTTS arises. The old criteria of more than a 20% discrepancy in weight and at least a 5 g/dL difference in haemoglobin in same-sex twins have been abandoned. Diagnosis now depends on finding polyhydramnios, cardiac hypertrophy and sometimes hydrops in the recipient twin; the donor twin develops oligohydramnios and can become a 'stuck' twin. The diagnosis of TTTS, particularly before 26 weeks, is very serious and there is a high risk of demise of one twin, with brain damage in the survivor. Current options include serial amniodrainage and laser ablation of the anastomotic vessels, of which the latter has been shown to have a better outcome in comparative studies. Even with laser ablation, there is a risk of severe cerebral lesions of around 16%, rising to 30% in those delivered before 30 weeks. If one MZ twin dies, the brain of the surviving twin should be monitored with serial ultrasound, with consideration of fetal MRI 4–6 weeks after the event because of the high risk (probably around 30%) of a significant cerebral lesion.

■ Immunological conditions

Rhesus haemolytic disease

See Chapter 23.

Neonatal alloimmune thrombocytopenic purpura

See Chapter 23.

■ Placental insufficiency

The use of Doppler ultrasound in combination with other tests to monitor fetal wellbeing is now an established and evidence-based practice, shown to reduce perinatal mortality. A poorly functioning placenta has an increased resistance to flow, which has an effect on the fetal umbilical blood flow velocity, particularly in diastole. Appropriate use of a combination of tests, including cardiotocogram (CTG), ultrasound imaging, measurement of liquor pools, and Doppler evaluation of blood flow in the umbilical artery and major fetal arteries including the middle cerebral artery, enables a distinction to be made between fetuses which are small because of placental insufficiency and those which are small for other reasons.

Absent or reversed end-diastolic flow (EDF) in the umbilical artery is seen in the worst-affected cases and is a predictor of adverse outcome, including neonatal necrotizing enterocolitis (see Chapter 21). This specific risk is sufficiently well established that most neonatologists would delay enteral feeds in intra-uterine growth restriction (IUGR) babies who were known to have reversed EDF in the umbilical artery before birth. Babies with placental insufficiency often have increased flow in the middle cerebral artery – a 'brain-sparing' effect – and middle cerebral artery flow is also increased in the presence of fetal anaemia.

■ Preterm membrane rupture

Preterm premature rupture of the membranes (PPROM) complicates ~2% of pregnancies but is associated with 40% of preterm deliveries and can result in significant neonatal morbidity and mortality. The three causes of neonatal death associated with PPROM are prematurity, sepsis and pulmonary hypoplasia. PPROM is diagnosed on the basis of maternal history, evidence of liquor in the vagina and ultrasound evidence of oligohydramnios. After diagnosis and the exclusion of infection the management is usually expectant; the mother has careful monitoring to look for signs of infection and delivery is planned for after 34 weeks, as below this the risks of prematurity are greater than those of the most common complication, chorioamnionitis. Maternal administration of oral erythromycin is associated with delayed delivery and decreased respiratory, cerebral and infective morbidity, and oral erythromycin is now routinely given to women with PPROM. Once the membranes have ruptured preterm, about 50% of women will go into labour within a week.

■ Prelabour rupture of the membranes at term

Women who suspect that their membranes have ruptured are offered an examination with a speculum in order to determine whether or not the fluid is indeed liquor, but those in whom the diagnosis is not in doubt do not need this examination. If the diagnosis is confirmed then 60% will go into labour within 24 hours; the risk of serious neonatal infection is estimated as 1%. Women who do not labour after 24 hours are usually offered induction, and in the interim are advised to check their own temperature every 4 hours while awake and to report change in the colour or smell of their vaginal loss. The National Institute for Health and Clinical Excellence (NICE) does not recommend that antibiotics be given to the mother or the baby, if both are well or that the baby should have blood/cerebrospinal fluid tests; it does recommend frequent observations of the baby's colour, temperature, respiration, feeding pattern and heart rate for 12 hours. Antibiotics are recommended if there is clinical chorioamnionitis; maternal pyrexia is usually defined as a temperature of more than 38°C on one occasion or more than 37.5°C on two occasions more than 2 hours apart.

Induction of labour

About 20% of labours are induced. Current NICE recommendations are to offer an induction of labour after 41 weeks in uncomplicated pregnancies. Women with prelabour rupture of the membranes at term are offered a choice of immediate induction or expectant management. The full guideline contains recommendations about the use of vaginal prostaglandins, monitoring and the dose of oxytocin. Induction of labour is easiest in women whose cervix is already 'ripe' and this is a gradual process in nature. The Bishop score is used to assess cervical ripening. Induction of labour is an uncertain process and has only around a 66% chance of ending with a normal vaginal delivery.

Intrapartum monitoring

The main method for assessing fetal wellbeing in labour is by assessing FHR. This can be done in three ways: by intermittent auscultation, counting the heart rate over a period of a minute at intervals, or by continuous estimation via a CTG using a Doppler transducer applied to the maternal abdomen, or via a fetal scalp electrode collecting a fetal electrocardiogram (ECG).

Current NICE guidance recommends intermittent auscultation every 15 minutes in the first stage and every 5 minutes in the second stage for low-risk women, with continuous CTG in those defined as 'high risk'. This category includes meconium-stained liquor, prior detection of a FHR abnormality, significant vaginal bleeding or maternal hypertension. CTG analysis can be supplemented with estimation of the fetal pH via fetal scalp sampling.

Cardiotocography

The FHR can be detected through the maternal abdomen via a Doppler transducer, basically a movement detector (Fig. 4.3). Alternatively a fetal ECG can be recorded directly via an electrode fixed onto the skin of the presenting part, usually the scalp. The latter is a more reliable method, although both are subject to artefact, either from inadvertent interrogation of the maternal aorta or because the scalp clip is dislodged and becomes affixed to the maternal cervix or vaginal wall. The FHR is averaged and displayed on one channel, with the other channel being used to show the uterine contractions recorded via a strain gauge (the tocograph). The conventional paper speed is 1 cm per minute. The main features are described below and the recommended categorization is given in Tables 4.2 and 4.3.

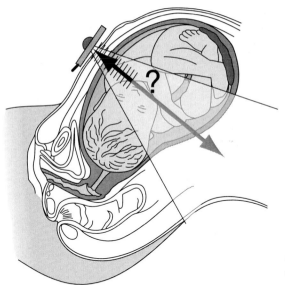

Fig. 4.3 Doppler transducer applied to the maternal abdomen, detecting movement of the fetal heart and estimating fetal heart rate

Table 4.2 Categorization of fetal heart rate traces (NICE guideline 2007)

Category	Definition
Normal	CTG with all four features in the reassuring category
Suspicious	CTG whose features fall into one of the non-reassuring categories with the remainder of the features reassuring
Pathological	CTG whose features fall into two or more non-reassuring categories or one or more abnormal categories

CTG, cardiotocogram.

Table 4.3 Categorization of fetal heart rate features (NICE guideline 2007)

Feature	Baseline bpm	Variability bpm	Decelerations	Accelerations
Reassuring	110–160	≥5	None	Present
Non-reassuring	100–109			
	161–180	<5 for 40–90 minutes	Early deceleration	The absence of accelerations with an otherwise normal CTG is of uncertain significance
			Variable deceleration	
			Single prolonged deceleration up to 3 minutes	
Abnormal	<100	<5 for more than 90 minutes	Atypical variables	
	>180		Late decelerations	
	Sinusoidal pattern ≥10 minutes		Single prolonged deceleration for more than 3 minutes	

bpm, beats per minute; CTG, cardiotocogram.

CTG assessment includes observation of the following four features:

1 heart rate (normally 110–160 beats per minute);
2 variability of baseline heart rate (normally 5–25 beats per minute);
3 the presence of accelerations (defined as a rise of baseline of more than 15 beats for more than 15 seconds);
4 whether or not there are decelerations (defined as a reduction in baseline of more than 15 beats over 15 seconds).

Decelerations are classified as:

- early – a slowing of the baseline FHR with onset early in the contraction and return to baseline at the end of the contraction;
- late – a slowing of the FHR with onset mid to end of the contraction and nadir more than 20 seconds after the peak of the contraction, returning to baseline after the end of the contraction;
- variable – intermittent periodic slowing of the FHR with variable relationship to the contraction cycle;
- atypical variable – variable decelerations with additional components, such as slow return to baseline at the end of the contraction, or loss of variability during the deceleration.

Fetal scalp pH estimation

The specificity of an abnormal CTG trace for fetal hypoxia is poor and hence on occasion it is necessary to sample fetal blood to check for the presence of acidosis. A result of pH >7.25 is considered reassuring, but should be repeated if the CTG abnormality persists. A result between 7.21 and 7.24 is borderline and should be repeated in 30 minutes, with consideration of delivery if there has been a fall since the last sample. A fetal scalp pH of <7.20 is an indication for urgent delivery.

Umbilical cord pH sampling

Many units routinely sample both the umbilical artery and vein at birth for the estimation of pH, but this is not recommended by NICE. The best quality results are obtained if a section of cord is 'double clamped'. Although the cord pH results are poor predictors of death or cerebral palsy, a normal paired cord gas result (with sufficient difference between the paired samples to show that two vessels were sampled) is strong evidence against intrapartum hypoxic ischaemia. The normal range is shown in Table 4.4.

■ Mode of delivery

Caesarean section

The rising caesarean section rate in developed countries has been the subject of much debate. The current caesarean section rate in the UK is between 15% and 30% depending on the population served by the reporting unit. The indications for an elective caesarean section include breech presentation and previous caesarean section. Many caesarean sections are emergency operations performed in the first or second stage of labour for indications such as suspected fetal compromise or failure to progress.

Table 4.4 Normal umbilical blood gas results; range derived from mean and two standard deviations (from Pomerance 2004)

	Venous blood	Arterial blood
pH	7.25–7.45	7.18–7.38
(H⁺) concentration	56–36	64–43
PCO_2 (mmHg)	26.8–49.2	32.3–65.8
(kPa)	3.57–6.56	4.30–8.77
PO_2 (mmHg)	17.2–40.8	5.6–30.8
(kPa)	2.29–5.44	0.74–4.1
HCO_3 (mmol/L)	15.8–24.2	17–27
Base excess	−8 to 0	−8 to 0

Instrumental delivery

The ventouse is the currently favoured method for assisted vaginal delivery, with approximately 8% of babies being delivered this way in the UK. Rotational forceps (Kjelland's forceps) have largely vanished from use. Ventouse is associated with a lower chance of successful vaginal birth than forceps.

From the neonatal point of view the rise in vacuum-assisted deliveries is important because the method involves the formation of an artificial caput, or chignon. This is associated with an increased risk of cephalhaematoma, and of bleeding into the subaponeurotic or subgaleal layer of the scalp, a large potential space into which more than 200 mL of blood can drain. This can have disastrous consequences for the baby unless the diagnosis is rapidly appreciated and blood transfused. Subgaleal haematoma, discussed on p. 224, can lead to difficulties in resuscitation (see p. 44).

References

National Institute for Health and Clinical Excellence (2007) *Intrapartum Care.* Clinical Guideline CGSS. Available from www.nice.org.uk.

Pomerance, JF (2004) *Interpreting Umbilical Cord Blood Gases.* Pasadena: BNMG (www.cordgases.com).

Further reading

James, DK, Steer, PJ, Weiner, CP, Gonik, B (eds) (2005) *High Risk Pregnancy: Management options.* Philadelphia: Saunders.

Kilby, M, Baker, P, Critcheley, H, Field, D (2006) *Multiple Pregnancy.* London: RCOG Press.

Kingdom, J, Baker, P (eds) (2000) *Intrauterine Growth Restriction.* London: Springer-Verlag.

Further information

UK National Screening Committee www.nsc.nhs.uk/

NICE guidance www.nice.org.uk
  Antenatal care 2008
  Diabetes in Pregnancy 2008
  The Use of Electronic Fetal Monitoring 2001
  Induction of Labour 2001, 2008
  Intrapartum Care 2007
  Maternity Matters DOH 2007
  Standards for Maternity Care RCOG 2008

5

Genetic disease

Key points

In any odd-looking baby:

- Compare his appearance with his next of kin.
- Carefully list his dysmorphic features and consult the computerized databases.
- Send blood for cytogenetic analysis.
- Consult an expert in dysmorphology if the suspicion remains high.

About 2–3% of babies are born with a malformation and malformation sequences are still a common cause of neonatal death. The diagnosis of genetic disease requires a high index of suspicion in the neonatal period, although some disorders, such as Down syndrome, are well known and easily recognized. Fetal medicine has changed the pattern of malformations which present in the neonatal period; for example, Patau syndrome (trisomy 13) and Edward syndrome (trisomy 18) are now rare because cases are diagnosed early in pregnancy and most parents choose termination. Some conditions are known to result from submicroscopic deletions of the genome, so that a specific request is required before the laboratory can help, by using fluorescent in-situ hybridization (FISH). If one of these conditions is suspected (e.g. a microdeletion of chromosome 22 in a child with congenital heart disease and an absent thymus – Di George syndrome or 'catch-22') it is always worth repeating a chromosome test which was thought to be normal antenatally. FISH-ing generally for microdeletions is not possible and a specific request is required.

The first clue to possible genetic disease is usually the appearance of the infant, who does not 'look right' – in other words, he is dysmorphic. This instant recognition, which is based partly on the examiner's experience, is often called 'gestalt' recognition, from the German word meaning shape or form. Infants appear dysmorphic for any of the following three reasons:

1 *Malformation.* A malformation is present when there is an anomaly in an organ or part of an organ. Examples include polydactyly, craniosynostosis, cleft lip, congenital heart disease or microcephaly. More subtle but equally important malformations are findings such as micropenis, hypertelorism, accessory nipples and misshapen digits. Multiple minor malformations are always suspicious.

2 *Deformation.* Deformation exists when the anatomy is normal but has been distorted by intra-uterine forces. The most common example is talipes secondary to oligohydramios.

3 *Disruption.* This is rare, but it occurs when there is an alteration of the normal process of development, such as from an amniotic band. Disruptions are non-genetic in nature.

When examining a baby with a possible malformation, always remember that any mention of a deviation from normal will be devastating to the parents. Sensitive handling is obviously essential, as is the provision of accurate information. Parent support groups are often excellent sources of information and support once a specific diagnosis has been made. The internet is another source (see the list of useful websites at the end of this chapter).

Experienced help from a clinical geneticist is required when considering the diagnosis of a baby who may have a genetic disorder. Once the baby has been examined thoroughly and carefully, and a detailed family history has been prepared, the combination of malformations can be entered into a computer program or looked up in a book with the appropriate tables to see whether a specific 'syndrome' diagnosis can be made. The number of 'hits' can be optimized by using a small number of the best 'handles'. This means choosing the abnormal features which are not common, such as imperforate anus, rather than those which are common in the general population (e.g. clinodactyly). Measurements, cranial imaging and X-rays may all contribute to a diagnosis.

Remember that apart from autosomal dominant and recessive inheritance, and X-linked disorders, genetic disease can be transmitted via mitochondrial DNA (exclusively from the female line, although both males and females can be affected) or by genetic imprinting. An imprinted gene has been marked during meiosis, to indicate the parent from whom it comes. For some genes it appears to be important not only to inherit two copies of that gene but also to inherit one from each parent. A good example is the presence of a small deletion of chromosome 15q, which has a different effect depending upon which chromosome 15 is deleted. If the deletion occurs on the chromosome inherited from a child's normal father, the child will develop Prader–Willi syndrome. If the deletion occurs on the chromosome inherited from a child's normal mother, the child will develop a completely different clinical condition, Angelman syndrome. Other conditions that show imprinting effects include Russell–Silver syndrome, Beckwith–Wiedemann syndrome, and the rare condition of transient neonatal diabetes mellitus.

Ophthalmological examination can be invaluable. One or two genetic diseases can be diagnosed with serum biochemical tests, perhaps the best-known example being Smith–Lemli–Opitz syndrome in which there is an elevated 7-dehydrocholesterol concentration. Some genetic disorders only ever occur as mosaics (e.g. Pallister–Killian syndrome), so that a skin biopsy has to be done to make the diagnosis because white cell chromosomes will be normal.

Malformations can result from fetal exposure to teratogens (e.g. fetal alcohol syndrome, rubella) and the cause of many malformations remains unknown. Photographs should be taken as a record because in many cases it is just not possible to reach a diagnosis in the nursery and follow-up and discussion with experts will be required.

■ Good 'handles' for genetic diagnosis

- Microcephaly
- Macrocephaly
- Polydactyly
- Syndactyly
- Cataract
- Hypertelorism

- Cleft lip and/or palate
- Small mandible
- Very short limbs
- Absent radius
- Anal atresia
- Skin abnormalities.

■ Further reading

Baraitser, M, Winter, RM (1996) *Colour Atlas of Congenital Malformation Syndromes.* London: Mosby-Wolfe.

Jones, KL (1997) *Smith's Recognizable Patterns of Human Malformation*, 5th edition. Philadelphia: WB Saunders.

Wiedemann, H-R, Kunze, J, Dibbern, H (1992) *An Atlas of Clinical Syndromes.* London: Wolfe.

■ Web links

www.ncbi.nlm.nih.gov/omim
http://rarediseases.info.nih.gov/
http://www.rarediseases.org/
www.cafamily.org.uk/

6

Neonatal resuscitation and stabilization

Key points

- Most babies do not need any resuscitation or suction.
- Most babies who are depressed at birth respond to ventilation given properly.
- Babies who are not responding quickly to ventilation (by 3 minutes) should be intubated and help will be required.
- Babies <30 weeks' gestation are at risk from respiratory distress syndrome, and unless they are vigorous at birth should be intubated for resuscitation and given surfactant prophylaxis as early as possible.
- 'Blind' drug therapy should not be given during resuscitation except in asystolic babies.
- Preparation and anticipation are the keys to successful resuscitation and stabilization.

Physiological adaptation at birth

During the final stages of labour and during the first few minutes of life a significant number of physiological adaptations have to occur in the baby to support the transition from fetal to neonatal life. An understanding of these changes helps to underpin our practices of neonatal resuscitation and to explain why sometimes 'things go wrong'. During fetal life gas exchange occurs in the placenta, the lungs are full of fluid and the fetal circulation diverts blood away from the lungs and through the placenta. During the transition to postnatal life the fluid in the lungs must be reabsorbed, gas exchange must transfer to the lungs, and the fetal circulation must change to that of the neonate. In the fetal lung the functional residual capacity (FRC) is maintained by lung liquid which is secreted by type II pneumocytes. This liquid is essential for prenatal growth and development of the respiratory system. In the late stages of a normal pregnancy, increasing glucocorticoid levels prepare the fetal lung, by increasing compliance, stimulation of surfactant production and preparation for lung liquid reabsorption. During labour there is a rise in the stress-related hormones adrenaline (epinephrine) and arginine vasopressin, which suppress fetal lung liquid production and stimulate its reabsorption. Normal babies take their first breath within a few seconds of delivery. Prior to the first breath the lungs are collapsed and have minimal FRC. The first two or three breaths expand the lungs and establish the normal FRC of approximately 30 mL/kg. To achieve this, extraordinarily high transpulmonary pressures are required to overcome the surface tension of the collapsed lung. Pressures of upwards of 60 cmH$_2$O are generated, compared with normal tidal breathing, which requires a peak transpulmonary pressure of approximately 10–15 cmH$_2$O.

A number of changes also need to occur in the circulatory system to help the newborn infant adapt to extra-uterine life. In the fetus blood is diverted away from the lungs through the patent foramen ovale (connection between the two atria) and the ductus arteriosus (connection between the aorta and the pulmonary trunk). In the fetal lung vasoconstriction results in high vascular resistance and hence high pressures within the pulmonary circulation. As this pressure exceeds that of the systemic circulation, blood moves across the foramen ovale and ductus arteriosus from 'right to left', that is, from the right to left atrium, and from the pulmonary trunk to the aorta. Following birth, as the lungs expand and the pulmonary arteries dilate, a fall in the pulmonary vascular resistance leads to increased blood flow into the lungs. The resultant increase in pulmonary venous return increases the pressure within the left atrium, which causes a functional closure of the foramen ovale. As respiration is established and the oxygen levels within the blood increase, there is a closure of the ductus arteriosus, which is mediated in part by a fall in local prostaglandin levels.

◼ Neonatal resuscitation

Neonatal resuscitation involves facilitation of the changes described above. It is reassuring that only a small percentage of newborn babies are not pink, vigorous and howling by 1–2 minutes of age. Furthermore, only about 5% of all babies born are still apnoeic at 1 minute of age, and only 0.5–1.0% will need intubation in the delivery room. Around 70% of babies requiring resuscitation at birth can be predicted from complications of pregnancy or labour. A skilled neonatal resuscitator should always be present at such deliveries (Table 6.1). This results in a neonatal attendance at 37% of all deliveries (Primhak *et al.* 1984). However, it follows that 20–30% of babies who require resuscitation at birth are unexpected. The implication of these data for those undertaking delivery without neonatal support, such as in isolated maternity units or at home, is clear.

◼ Resuscitation equipment

The following equipment is required for neonatal resuscitation:

1. An adequate surface on which to resuscitate the baby, with an overhead radiant heat source and sides to minimize the convective and radiant heat losses.
2. A gas supply of up to 5 L/min. Ideally both air and oxygen should be available with a blender to achieve different oxygen concentrations. It is now clear that most babies can be resuscitated adequately with air, and air is the

Table 6.1 Deliveries which should be attended by an experienced neonatal resuscitator

Gestation less than 36 weeks
Instrumental or surgical deliveries (excluding 'lift-out' forceps or elective caesarean section under epidural anaesthesia)
Malpresentations
Twins and higher multiple deliveries
Evidence of fetal compromise on cardiotocogram or fetal scalp pH
Meconium staining of the liquor
Antenatal diagnosis of fetal malformation
Antenatal diagnosis of blood group incompatibility, e.g. rhesus
The attending obstetrician requests the presence of a paediatrician

first-choice gas for resuscitation in order to avoid 'free radical' damage. However, oxygen is sometimes required and must always be available. A bag and mask system can deliver air if not connected to an oxygen supply, 40% oxygen if attached to an oxygen supply at 5 L/min and 60–70% oxygen if a reservoir is also used (Hermansen and Prior 1993). Whichever method of administering positive pressure ventilation is used, the gas *must* be passed through a suitable pressure-reducing system and via a blow-off valve set at 30 cmH$_2$O. Gas supplied at high pressure (the standard 'hospital' supply) must never, ever be used directly to resuscitate a baby.

3. Adequate suction with a soft end on the sucker. The suction should not exceed 200 mmHg and, for routine use, should be set at 100 mmHg ($\cong$ 136 cmH$_2$O) to prevent damage to the oropharyngeal mucosa. FG3–4 suction tubes are needed to clear the endotracheal tube (ETT) and FG8–10 tubes to clear the airway and occasionally to empty the stomach.
4. A clock with a second timer, since time passes very quickly in any emergency procedure.
5. A face mask to administer ambient oxygen to the cyanosed but breathing baby.
6. Varying sized face masks for administration of mask ventilation. Round, soft and flexible semitransparent autoclavable face masks are ideal.
7. A device for administering positive pressure ventilation. Traditionally a bag/valve system which can connect either to a mask or an ETT has been used. Increasingly, T-piece systems are used which allow the administration of a prolonged inspiratory time, and the provision of positive end expiratory pressure.
8. A selection of baby-size oropharyngeal airways (sizes 00 and 000).
9. At least two laryngoscopes (since one may fail at the crucial moment). Which blade to have on the laryngoscope is a matter of individual preference, but generally speaking a straight-bladed Wisconsin, Magill or Oxford Infant type are the best.
10. A selection of ETTs (2.0–3.5 mm), with an introducer as appropriate. The use of straight/shouldered oral tubes or nasal tubes is personal preference; however, if nasal intubation is to be performed, a set of Magill forceps is also needed.
11. Appropriate devices for ETT fixation.
12. A stethoscope.
13. Equipment for emergency cannulation of the umbilical vessels and thoracocentesis.
14. A selection of syringes, needles and specimen bottles.

The only drugs currently included in neonatal life support algorithms can be remembered by the mnemonic BAD (and things are indeed bad if these are required):

- 4.2% sodium **B**icarbonate;
- **A**drenaline 1:10,000 (100 µg/mL);
- 10% **D**extrose, 0.9% saline.

Additionally, volume in the form of both normal saline and O-negative emergency blood should be available.

Preparation

The key to any successful resuscitation is preparation. This includes ensuring that both the appropriate personnel and equipment are available. Essential to this is to always ask for help: do not be proud. If a very sick baby or several babies are expected, call for help before the baby is born. When preparing for resuscitation, wherever possible run through the following checklist:

1. Introduce yourself to the mother and her partner; the sudden arrival of an unknown crowd of people into the delivery room after a long day in labour can be unnerving for the mother.
2. Read the mother's notes or get a history from the midwife or obstetrician about her medical/obstetric past, including the reasons for any interventional delivery and what drugs she has received during labour.
3. Send for help straight away if you assess the situation as being likely to result in a severely depressed or malformed baby.
4. Turn on and test equipment, including heater and oxygen/air. Test positive pressure device: if using a bag, check that the blow-off pressure is set at 30 cmH$_2$O; if using a T-piece check peak and end expiratory pressures. Check that the suction is working at appropriate pressure and a suction catheter is attached.
5. Go round and close all the doors and windows and turn off fans near the resuscitation trolley. The labour ward staff will hate you, but it is important to do this to prevent the baby becoming profoundly hypothermic, particularly if premature. The ideal room temperature is 25°C, uncomfortable for most adults.
6. Make sure there are warmed, dry towels to wrap the baby in during resuscitation and a plastic bag/wrap and hat for premature babies.
7. Wash hands and put on gloves (plus goggles for high-risk cases).

Physiology of neonatal resuscitation

Fundamental to an understanding of the physiology of neonatal resuscitation is an appreciation of what makes the neonate different:

- Neonates are small and wet and they therefore get cold very quickly.
- Neonatal lungs are not expanded and are filled with fluid.
- Neonates, like children, have primary respiratory arrests with cardiac arrest occurring as a secondary phenomenon, so management of airway and breathing is usually all that is required for a successful resuscitation.

The strategy for resuscitation of the newborn follows the familiar A, B, C, D or 'airway, breathing, circulation, drugs' algorithm which is taught for resuscitation at all ages.

To understand the rationale for the interventions in neonatal resuscitation it is important to have an appreciation of the sequence of events that occur in acute asphyxia. This sequence of events was demonstrated in experimental animals in the early 1960s. When placental oxygen supply is interrupted, the fetus attempts to breathe. Should these attempts fail to inflate the lung with air (for example if this occurs *in utero* or with an obstructed airway), the baby will lose consciousness. Continued hypoxia of the respiratory centre within the brain results in the cessation of breathing usually within 2–3 minutes; this is termed primary apnoea (Fig. 6.1). After 1–2 minutes of primary apnoea most animals start to gasp with increasing frequency and vigour, and then decreasing frequency and vigour until they literally reach the last gasp. Gasping lasts for 5–10 minutes, after which the animal is again apnoeic (Fig. 6.1) – terminal apnoea. The whole process lasts about 20 minutes. The accompanying changes in blood pressure and blood gases are also illustrated in Fig. 6.1.

The animal studies demonstrate that it is possible to survive for more than 20 minutes of complete asphyxia. This is due to the large stores of glycogen in the brain, liver and myocardium, which can produce energy by anaerobic glycolysis, and also to the ability of the neonatal brain to metabolize lactate and ketones rather than glucose during hypoxia (Volpe 2008), although, in the same experiments, brain damage affecting primarily the basal ganglia and brainstem appears within 10–12 minutes.

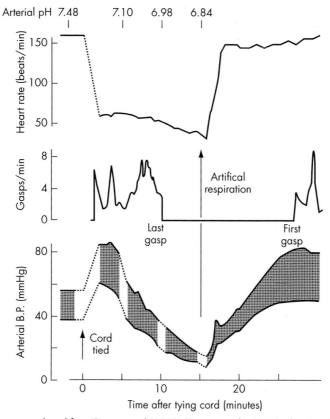

Fig. 6.1 Figure reproduced from Dawes et al (1963) (Dawes et al., 1963), showing the response of an asphyxiated monkey to asphyxia and resuscitation. Reproduced from the *Journal of Physiology* with permission.

The response to removing the airway obstruction during the above experiment depends on the state of asphyxia. In primary apnoea, the apnoea will persist until some stimulus provokes gasping, when the animal will inhale air or oxygen and soon develop regular respiration. If the animal is gasping when the obstruction is removed, air or oxygen enters its lungs and a regular respiratory pattern develops. If the obstruction is removed in terminal apnoea, respiration will never occur. To resuscitate such an animal, positive pressure ventilation must be used. Furthermore, if the heart rate is very low (or has stopped), external cardiac massage will be necessary. There is no reason to suppose that the human neonate will respond to asphyxia differently to experimental animals.

The animal experiments have also demonstrated that the onset of gasping, and therefore regular respiration, can be expedited in primary apnoea by peripheral stimulation, including rubbing the baby with a warm towel or giving him an intramuscular injection. Additionally, drugs administered to the mother, including all commonly used sedatives, analgesics and all anaesthetics, can pass to the fetus and may prolong primary apnoea to such an extent that the acidaemia becomes severe and the phase of gasping may never occur. In babies resuscitated from terminal apnoea, the time from the onset of artificial ventilation to either the first gasp or regular respiration is proportional to the severity of the asphyxia before ventilation was started. If artificial ventilation is started before the pH becomes too depressed, the baby may be expected to gasp and start regular respiration after 3–4 minutes of intermittent positive pressure ventilation (IPPV), whereas if resuscitation is started well into terminal apnoea when the arterial pH is <6.8, gasping may be delayed for 20 minutes and regular respiration for more than half an hour.

◼ Practice of neonatal resuscitation

Assessment of the newborn

Assessment of the neonate involves evaluation of the respiratory activity, heart rate, colour and muscle tone. The most commonly used assessment tool is the Apgar score described by Virginia Apgar in 1952 (Table 6.2). It is usual to assign a score at 1, 5 and 10 minutes. In the practice of neonatal resuscitation, assessment of respiration, heart rate, colour and tone is made immediately and after every 30 seconds of resuscitation.

It should be remembered that factors other than asphyxia can result in a depressed Apgar score (Table 6.3) and that several of these may be present in a single baby. It is crucial to recognize that even if the failure of regular respiration is *not* the result of asphyxia, adequate resuscitation must nevertheless be carried out or all the biochemical and clinical consequences of asphyxia will develop very quickly.

Cord blood gas analysis

Another way of assessing whether or not a baby is asphyxiated at the moment of birth is to measure the blood gases and pH in a sample drawn from the umbilical artery

Table 6.2 Apgar score

	Score	0	1	2
A	Appearance (colour)	Pale or blue	Body pink but extremities blue	Pink
P	Pulse rate	Absent	<100	>100
G	Grimace (response to suction catheter)	Nil	Some	Cry
A	Activity (muscle tone)	Limp	Some flexion	Well flexed
R	Respiratory effort	Absent	Hypoventilation	Good

Table 6.3 Factors other than asphyxia which may depress the Apgar score after birth

Drugs depressing the CNS
Trauma – especially of the CNS
Prematurity – in particular surfactant-deficient, stiff lungs
Sepsis – classically early-onset group B streptococcal sepsis (see p. 197)
Maternal or neonatal hypocapnia from overbreathing
Muscle weakness, due to prematurity or primary muscle disease
Anaemia (e.g. fetal haemorrhage)
Previous neurological damage *in utero*
Congenital malformations affecting the airway or preventing lung expansion

CNS, central nervous system.

in a section of the umbilical cord clamped immediately after delivery. These data are usually available within 5–10 minutes and then can be extremely useful in guiding the baby's subsequent management. Umbilical vein gases are less accurate than umbilical arterial pH. The umbilical vein pH is 0.01–0.1 pH points better than the umbilical artery result (see Table 4.4), and in acute cord occlusion the umbilical venous pH may be normal, representing blood leaving the placenta, but the fetus distal to the cord obstruction may be severely acidaemic.

Initial assessment

- Whatever the problem, first make sure the cord is securely clamped. In sick and preterm infants where catheterization of the umbilical vessels can be anticipated, leaving a short length of cord (approximately 5–10 cm) facilitates catheter insertion.
- In term infants, dry with a towel, then remove the wet towel and cover the baby with fresh dry towels. Drying the baby will provide significant stimulation and will allow time to assess colour, tone, breathing and heart rate. In infants suspected of having had a severe hypoxic ischaemic insult, e.g. still requiring active resuscitation at 10 minutes, it may be prudent to switch off any radiant heating device before considering total body cooling once the initial resuscitation and stabilization have occurred.
- Reassess colour, tone, breathing and heart rate regularly (particularly the heart rate) – every 30 seconds or so throughout the resuscitation process. The first sign of any improvement in the baby will be an increase in heart rate. At all stages consider the need for help and if in doubt request support immediately.
- A healthy baby will be born blue but will have good tone, will cry within a few seconds of delivery, will have a good heart rate (the heart rate of a healthy newborn baby is about 120–150 beats/min) and will rapidly become pink during the first 90 seconds or so. A less healthy baby will be blue at birth, will have less good tone, may have a slow heart rate (less than 100 beats/min) and may not establish adequate breathing by 90–120 seconds. An ill baby will be born pale and floppy, not breathing and with a slow or very slow heart rate.
- The heart rate of a baby is best judged by listening with a stethoscope, or attaching a pulse oximeter.

Airway

Before the baby can breathe effectively the airway must be open.

- The best way to achieve this is to place the baby on his back with the head in the neutral position, i.e. with the neck neither flexed nor extended. Most newborn babies have a relatively prominent occiput, which will tend to flex the neck if the baby is placed on his back on a flat surface. This can be avoided by placing some support under the baby's shoulders, but be careful not to overextend the neck.
- If the baby is very floppy it may also be necessary to apply chin lift or jaw thrust.
- A resuscitator skilled in intubation may elect to intubate early in resuscitation to achieve rapid control of the airway, e.g. immediately in a baby born with no heart rate or in a very preterm infant. To intubate a baby, lie him flat or slightly extend his neck. Even moderate flexion pushes the larynx into a very anterior position that makes it difficult to visualize. Insert the blade of the laryngoscope into the vallecula and pull the epiglottis forward to reveal the larynx. Press lightly on the cricoid cartilage (with the fifth finger of the hand holding the laryngoscope) and the view of the larynx is improved. See Procedures (p. 358) for more detail.

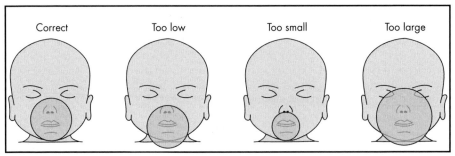

Fig. 6.2 Correct position and size of face mask. Source: Resuscitation Council Neonatal Life Support Guidelines 2005

Breathing

- If the baby is not breathing adequately by about 90 seconds, give five inflation breaths. Until now the baby's lungs will have been filled with fluid. In a term baby, initial aeration of the lungs is likely to require sustained application of pressures of about 30 cmH$_2$O for 2–3 seconds – termed 'inflation breaths'. For mask ventilation to be effective there must be a tight seal between the mask and the baby's face. Use the correct size of face mask and position it over the baby's mouth and nose (Fig. 6.2). Slightly extend his neck (chin lift) and hold his jaw forward ('jaw thrust'). An oropharyngeal airway may help but will not substitute for incorrect positioning.

- Growing evidence suggests that initial resuscitation should be with air if available. The fraction of inspired oxygen should be increased if the baby does not respond rapidly to adequate inflation breaths with air.

- If the heart rate was below 100 beats/min initially then it should rapidly increase as oxygenated blood reaches the heart. If the heart rate does increase then you can assume that you have successfully aerated the lungs. If the heart rate increases but the baby does not start breathing for himself, continue to provide regular breaths at a rate of about 30–40/min until the baby starts to breathe on his own.

- If the heart rate does not increase following inflation breaths, then either you have not aerated the lungs or the baby needs more than lung aeration alone. By far the most likely reason is that you have failed to aerate the lungs effectively. If the heart rate does not increase and the chest does not passively move with each inflation breath, you have not aerated the lungs. Consider:
  - Is the baby's head in the neutral position?
  - Do you need jaw thrust?
  - Do you need a longer inflation time or higher pressure?
  - Do you need a second person's help with the airway?
  - Is there an obstruction in the oropharynx (laryngoscope and suction)?
  - What about an oropharyngeal (Guedel) airway?

- Check that the baby's head and neck are in the neutral position, that your inflation breaths are at the correct pressure (30 cmH$_2$O for a term infant) and applied for the correct time (2–3-second inspiration) and that the chest moves with each breath. If the chest still does not move, ask for help in maintaining the airway and consider an obstruction in the oropharynx, which may be removable by suction under direct vision. An oropharyngeal (Guedel) airway may be helpful.

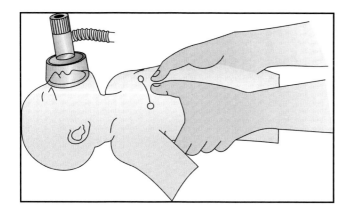

Fig. 6.3 Technique of encircling the chest to give cardiac massage

- If the heart rate remains slow (less than 60 beats/min) or absent following five inflation breaths, despite good passive chest movement in response to inflation efforts, start chest compression.

Chest compression

Almost all babies needing help at birth will respond to successful lung inflation with an increase in heart rate followed quickly by normal breathing. However, in some cases chest compression is necessary.

- Chest compression should be started only when you are sure that the lungs have been aerated successfully.
- In babies, the most efficient method of delivering chest compression is to grip the chest in both hands in such a way that the two thumbs can press on the lower third of the sternum, just below an imaginary line joining the nipples, with the fingers over the spine at the back (Fig. 6.3).
- Compress the chest quickly and firmly, reducing the anteroposterior diameter of the chest by about one-third.
- The ratio of compressions to inflations in newborn resuscitation is 3:1.
- Chest compressions move oxygenated blood from the lungs back to the heart. Allow enough time during the relaxation phase of each compression cycle for the heart to refill with blood. Ensure that the chest is inflating with each breath. In a very few babies, inflation of the lungs and effective chest compression will not be sufficient to produce an effective circulation. In these circumstances drugs may be helpful.

Drugs

Drugs are needed only if there is no significant cardiac output despite effective lung inflation and chest compression. The drugs used are adrenaline (1:10,000), sodium bicarbonate (ideally 4.2%) and dextrose (10%). They are best delivered close to the heart, usually via an umbilical venous catheter (UVC).

- The recommended dose for adrenaline is 10 µg/kg = 0.1 mL/kg of 1:10,000 solution). If this is not effective, a dose of up to 30 µg/kg (0.3 mL/kg of 1:10,000) may be tried.
- The dose for sodium bicarbonate is between 1 and 2 mmol of bicarbonate/kg (2–4 mL/kg of 4.2% bicarbonate solution).
- The dose of dextrose recommended is 250 mg/kg (2.5 mL/kg of 10% dextrose).

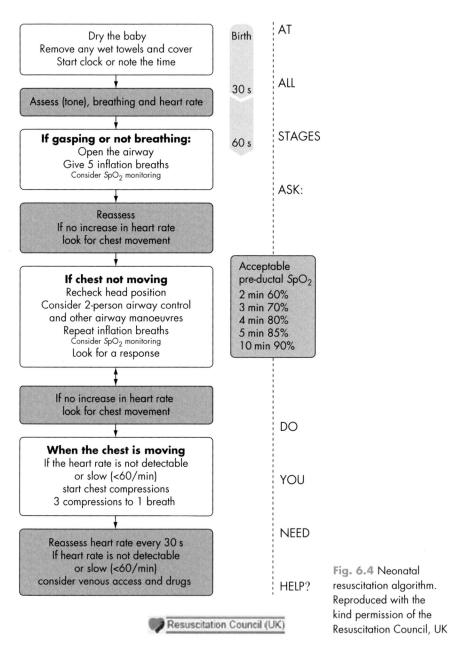

Dry the baby Remove any wet towels and cover Start clock or note the time	Birth AT
Assess (tone), breathing and heart rate	30 s ALL
If gasping or not breathing: Open the airway Give 5 inflation breaths Consider SpO₂ monitoring	60 s STAGES
Reassess If no increase in heart rate look for chest movement	ASK:
If chest not moving Recheck head position Consider 2-person airway control and other airway manoeuvres Repeat inflation breaths Consider SpO₂ monitoring Look for a response	Acceptable pre-ductal SpO₂ 2 min 60% 3 min 70% 4 min 80% 5 min 85% 10 min 90%
If no increase in heart rate look for chest movement	
When the chest is moving If the heart rate is not detectable or slow (<60/min) start chest compressions 3 compressions to 1 breath	DO YOU
Reassess heart rate every 30 s If heart rate is not detectable or slow (<60/min) consider venous access and drugs	NEED HELP?

Resuscitation Council (UK)

Fig. 6.4 Neonatal resuscitation algorithm. Reproduced with the kind permission of the Resuscitation Council, UK

■ Very rarely, the heart rate cannot increase because the baby has lost significant blood volume. If this is the case, there is often a clear history of blood loss from the baby, but not always. Blood loss should be replaced with uncross-matched O-negative blood. If this is not available, isotonic crystalloid rather than albumin is preferred for emergency volume replacement. A bolus of 10 mL/kg of 0.9% saline or similar given over 10–20 seconds will often produce a rapid response and can be safely repeated if needed.

Babies who are active, breathing easily and pink by 10 minutes can go to the postnatal ward with their mother unless there was a long history of fetal distress or a very low cord pH, when a period of observation on the neonatal intensive care unit is wise in case hypoxic ischaemic encephalopathy develops (see p. 220). Early feeds and glucose monitoring are important.

Conversely, if there is no response at all without any cardiac output by 15 minutes of continuous and adequate resuscitation, consideration should be given to stopping the resuscitation. If there are no regular respirations by 30 minutes, the outlook is poor.

Special situations in neonatal resuscitation

Meconium staining

It has now been demonstrated that intrapartum suctioning, i.e. with the head on the perineum, does not prevent meconium aspiration syndrome and this practice is no longer recommended.

Equally, attempts to remove meconium from the airways of vigorous babies is also futile. However, if babies who are born through thick meconium are unresponsive or not vigorous at birth, the oropharynx should be inspected and cleared of meconium. If intubation skills are available, the larynx and trachea should also be cleared by direct suctioning.

Preterm

The basics of assessment and resuscitation, i.e. ABC, are similar, but a number of important differences require highlighting:

- When the birth of a significantly preterm infant is expected, provisions should be made to ensure an experienced neonatologist attends the delivery.
- At birth, preterm babies 30 weeks and below should be placed under a radiant heater, a hat should be applied and, without drying the body, place the baby immediately into a food-grade plastic bag to keep them warm during resuscitation and/or stabilization.
- Babies <30 weeks' gestation are at risk from respiratory distress syndrome. Unless they are vigorous at birth they should be intubated immediately for resuscitation and given surfactant prophylaxis as early as possible.
- When giving positive pressure ventilation, the lowest possible pressures should be used to avoid damage to the lungs. You should not expect to see large chest excursions, and if these are present the peak inspiratory pressure should be reduced. Similarly, the minimum pressures possible should be used on the transport incubator when transferring from the delivery room to the neonatal unit (NNU).
- It is generally accepted that the use of drugs in the resuscitation of babies at the threshold of viability is not appropriate. Continued resuscitation of babies who fail to respond to appropriate airway management, positive pressure ventilation and possibly a short period of cardiac massage is not appropriate.

Problems with resuscitation

The baby who goes pink but does not start to breathe

If, by 20 minutes of age, the baby has made no spontaneous respiratory effort – despite adequate oxygenation and correction of acidaemia and hypoglycaemia – further therapy should be delayed until the baby is transferred to the NNU. Once there, further blood gas analysis, blood glucose measurements and a chest X-ray should be carried out.

If these tests show some persisting abnormality, appropriate therapy can be given. If they are normal, yet apnoea persists, this suggests profound asphyxia with severe neurological damage and a grave prognosis. Alternatively, if the evidence for pre-delivery asphyxia is unimpressive, consider some underlying neurological disorder such as cervical cord transection, *in-utero* neurological damage or a primary muscle disease (see p. 231).

The baby with no response to intermittent positive pressure ventilation

A few babies will remain blue, apnoeic and bradycardic. In some cases the reasons will be obvious (e.g. severe skeletal abnormalities in thanatophoric dwarfism). However, in babies who look normal, the reason for the poor response is commonly some technical error in resuscitation. Therefore check the following:

1. If a bag and mask system is being used, is there a poor seal around the face and is the baby's chest moving?
2. If the baby is intubated, is the endotracheal tube in the trachea and not in the oesophagus?
3. Is the endotracheal tube too small (a common mistake)? A 3.0 or 3.5 mm tube should always be used except in babies <1 kg. Smaller tubes have a big internal resistance, allow a big air leak and very easily get pushed in too far so that they lodge in a main-stem bronchus. This is not only bad for overall ventilation but carries the risk of rupturing the lobe and causing a pneumothorax.
4. Is an adequate inflation pressure being applied? The blow-off valve may have become inadvertently reset at a low pressure.
5. Is enough oxygen being given? Has the supply been disconnected or the reservoir removed from a bag and mask system? Should 80–100% oxygen be given by using a T-piece or connecting the baby to a ventilator or continuous positive airways pressure (CPAP) device?

If technical errors can be excluded, check the following:

1. Is the asphyxia more severe than the initial clinical assessment suggested? Check blood gases and blood glucose and intervene further based on the results. It may be appropriate to transfer the baby to the NNU for further evaluation.
2. Is the baby premature and developing severe respiratory distress syndrome (RDS), or could he have congenital group B beta-haemolytic *Streptococcus* pneumonia? Increase the inflating pressure to 35 cmH$_2$O if possible, give high FiO$_2$ and surfactant, and increase the ventilation rate. This virtually always improves the baby enough to allow transfer to the NNU.
3. Has the baby developed a pneumothorax during resuscitation?
4. Is the baby very pale? Consider fetal haemorrhage (p. 306). Such babies may have lost more than half their blood volume. If the history is suggestive and the pallor seems due to anaemia, give 15–20 mL/kg of fresh uncrossmatched O-negative blood at once over 10 minutes; repeat this if necessary. Blood is much better than saline because blood carries oxygen. This will usually improve the baby enough for him to be transferred to the NNU where a more accurate assessment of the anaemia can be made (see p. 307).

The vigorous but cyanosed baby

A few babies are fairly vigorous and active with a normal heart rate, often marked respiratory distress, yet remain very cyanosed. This situation strongly suggests some underlying structural problem in an (initially) unasphyxiated baby. Consider the following:

1. Is there a diaphragmatic hernia, suggested by mediastinal shift, poor air entry on the left side (the usual side of the hernia) and a scaphoid abdomen? Intubate the baby, transfer him to the NNU and X-ray him.
2. Is there a pneumothorax? This can be spontaneous, or the result of overvigorous positive pressure respiration, especially with bag and mask systems or if too small an endotracheal tube has been pushed down into a segmental bronchus. The clinical signs are given on p. 157. There is rarely time to confirm the diagnosis radiologically, but a cold (fibreoptic) light source may help. If the baby is deteriorating quickly, insert a wide-bore needle into the second intercostal space in the mid-clavicular line. If you are right, there will be a gratifying hiss of escaping air, the baby's condition will improve and the needle can be followed by insertion of a chest drain.
3. Is there lung malformation or pulmonary hypoplasia? Airway, lung or cardiac malformations which make it impossible to resuscitate the baby are rarely surgically correctable and therefore are usually fatal.

First-hour care after resuscitation

It is not possible to overemphasize the importance of the 'golden hour', especially in the premature baby at risk from RDS, in whom failure to control clinical, biochemical and physiological abnormalities results in severe surfactant depletion and clinical deterioration. Put simply, sloppy first-hour care can convert mild RDS into severe or fatal RDS, or a treatable case of septicaemia into a fatal one. Equally important is the immediate care of the baby who has required resuscitation for birth depression. Not all babies with low Apgar scores have suffered *in-utero* hypoxia (Table 6.2), but some will develop hypoxic ischaemic encephalopathy requiring close monitoring (see p. 220); others need investigation to exclude sepsis, myopathy or some other pre-existing central nervous system disorder.

Preparation

Good communication between obstetric and paediatric teams allows preparation to be made for an admission and prevents ghastly and life-threatening delays while appropriate staff and equipment are found. Having an intensive care cot kitted out and ready is ideal but not always possible in busy units running at full capacity. When an admission can be anticipated, such as the expected preterm delivery or a surgical case, e.g. congenital diaphragmatic hernia, the setting up of appropriate equipment prior to delivery can save valuable time once the baby is born. For example, laying out the equipment for umbilical lines, peripheral canulation and collecting the blood bottles required for initial tests can all potentially be completed prior to the delivery. Additionally, the maternal notes can be reviewed and the maternal medical, obstetric and pregnancy details can all be documented before the birth of a baby, saving valuable time in the postnatal period.

Transfer from the labour ward

This is where the control and care of the sick neonate often starts to go awry. It is essential that the neonate has been adequately and appropriately resuscitated prior to transfer to the NNU. The exact nature of transfer from delivery room to NNU will depend on the individual hospital, but in general the baby should be placed in a warmed transport incubator and transferred with appropriate ventilatory support and monitoring. Usually, if intubation has been needed for resuscitation, it is sensible to keep the baby intubated and ventilated during transport and until baseline blood gases have been obtained after admission to the NNU. The baby must be accompanied on transfer by the neonatologist responsible for resuscitation and a trained neonatal nurse who will also ensure that the baby is labelled. A copy of the maternal notes or a good history is vital so that important diagnoses such as maternal HIV or hepatitis are known and appropriate treatment can be commenced without delay.

Admission routine

Immediate care is then usually provided by the nursing staff and it is important not to get in their way while the following occur:

- As soon as an ill baby arrives in the NNU, he should be weighed and placed in a warmed incubator or under a suitable radiant heater.
- If he was ventilated during transfer, this should be continued. Unventilated babies with respiratory distress should be given CPAP or oxygen as appropriate. Attach a pulse oximeter and give enough oxygen (by IPPV if necessary) to keep the SpO_2 > 90% in a term infant and 85–92% in a preterm.
- The baby should be connected to appropriate monitoring, which may include an electrocardiogram monitor, an apnoea monitor and transcutaneous monitoring of oxygen and carbon dioxide.
- A baseline set of observations should be taken, including heart rate, four-limb blood pressure and admission temperature.
- It is usual practice to obtain surface swabs for culture from ear and throat.
- Organize vitamin K if it was not given in the labour ward.

Once the baby is safely in an incubator and the nursing staff have completed their initial care, quickly and accurately examine the baby and measure the head circumference. A decision should then be made as to the type of intravenous and arterial access that is required. In a very preterm infant, and if sufficient skill is present to obtain umbilical arterial and venous access quickly, it may be preferable to site these immediately without first obtaining peripheral venous access.

Immediate care

All ill babies admitted directly from the delivery suite should have the following investigations set in train within 30 minutes of admission:

1. Arterial blood gases.
2. Blood glucose.
3. Haemoglobin (packed cell volume), full blood count with differential white blood cell count.
4. Blood culture.
5. Group and crossmatch.
6. C-reactive protein. Urea and electrolytes are often sent but will reflect maternal values immediately after birth. It may therefore be sensible to delay this until 4–6 hours.
7. One spot on the Guthrie card.

A chest X-ray will be required but can wait if the baby is clinically stable, especially if arterial lines are to be inserted. Coagulation studies may be indicated and should be taken from the umbilical arterial line before the heparinized saline is connected.

Once heparin has been commenced, coagulation samples must be obtained peripherally. Also think about collecting blood for chromosomes if you need to give a blood transfusion urgently.

An indwelling umbilical artery catheter (UAC) provides the most satisfactory way of monitoring sick babies with RDS (p. 127). Umbilical catheterization should be attempted in all very low birth weight babies requiring ventilation, in any other ventilated baby requiring more than 30% oxygen and not rapidly weaning, and in any shocked or very ill baby of any gestation. The risk of complications is low (p. 357). The catheter can always be removed later if it is not needed and the chance of success is high if you try while the cord is fresh. A UVC should be inserted in babies <1 kg at the same time as the UAC. This helps to achieve minimal handling and can be replaced with a silastic 'long' line after a few days when the baby is more stable. If insertion of the UAC fails, consider peripheral arterial cannulation (p. 355). If all attempts fail, obtain the first blood gas by arterial puncture; capillary blood gases from sick underperfused babies at any gestation are often misleading.

On the basis of the initial investigations, a working differential diagnosis must be made and appropriate treatment started without delay. If RDS is present, surfactant should be given if not already administered in the delivery room (p. 137). On the basis of the first set of blood gases, appropriate changes in the ventilator settings or inspired oxygen concentration can be made. Although large vigorous babies have a considerable capacity for correcting metabolic acidaemia spontaneously, small sick ones do not, and acidaemia depresses surfactant synthesis and function. Base deficits above 8–10 mmol/L present in symptomatic babies less than 60 minutes old often need correction by infusing an appropriate dose of base.

All sick babies should be started on intravenous dextrose at once through a peripheral line or UVC. The rate of infusion is dependent on the gestation and clinical situation. Term babies require 40–60 mL/kg/day of 10% dextrose; extreme preterm infants lose copious amounts of fluid and may need 100 mL/kg/day (which may need to be 5% dextrose to avoid hyperglycaemia). Babies with hypoxic ischaemic encephalopathy should be restriced to 40 mL/kg/day with close monitoring of blood glucose. Anaemia should be corrected by transfusion, urgently if appropriate.

Hypotension accompanied by poor capillary refill and/or an acidosis should always be treated. A useful rule of thumb is that the mean blood pressure roughly equates to the baby's gestational age in weeks, but what matters most is any evidence of poor tissue perfusion. In babies with continuous arterial pressure monitoring, gentle pressure over the liver will result in a rise in blood pressure in the hypovolaemic neonate due to increased venous return. This can be a useful bedside test to guide the treatment of hypotension. If hypotension is accompanied by anaemia, packed red cells should be transfused (10–15 mL/kg). However, if the haematocrit is greater than 45%, then infuse 10–15 mL/kg of normal saline. If the hypotension persists despite correction of hypovolaemia, acidaemia and hypoxia, or if there are signs of heart failure, ionotropic support is required.

Since it is impossible to exclude serious infection – especially with group B *Streptococcus* – as the cause of any illness presenting in the first hour, start the baby on antibiotics after taking cultures. Give penicillin and an aminoglycoside to all seriously ill babies, including any baby requiring IPPV. Consider a lumbar puncture if there is a high index of suspicion of sepsis, for example prolonged rupture of membranes or known maternal infection.

As a standard of care, all infants admitted to intensive care should have a cranial ultrasound scan as soon as possible after admission to the unit. This allows timing of intracranial haemorrhage (p. 224–230) and early identification of other intracranial pathology. In infants suspected of having experienced a hypoxic ischaemic insult, the ultrasound should include assessment of the resistance index in the anterior cerebral artery (p. 222). Such infants should commence cerebral function monitoring as early as possible and be considered for therapeutic hypothermia to minimize brain injury.

The baby will now be an hour old. If the above routines have been carried out correctly, even the sickest baby should now be in the optimal condition possible. At this stage make detailed notes, see the parents, explain what is happening and encourage them to visit the ward. If possible, take a photograph of the baby for the mother to keep with her on her bedside table.

■ References

Apgar, V (1952) Proposal for a new method of evaluation of newborn infants. *Anaesthesia and Analgesia* **32**: 260–7.

Hermansen, MC, Prior, MM (1993) Oxygen concentrations from self-inflating resuscitation bags. *American Journal of Perinatology* **10**: 79–80.

Primhak, RA, Herber, SM, Whincup, G, Milner, RDG (1984) Which deliveries require paediatricians in attendance? *British Medical Journal* **289**: 16–18.

Resuscitation Council UK (2005) Newborn Life Support (NLS), www.resus.org.uk

Volpe, JJ (2008) Hypoxic ischaemic encephalopathy: biochemical and physiological aspects. Chapter 6 in Volpe, JJ, *Neurology of the Newborn*, 5th edition. Philadelphia: WB Saunders, pp. 247–324.

■ Further reading

Adamsons, K, Behrman, R, Dawes, GS, *et al.* (1964) Resuscitation by positive pressure ventilation and tris-hydroxymethyl-aminomethane of rhesus monkeys asphyxiated at birth. *Journal of Pediatrics* **65**: 807–18.

Casalaz, DM, Marlow, N, Speidel, BD (1998) Outcome of resuscitation following unexpected apparent stillbirth. *Archives of Disease in Childhood. Fetal and Neonatal Edition* **78**: F112–15.

Dawes, GS, Jacobson, HN, Mott, JC, *et al.* (1963) Treatment of asphyxia in newborn lambs and monkeys. *Journal of Physiology* **169**: 167–84.

Field, D, Milner, AD, Hopkin, IE (1986) Efficacy of manual resuscitation at birth. *Archives of Disease in Childhood* **61**: 300–2.

Helwig, JT (1996) Umbilical blood acid-base state – what is normal? *American Journal of Obstetrics and Gynecology* **174**: 1807–14.

Kleinman, ME, Oh, W, Stonestreet, BS (1999) Comparison of intravenous and endotracheal epinephrine during cardiopulmonary resuscitation in newborn piglets. *Critical Care Medicine* **27**: 2748–54.

Low, JA (1993) The relationship of asphyxia in the mature fetus to long-term neurologic function. *Clinical Obstetrics and Gynecology* **36**: 82–90.

Milner, AD, Vyas, H, Hopkin, IE (1984) Efficacy of face mask resuscitation at birth. *British Medical Journal* **289**: 1563–5.

Palme, C, Nystron, B, Tunell, R (1985) An evaluation of the efficiency of face masks in the resuscitation of newborns. *Lancet* **i**: 207–10.

Resuscitation Council UK (2010) Newborn Life Support (NLS), www.resus.org.uk

Royal College of Paediatrics and Child Health (1997) *Resuscitation of Babies at Birth*. London: British Medical Association.

Scott, HM (1976) Outcome of very severe birth asphyxia. *Archives of Disease in Childhood* **50**: 712–16.

7

Nursing, monitoring and transport of the sick neonate

Key points

- Under normal circumstances babies should be kept in the thermoneutral range, with a core body temperature as close to 37°C as possible.
- Respiration (apnoea), heart rate (electrocardiogram), blood pressure and blood gases should be monitored in critically ill neonates on ventilatory support.
- Arterial PaO_2 is the gold standard method to avoid hyperoxaemia and minimize the risk of retinopathy of prematurity; capillary samples and intermittent arterial puncture are useless.
- Fluid balance must be monitored by daily weighing, continuous records of fluid input and output, and frequent estimations of the serum sodium and creatinine.
- In very low birth weight babies in intensive care, blood electrolytes, creatinine and full blood count should be monitored daily, with more frequent estimations in extremely low birth weight babies in the first few days.

Thermal control

In the era of sophisticated incubators and complex infant care centres with overhead radiant heaters, it should not be assumed that the control of a premature infant's thermal environment is either unimportant or easy. The neonate has a huge surface area to volume ratio and therefore loses heat rapidly. The smaller the baby, the greater this loss, particularly if he is naked. Heat is lost in four ways:

1. Conductive losses should be small. However, placing a baby in a cold incubator will lead to rapid heat loss through conduction. Conversely, self-heating gel-filled mattresses can be useful for thermoregulation, particularly during transport.
2. Evaporative heat loss is due to the latent heat of evaporation of water on the baby's skin and is dependent on how wet the baby is, how immature and water permeable is the skin, and exposure to drying factors such as air movement or radiant heaters. Babies are often nursed in a closed incubator in which it is possible to attain a high level of humidification; however, it is essential to remember that these levels drop rapidly when incubator doors are opened.
3. Convective heat loss is due to the cooling effect of air currents around the baby and is normally small, unless the baby is in a cool draught.
4. The baby also loses heat by radiation onto nearby objects. When this is the incubator wall, the effective temperature is a function of the temperature inside and outside the incubator. To obtain the 'operative' temperature, 1°C needs to be deducted from the incubator temperature for every 7°C the room temperature

falls below the incubator temperature. This form of heat loss is much greater when the baby, particularly if naked, is outside an incubator and is radiating heat onto the walls and windows of a labour ward or a neonatal unit (NNU).

Clinical effects of cold

The deleterious effects of cold on the premature baby are listed in Table 7.1. Even without the neonate's temperature falling, cooling can cause problems, but once his physiological responses to cold are overcome and his body temperature falls, the effects of a cool environment become much more serious. The most dramatic effect of allowing babies to get cold is the increase in morbidity and mortality. Blackfan and Yaglou (1933) showed that keeping babies warmer significantly reduced mortality, and this has since been reconfirmed in a number of studies.

Clinical effects of overheating

There are also dangers from overheating (Yashiro *et al.* 1973). Although the exact mechanisms are not clear, the various associations which have been reported are listed in Table 7.1.

Management of temperature control

Since babies who get cold or who are overheated have a much higher morbidity and mortality, it is essential to make every effort to keep their core temperature as close to 37°C as possible. The following five practices should be routine in all maternity hospitals and all NNUs:

1. Keep labour wards as warm and as draught-free as possible, and make special efforts when a premature baby is being delivered. Ideally the room should be warmed to 23–25°C. The resuscitation area must be draught-free, away from

Table 7.1 Deleterious effects of thermal stress on low birth weight babies

Cold	Heat
↓ Surfactant synthesis	↑ Fluid loss (evaporative, sweating)
↓ Surfactant efficacy	↑ Postnatal weight loss
↓ pH	Hypernatraemia (hyperosmolarity)
↓ PaO_2	↑ Jaundice
Hypoglycaemia	Recurrent apnoea
↑ O_2 consumption	↑ NEONATAL MORTALITY
Diversion of cardiac output to brown fat	
↑ Utilization of calorie reserves	
↑ Postnatal weight loss	
↓ Later weight gain	
Neonatal cold injury (?sclerema)	
↓ Blood coagulability	
↑ NEONATAL MORTALITY	

windows and air conditioning, and the resuscitation must be carried out under an overhead radiant heater.

2. Dry all term babies after delivery with a warm towel and thereafter keep them either wrapped up or under the radiant heat source. Very small or preterm infants should not be dried but placed immediately after delivery into a food-grade plastic bag, leaving just their head exposed – to which a bonnet should be applied. They should remain in the bag until safely in a humidified incubator. It is often useful to maintain them in the bag until after any umbilical lines have been sited as this is often a time when babies get cold. Small holes can be made in the bag to allow access to limbs or the umbilicus for cannulation.

3. Keep nurseries and NNUs hot enough (26–28°C) to minimize radiant heat loss.

4. Nurse babies in incubators and minimize radiant, evaporative and convective heat loss.

5. Warm and humidify all medical gases administered to babies.

Pyrexial babies

A temperature of 37.5°C, or sometimes even higher, in a baby in an NNU or on a postnatal ward is usually due to:

1. incubator/room temperature being too high;
2. lying in direct sunlight or phototherapy – effectively a radiant heat source;
3. overswaddling the baby;
4. some combination of all three (common).

These simple errors should be remedied, and, if the temperature falls rapidly, no further action is usually required. However, if none of them is present and the baby looks unwell, or if he is still febrile 60 minutes later, the following three important conditions should be considered:

1. Infection (see Chapter 16). A full infectious disease workup should be carried out. The normal core–peripheral temperature difference is 2°C and a higher difference suggests sepsis.
2. Dehydration fever (usually a term baby who has fed poorly and lost more than 10% of his birth weight). His serum osmolarity will exceed 300 mOsmol/ kg water, and rehydration with milk or intravenous or oral glucose electrolyte solution rapidly restores the temperature to normal.
3. Brain damage with injury to hypothalamic centres.

▮ Minimal handling

An extremely important basic tenet of neonatal intensive care is that handling and disturbing a sick neonate in any way may cause their condition to deteriorate, usually by making them hypoxic. Anything that makes an infant cry, by making respiration irregular, will compromise ventilation (even if ventilated), increase pulmonary artery pressure, increase the right to left shunt (pp. 162–165) and thus lower the PaO_2. Complex manoeuvres, such as a chest X-ray or a lumbar puncture, disconnecting the oxygen supply when sucking out the endotracheal tube, or giving chest physiotherapy, are other potent causes of hypoxia.

Many spontaneously breathing low birth weight babies, when handled or made to cry, start to writhe about, take a deep inspiration, stop breathing, remain apnoeic and become cyanosed with a bradycardia.

Points to remember

■ The less you touch a baby, the less likely you are to transmit infection. Always wash and gel your hands before and after handling a neonate.

■ Heel pricks, venous and arterial punctures are painful and make infants cry. This not only gives incorrect results for blood gases but causes clinical deterioration. If blood sampling for biochemistry, blood gases or haematology is going to be frequent, an intra-arterial sampling line is essential.

■ Electrocardiogram (ECG), respiration, temperature, blood pressure, oxygen saturation and blood gases should be monitored continuously by electronic means. Continuous monitoring is, in any case, always superior to intermittent monitoring.

■ Getting arterial lines and monitors in place does mean one intense period of activity and interference immediately after admission. Do these procedures within the incubator or under a radiant heat source, and ensure that the infant's oxygenation is sustained throughout.

■ Use analgesic for painful procedures; there is no doubt that neonates feel pain.

■ Oropharyngeal suction, and in particular suction down an endotracheal tube (ETT) during assisted ventilation, is notorious for causing deterioration. ETT suction is overdone and with rare exceptions is not indicated at all in the first 24 hours of ventilation, and then not more than 12 hourly unless there is infection or bronchorrhoea. If the PaO_2 falls below 6.6 kPa (50 mmHg), stop suctioning at once and reconnect the intermittent positive pressure ventilation.

■ If a lumbar puncture needs to be done or an intravenous line resited, do it as expeditiously as possible without moving the infant from his incubator and interfering with oxygen administration.

■ If anyone fails on any procedure more than twice, *stop*. Let the infant recover, then get someone else to try.

■ X-rays involve major handling of the infant if the incubator does not have a film cassette. A member of the medical or nursing staff must always help the radiographer. Take great care to sustain oxygenation during the procedure.

■ If you are doing an X-ray to exclude pneumothorax or to ensure that an ETT is properly sited – and if the X-ray gives you that information even if it is blurred, rotated, expiratory or overpenetrated – do not repeat it. A surfeit of technically poor films may stop the X-ray department sending inexperienced staff to take X-rays on very sick infants!

■ Does the infant's incubator really need a spring clean and does he really mind that small amount of meconium in his nappy or the crusted blood on his scalp? The nursing staff may feel that a clean baby in a clean incubator is a healthy baby, but the neonate will not share their enthusiasm if they make him hypoxic and apnoeic.

■ Does the baby perhaps need a rest? Studies have shown that infants in intensive care are never left alone for more than a few minutes. They certainly do not often get the chance to sleep without someone stuffing a suction tube up their nose, a thermometer under their armpit or a needle into their skin.

Analgesia

Opioids

Morphine and fentanyl are the most commonly used opioids in the UK. All can cause ventilatory depression, urinary retention and decreased intestinal motility, leading to delayed feeding after abdominal surgery. Fentanyl provides intense analgesia and relative cardiovascular stability. Morphine has both slower onset and offset than fentanyl after a single dose, but after long-term infusion this effect is reversed. While initial doses of opioid infusions needed for analgesia and sedation are low, the dose requirements increase rapidly as babies become tolerant. In long-term use, withdrawal can become a problem if infusions are stopped too rapidly (see Chapter 28).

Paracetamol

Paracetamol is a widely accepted treatment for moderate pain in neonates. Current data suggest that its short-term use in term and preterm neonates is safe and efficacious. Intravenous paracetamol is available, although the dose regimens for neonates vary throughout the world.

Local anaesthetics

The use of local and regional anaesthesia/analgesic techniques has a significant role in the treatment of neonatal pain. Single-dose local anaesthetic is especially useful for painful procedures such as insertion of chest drains. Topical anaesthetic creams have not been found to be effective for reducing pain from heel-pricking.

Environmental and behavioural interventions

There is a growing body of evidence that environmental, behavioural and non-pharmacological strategies can reduce the behavioural and physiological indicators of pain and stress in the newborn. These principles are encompassed in the concepts of developmental care and minimal handling. Minimizing painful procedures to those absolutely necessary and clustering them together can reduce the frequency of noxious stimuli. Oral sucrose and sweet compounds are safe and effective in reducing pain scores during invasive procedures.

■ Monitoring

Even the most sophisticated monitor is no substitute for a good intensive care nurse. The equipment outlined in this chapter is there to assist minimal handling (p. 53). Equipment can achieve these aims only if it is maintained and used properly.

Respiration monitoring

Apnoea monitoring

Various systems are available for monitoring respiration. They all have the problem that, if the baby gasps or moves when apnoeic, they fail to alarm. Nevertheless, some form of apnoea monitor should be attached to all spontaneously breathing babies at risk of apnoea. The most widely used device (Valman *et al.* 1983) consists of a pressure-sensitive capsule (Graseby monitor) which is attached to the baby's abdominal skin, close to the umbilicus or on the lower abdomen. The movements of the abdominal wall distort a membrane which is covering the capsule, producing pressure changes. Modern multichannel monitors have built-in impedance monitors, detecting respiration by using a high-frequency oscillator to send a small current across conventional ECG electrodes on the chest wall. The volume alterations during breathing produce tiny changes in electrical resistance, which are detected and recorded electronically.

Dual monitoring of heart rate and oxygen saturation for apnoea

The best and most widely used method to detect apnoea in routine clinical care is to use the Graseby monitor plus heart rate, detected by ECG, or oxygen saturation by pulse oximetry. This allows detection of the two consequences of apnoea which may be harmful: bradycardia and hypoxaemia.

Respiratory pattern and waveform

A large number of devices are now commercially available which, in addition to detecting apnoea, display the baby's respiratory rate and combine this with a visual display of the respiratory waveform and trend recording.

Blood gases

The target range for PaO_2, $PaCO_2$ and pH, and the physiological justification for the tight control required, is given in Chapter 13.

To monitor blood gases adequately it is necessary to have an indwelling arterial line and ideally some device for continuous oxygen (and occasionally CO_2) monitoring. It must be emphasized that only arterial blood gases can be relied on to give accurate analysis of the baby's oxygenation, particularly in those babies at risk from retinopathy of prematurity (ROP). An indwelling arterial line also enables the neonatologist to take frequent samples without contravening the minimal handling rule.

Arterial blood gases must be measured at least 4–6 hourly during the acute phase of any respiratory illness, even in the presence of continuous oxygen monitoring. Arterial sampling is also necessary to calibrate the continuous PaO_2 or transcutaneous PO_2(TcPO_2) monitoring device and to measure the $PaCO_2$ and acid–base status. If continuous PaO_2 catheters or TcPO_2 monitors are being used, are found to be accurate in an individual baby and the neonate is otherwise stable, the frequency of direct blood gas sampling can be reduced to 6–8 hourly after 2–3 days of age or sooner if the baby is in less than 30% oxygen.

Umbilical arterial catheters

The umbilical arteries are easily cannulated for 4–5 days after birth (Chapter 29). The catheter should be FG3.5 or FG4.0 for babies <1500 g and FG5.0 for larger ones. The Cochrane Review concludes that the evidence is strongly in favour of a high catheter position and all agree that the area of T12–L3/4 should be avoided (Fig. 7.1, derived from Phelps et al. 1972) as this is where the renal, coeliac and mesenteric vessels arise from the aorta. The optimal position is with the tip opposite T7–9; a 'low' catheter should have the tip opposite L3–5. The accuracy of positioning has been shown to be improved, so reducing significantly the need for further manipulation of the line, using the formula (Wright et al. 2008):

$$\text{insertion length (cm)} = (4 \times \text{birth weight [kg]}) + 7$$

Once in situ, blood can be taken from the umbilical artery catheter (UAC) as required for PaO_2, $PaCO_2$ and acid–base estimations as well as other laboratory investigations: even blood cultures can be taken from them under appropriate circumstances (Pourcyrous et al. 1988). Only coagulation studies present a problem; because of heparinization of the fluid infused through the catheter, more accurate

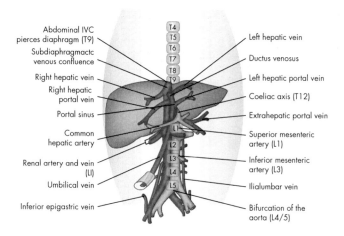

Fig. 7.1 Positions of important branches of the abdominal aorta which should be avoided by umbilical artery catheter tips. Reproduced with permission from Rennie and Robertson (2012)

data are obtained from a peripheral venous sample. Blood pressure can be measured continuously via a transducer connected to the catheter.

Peripheral arterial cannulae

If a UAC cannot be inserted (and the success rate is more than 90% in experienced hands) then a peripheral site should be cannulated to allow for frequent arterial sampling without disturbing the baby. These cannulae can be used for continuous measurement of blood pressure, and withdrawing samples for biochemical and haematological monitoring, but they must not be used for infusions, other than the 0.5–1 mL/h of heparinized saline used to keep them patent. The preferred arteries are the radial and posterior tibial since they have good collateral supplies. The ulnar artery should not be cannulated unless the radial artery is patent (and vice versa).

Horrific complications from arterial cannulation have been reported (Chapter 29). The complication rate with UACs is no greater than that with peripheral arterial lines. Umbilical catheters can be left in situ for at least 2 weeks, whereas peripheral arterial lines rarely last for more than 6–7 days. The complications of either type of cannula can be reduced to a minimum if the following rules are observed:

- maintain a continuous infusion of heparinized saline with 1 unit of heparin/mL;
- remove all arterial lines immediately if they show signs of partial or complete blockage (i.e. if there are other than transient vascular changes in the area supplied);
- remove all central lines (venous or arterial) if septicaemia is not responding rapidly to treatment.

Capillary blood gases

Capillary PO_2 cannot be relied on to detect hyperoxaemia, and in the first few days after birth capillary acid–base values are also less reliable, tending to read high for PCO_2 and low for pH. Therefore babies requiring significant ventilatory support, especially if this includes supplemental oxygen, should ideally by monitored using arterial gases, as above. Capillary gas analysis is of greatest value in babies with chronic lung disease. In such babies, who are usually sufficiently mature not to be at risk from ROP, oxygenation is effectively monitored by oximetry. However, it is important to know the degree of carbon dioxide retention in such cases and capillary blood gas analysis achieves this.

Continuous transcutaneous monitoring

Transcutaneous monitoring for $PO_2(TcPO_2)$ and $PCO_2(TcPCO_2)$ is possible using appropriately adapted electrodes accurately applied to the skin. Transcutaneous devices work on the principle that the partial pressure of oxygen and carbon dioxide diffusing from the capillaries through skin heated to 44°C is very close to true arterial PO_2. Great care has to be taken with the in-vitro calibration of these devices and with how they are attached to the skin. To ensure accuracy and to prevent skin damage from prolonged exposure to the temperature of 44°C, the electrode site should be changed every 4 hours.

Transcutaneous devices give an instantaneous measure ($\pm15\%$) of PaO_2 in most babies. However, in routine clinical use they are not predictably accurate, particularly at higher PaO_2 values, or in ill hypotensive neonates following vasodilator therapy, or in mature babies with a thick skin. The accuracy of $TcPO_2$ monitors must always be checked by intermittent arterial blood gas analysis. Continuous $TcPO_2$ monitoring, used in association with blood gas analyses on blood drawn from an indwelling arterial line, is an acceptable way of monitoring the critically ill neonate. $TcPCO_2$ monitors are useful when adjusting ventilator settings in critically ill ventilated babies and may give early warning of a blocked ETT or pneumothorax.

Continuous pulse oximetry

The correct shorthand for a pulse oximeter reading is SpO_2. Pulse oximetry is easy to use, requires no calibration and gives immediate information. The technique has revolutionized oxygen monitoring and is extremely valuable during resuscitation. Oximetry estimates the percentage oxygen *saturation* of haemoglobin in arterial blood (SpO_2), not the partial *pressure* of oxygen (PaO_2); it is not the same as true saturation (SaO_2) measured in vitro with a co-oximeter. The technique of oximetry is dependent on the differential absorption of red (circa 660 nm) and infra-red (circa 940 nm) light by deoxyhaemoglobin and oxyhaemoglobin, respectively.

The SpO_2 in pulse oximeters has a standard error of about ±2–3% from true SaO_2 in the range of saturation between 70% and 100%. Thus at a SpO_2 read-out of 92%, the true saturation (SaO_2) could be anywhere between 88% and 96% (±2 standard errors). It has been shown that, at a SpO_2 of 92%, the arterial oxygen tension can be anywhere between 5.3 and 13 kPa; the errors get bigger with underperfusion (Clayton *et al*. 1991). The results are not affected by racial pigmentation of the skin or staining from bilirubin, but extraneous light can affect the reading.

Pulse oximetry must never be relied upon to prevent hyperoxaemia in at-risk babies since PaO_2 values may be unacceptably high even at a saturation of 95%. Pulse oximetry is invaluable in the very preterm infant, in whom it is not possible to maintain arterial access during the many weeks of oxygen therapy many require to treat their chronic lung disease. The Support study reported the outcome of 1316 babies between 24 and 27 weeks' gestation nursed to achieve oxygen saturation targets of either 85–89% or 91–95%. There was no difference in the composite outcome of severe retinopathy or death, but the group in the lower saturation range had significantly less retinopathy but there was evidence of a higher mortality (p=004) (Support Study Group 2010).

Oximeters are popular because they are easy to use. Oximetry can be very helpful in confirming or refuting hypoxia in babies suspected of having cyanotic congenital heart disease, although the proposal that it should be used as a screening tool has not yet reached acceptance. The non-invasive nature of the sensors means that two can be applied easily to measure pre- and post-ductal oxygen saturation in pulmonary hypertension (pp. 162–165). Table 7.2 gives our current guidance for oximeter alarm settings.

Heart rate monitoring

As part of intensive care an ECG should be continuously recorded and displayed. Small pre-gelled electrodes suitable for use in the preterm neonate are widely available. Some thought should be given to positioning the electrodes to minimize the effect of the inevitable shadow they will cause on a chest X-ray. The pattern of the ECG may alert the clinician to electrolyte disturbances, myocardial hypoxia or even a pneumothorax. Regularity of the heart rate is a sign of severe respiratory disease. A fixed slow heart rate is a sign of central nervous system depression. Tachycardia can be an early warning sign of haemorrhage, inadequate analgesia or drugs, e.g. methylxanthines. Bradycardia can be an early sign of a blocked ETT or raised intracranial pressure.

Blood pressure monitoring (normal ranges in Appendix 3)

Oscillometry

Oscillometry detects movement (oscillations) within the limb caused by the inflow of blood. A small plastic sphygmomanometer-type cuff is inflated and automatically deflated

Table 7.2 Guidance for oximeter alarm settings

Gestation at birth	Postmenstrual age	Status	Target saturation %	Alarm limits
≤32 weeks	<36 weeks	In oxygen	91–93	88–95
≤32 weeks	<36 weeks	In air	91–93	88–100
≤32 weeks	>36 weeks	In oxygen	91–93	88–95
≤32 weeks	>36 weeks	In air	>91	88–100
≤33 weeks	Any	Ventilated for significant lung disease	>94	94–100
≥33 weeks	Any	In oxygen	91–97	88–97
≥33 weeks	Any	In air	>91	88–100

Cyanotic congenital heart disease: settings to be individualized and agreed with cardiologists, alarm limits set at 4% above and below agreed target.

Pulmonary hypertension: settings to be individualized and agreed with neonatologist, generally target >95%, alarm settings 94–100. Pre-ductal and post-ductal saturations to have a difference of less than 10%.

at regular intervals. When the air pressure within the cuff is above systolic pressure, no movement is detected; when the cuff pressure is reduced, blood enters the limb, increasing the limb volume and compressing the cuff, thus oscillating the pressure within it. These devices can be relied upon only if a suitably sized cuff is carefully applied (two-thirds of the length of the upper arm), the baby weighs more than 1 kg and the blood pressure is reasonable. In the shocked extremely low birth weight baby these devices overestimate systolic blood pressures in the 35–45 mmHg range by as much as 5–10 mmHg.

Invasive blood pressure monitoring

Direct recording from an indwelling arterial cannula is the preferred method of monitoring blood pressure in sick very low birth weight neonates. It is important to avoid common mistakes in using pressure transducers, in particular ensuring that the apparatus is at the same level as the neonate's heart and that there is no damping due to bubbles in the connecting lines. Having a visual display of the blood pressure waveform which should show a good pulse pressure and a dichrotic notch is a check on the presence of damping, as well as on the state of the cardiac output in the patient.

Central venous pressure monitoring

Although widely used in babies and older children, central venous pressure (CVP) monitoring has not caught on in neonatology. Yet it is clear that ventilated neonates with low CVP do badly (Skinner *et al.* 1992). The pressure in the inferior vena cava does give clinically useful information (Lloyd *et al.* 1992). To monitor CVP the transducer should be attached to the end of the umbilical venous catheter and the techniques used are identical to those of blood pressure monitoring.

Temperature monitoring

Temperature can be monitored either by 4-hourly use of a rectal or axillary thermometer, or by the use of a rectal or skin thermistor left in place to minimize handling. Measuring the central/peripheral temperature difference can provide useful information about the state of the circulation, particularly circulating blood volume. Continuous skin or core temperature monitoring will need to be used if the incubator or radiant heat cradle is used in servo mode.

■ Clinical and laboratory monitoring

Fluid balance

A fluid balance chart is an integral part of the monitoring of all ill babies, although it is difficult to record accurately all the fluid infused, including that given as drugs or for flushing catheters after sampling. Boluses of saline, blood and bicarbonate must always be included. Urine output should be checked regularly. Critically ill neonates should have an absolute measure of urine output daily, together with urinalysis for protein, blood and glucose. Since catheterization carries the risk of infection, and adhesive urine bags frequently damage the thin, frail skin of preterm newborns, the most effective way of measuring urine output is to weigh disposable nappies (or cotton wool balls placed within them). These items must be weighed as soon as possible after voiding to avoid evaporative loss.

Weighing is the single most important investigation in assessing fluid balance in the critically ill neonate and should be done at least once a day. In very preterm babies who have an enormous transepidermal water loss, 12-hourly weighing may be indicated.

Nursing, monitoring and transport of the sick neonate

Bacteriological monitoring

As part of the workup to exclude infection, all neonates with respiratory distress will have a full set of swabs and a blood culture taken. Thereafter we find surface swabs once per week useful. Such surveillance enables identification of colonization with serious pathogens and can help to target therapy should such babies develop a deteriorating chest X-ray, a rise in C-reactive protein and/or white cell count. Surveillance also helps monitoring of the NNU flora, including MRSA.

Biochemical monitoring (Table 7.3)

It is impossible to predict hypo- or hyperglycaemia, hypo- or hypernatraemia, hypo- or hyperkalaemia, hypocalcaemia or hypoalbuminaemia in ill babies despite meticulous attention to the content and volume of the intravenous fluid therapy. It is more difficult when total parenteral nutrition is used. Bilirubin must be checked frequently in jaundiced babies (see Chapter 20).

Haematological monitoring (Table 7.3)

Ill babies, in particular those <1.50 kg, tolerate anaemia badly and are also subject to large blood losses from monitoring. Such babies should have regular haemoglobin and packed cell volume estimation. The white cell count should always be checked as part of the initial evaluation when a baby is admitted to the NNU. Thereafter daily white cell counts in acutely ill babies can help in the detection of early sepsis and in the evaluation of antibiotic therapy in established sepsis.

Monitoring infusion pressures

Modern infusion pumps are fitted with devices which continuously monitor the pressure required to deliver the infusion and these can be set to alarm. Accuracy of delivery at small volumes is now taken for granted, but there is little information on which to base a decision regarding setting pressure alarm limits for infusions in neonatal intensive care units. The UK Department of Health standard of

Table 7.3 Routine monitoring of the ill neonate

4-hourly	Daily
Temperature, pulse and respiration rate Glucose * Bilirubin * Blood gases (see p. 146)	Haemoglobin, packed cell volume, white blood cells, platelets ^Na, K, creatinine, calcium, phosphate, Glucose, C-reactive protein
2 or 3 times per week	**Weekly**
Albumin Surface swabs	Liver enzymes (when on TPN) Triglycerides (when on TPN) Alkaline phosphatase (for osteopenia) Reticulocytes (for anaemia of prematurity)

* In babies with appropriate diagnoses. In stable babies glucose need only be checked daily. Bilirubin need not be measured in the absence of clinical jaundice.

^ Electrolytes may need to be measured two or three times per day in extreme preterm/very low birth weight or very sick babies.

TPN, total parenteral nutrition.

300 mmHg is well above the operating pressure of most neonatal infusions. For peripheral venous infusions and silastic 'long lines', 40 mmHg is a suitable choice for general purposes. This provides an acceptable compromise between the number of nuisance alarms from self-clearing occlusions and detecting genuine blockages quickly. Suitable settings for UACs are 100 mmHg.

Neonatal transport

Neonatal transport forms a vital component of the network system of neonatal intensive care delivery used in the UK. Recent changes in the UK have seen the evolution of dedicated transport teams to improve the retrieval and repatriation of sick neonates. The process of transport has the potential to cause further disruption of the neonate's physiological balance, at a time when they are often critically ill. In an attempt to minimize these changes, transport needs to be undertaken with care. The process of transport can be divided into various phases:

■ Handover 1: on arrival of the transport team a detailed handover of the history and clinical condition of the baby is essential. This should, ideally, be a joint handover between both medical and nursing staff, to aid good communication.
■ Stabilization: a variable period is required to optimize the infant's condition prior to transport. The baby's stability should be assessed systematically, evaluating respiratory, cardiovascular, gastrointestinal, renal, metabolic, neurological, septic, haematological and biochemical parameters as well as checking fluid status and the adequacy of vascular access. Particular care must be taken with temperature management in premature or low birth weight infants. It can be difficult to know how long to continue stabilization at the referring hospital and when to 'scoop and run'. However, much of this decision-making is based on communication with the receiving unit and an assessment of whether stability may be achieved only on instigation of treatments not available in the referring unit.
■ Transfer: the baby will generally need to be moved from his own incubator to a transport incubator while maintaining appropriate physiological monitoring (heart rate, oxygen saturation, blood pressure and temperature). A final checklist of physiological parameters prior to leaving the referring unit can be valuable. During the transfer itself the health and safety of the staff, as well as the baby, are essential. Although 'on transport' incidents are minimized by pre-transfer stabilization, a rapid troubleshooting approach is required for solving problems. Any intervention or evaluation necessitating unfastening of staff seatbelts requires the ambulance to be stopped. All emergency equipment and drugs should be kept close to hand to deal with emergencies such as displaced tubes, pneumothorax or cardiac arrest.
■ Handover 2: on arrival at the receiving unit a second, joint, detailed handover of the baby's history and condition and the transport itself is required.
■ Careful consideration must be given to parents already facing distress over their baby's illness. Here again good communication is essential. An assessment should be made as to whether allowing parents to travel in the ambulance is safe and appropriate. Alternatively, where appropriate the parents should be helped with transport to the receiving unit.

References

Blackfan, KD, Yaglou, CP (1933) The premature infant: a study of the effects of atmospheric conditions on growth and on development. *American Journal of Diseases of Children*, **46**: 1175.

Clayton, DG, Webb, RK, Ralston, AC, Duthie, D, Runciman, WB (1991) A comparison of the performance of 20 pulse oximeters under conditions of poor perfusion. *Anaesthesia*, **46**: 3–10.

Lloyd, TR, Donnerstein, RL, Berg, RA (1992) Accuracy of central venous pressure measurement from the abdominal inferior vena cava. *Pediatrics*, **89**: 506–8.

Phelps, DL, Lachman, RS, Leake, RD, Oh, W (1972) The radiologic localisation of the major aortic tributaries in the newborn infant. *Journal of Pediatrics*, **81**: 336–9.

Pourcyrous, M, Korones, SB, Bada, HS, *et al.* (1988) Indwelling umbilical arterial catheter: A preferred sampling site for blood culture. *Pediatrics*, **81**: 821–5.

Skinner, JR, Milligan, DWA, Hunter, S, Hey, EN (1992) Central venous pressure in the ventilated neonate. *Archives of Disease in Childhood*, **67**: 374–7.

Support Study Group of the Eunice Kennedy Shriver NICHD Neonatal Research Network (2010) Target ranges of oxygen saturation in extremely preterm infants. *New England Journal of Medicine*, DOI: 10.1056/NEJMoa0911781.

Valman, HS, Wright, BM, Lawrence, C (1983) Measurement of respiratory rate in the newborn. *British Medical Journal*, **286**: 1783–4.

Wright, IM, Owers, M, Wagner, M (2008) The umbilical arterial catheter: a formula for improved positioning in the very low birth weight infant. *Pediatric Critical Care Medicine*, **9**: 498–501.

Yashiro, K, Adams, FH, Emmanouilides, GC, Mickey, MR (1973) Preliminary studies on the thermal environment of low birthweight infants. *Journal of Pediatrics*, **82**: 991–4.

8

Physical examination of the newborn

Key points
- All babies should have a routine head to toe examination by a sufficiently qualified health professional within 72 hours of birth.
- Measurement of head circumference at birth is a crucial part of first-hour care.

The postnatal examination of the newborn is an important routine screening tool carried out to identify any problem or abnormality that the newborn infant may exhibit. Despite it being a comprehensive examination there are some abnormalities that are not possible to detect immediately after birth and some may not be apparent until the infant is several days or weeks old. During the examination problems can be identified and, if appropriate, referral made for investigation, specialist assessment and treatment and the findings can be fully discussed with the parents. Helpful information can be obtained from the UK Newborn and Infant Physical Examination (NIPE) website (http://newbornphysical.screening. nhs.uk/).

The purposes of the newborn examination include:

- review of any problems arising or suspected from antenatal screening, family history or the events in labour;
- ascertaining whether or not the family have any worries about the baby and trying to address them;
- initiating appropriate treatment and following up where indicated (e.g. hepatitis vaccination, phototherapy for jaundice, special teat for cleft palate);
- screening for the four specific NIPE target conditions including developmental dysplasia of the hips, cataract and retinoblastoma, undescended testes in boys, and congenital heart disease;
- diagnosing congenital malformations and common neonatal problems, and giving advice about management;
- detecting the occasional baby who is obviously ill and requires urgent treatment;
- collecting baseline information about weight and head circumference;
- identifying parents who may have problems in caring for their baby due to substance abuse, mental health problems, learning difficulties or very poor housing and alerting the appropriate professional groups;
- beginning to provide health education advice, e.g. regarding breastfeeding, cot death prevention, safe transport in cars.

Timing of the examination

An examination should be carried out by trained personnel before 72 hours of age, and ideally before the baby leaves hospital. Early discharge, combined with an increasing number of home births, makes it more difficult to organize routine examination of the newborn. As a result there is a need to involve other professional groups in this task, and studies have shown that advanced neonatal nurse practitioners and midwives with special training can be effective in this role. A baby who is well can be allowed to leave the hospital prior to a full examination being carried out; however, an arrangement must be made for the baby to be examined by a sufficiently competent practitioner within 72 hours of birth. Criteria for early discharge may include the following:

- Mother has no medical complications in pregnancy, e.g. diabetes, epilepsy, heart condition, mental health concerns.
- Mother is fit for discharge, is supported at home and received all appropriate treatment.
- Singleton, 37–42 weeks of gestation with an appropriate weight for gestation (i.e. between 2.5 kg and 4 kg) and not clinically growth restricted.
- Baby well at birth without the need for resuscitation.
- No thick meconium (grade 2 or 3) in the liquor requiring a period of respiratory observations.
- No risk factors for infection requiring observation (premature rupture of membranes, fetal tachycardia, group B beta-haemolytic *Streptococcus* (GBS) on maternal swabs, previous infant with GBS sepsis).
- Not at risk of hypoglycaemia (see Chapter 18).
- Axillary temperature >36.7°C without additional thermoregulatory support.
- Initial physical examination and fetal history reveals no abnormalities that require continued investigations or treatment.
- Baby pink in air with a respiratory rate of <60 breaths/min, no respiratory distress and has a heart rate of 100–160 beats/min and with normal tone.
- No suspicion of jaundice or family history of early jaundice in siblings.
- Completed at least one effective feed.
- No unresolved issues regarding safeguarding the baby.

The mother must have been told where and how to access help and there must be a follow-up plan in place. Babies born at home also require a full examination within 72 hours of birth. This can be performed by the midwife present at birth if she has the relevant training or arrangements must be made with the GP or with the local hospital for the examination to be carried out.

The examination should take place in a safe, warm, private environment, and the findings should be documented appropriately including in the parent-held, child health record. All new parents should receive an 'NHS Antenatal and Newborn Screening Programmes' booklet. This gives information about the reason for the examination and its extent. The person undertaking the examination should also explain to the parents the rationale for the examination of the baby and gain verbal consent. Communication should be clear and appropriate throughout the examination and findings explained afterwards, including appropriate information and advice. Time should always be included for the parents to ask questions.

The examination

There are no absolute standards that define what should be included within the examination; however, a top to toe approach is helpful and guidance can be found on the NIPE website and in the chapter by Rennie (2012).

1. The weight and head circumference of the baby should be documented.
2. Throughout the consultation observations of the general appearance, colour, position, respiration, behaviour, activity and posture of the baby should be made. It may be advantageous to listen to the heart while the baby is quiet and settled.
3. Examine the scalp, head, face, nose, mouth (including visualizing the hard and soft palate), ears, neck and general symmetry of head and facial features.
4. Check the eyes with an ophthalmoscope and test for the 'red reflex'.
5. If exposed, the hands, feet, limbs and digits can be examined at this point.
6. The baby should then be fully undressed and the rest of the examination performed.
7. Cardiovascular system – this includes colour, heart rate (normal 100–160 beats/min), rhythm and femoral pulse volume as well as listening to the heart for a murmur. The cardiovascular assessment should also include palpation of the abdomen to identify any organomegaly. If there is any concern about cardiac disease then check saturation with a pulse oximeter.
8. Respiratory effort should be assessed in conjuction with other signs of respiratory problems such as tachypnoea at rest, retraction, grunting and nasal flaring. Observe the rate (normal 30–60 breaths/min) and pattern of chest movement. Auscultate to check for crackles and stridor.
9. Clavicles and upper limbs – observation, palpation and examination to identify any abnormalities, e.g. Erb's palsy.
10. Abdomen – observe colour and shape and palpate to identify any organomegaly. The condition of the umbilical cord should be assessed and the number of cord vessels should be included in the notes.
11. Renal area – bimanual palpation of the renal area should be performed to identify any masses.
12. Genitalia and anus – assess gender and appearance of genitalia. Patency of the anus is examined.
13. Spine – with the baby prone inspect for completeness of bony structures and skin. Observe the coccygeal area and note any abnormal pigmentation or sacral dimples.
14. Skin – the examination of the skin will include any variations from normal skin colour, e.g. jaundice and cyanosis, and also any birthmarks, e.g. Mongolian blue spots, café au lait spots or rashes.
15. Reflexes – the Moro, grasp, rooting and sucking reflexes are assessed.
16. Hips – the proportions and symmetry of the lower limbs and skin folds are examined before testing hip stability. It is important to view the skin creases from the posterior aspect of the thigh. The hips are then tested using both the Barlow and Ortolani tests to ensure they are neither dislocated nor dislocatable.
17. Feet – observe and examine to identify postural abnormalities, e.g. talipes.

■ Reference

Rennie, JM (2012) Examination of the newborn. In Rennie, JM (ed.) *Rennie & Roberton's Textbook of Neonatology*, 5th edition. Edinburgh: Elsevier, pp. 247–262.

■ Further reading

Lee, TW, Skelton, RE, Skene, C (2001) Routine neonatal examination: effectiveness of trainee paediatrician compared with advanced neonatal nurse practitioner. *Archives of Disease in Childhood. Fetal and Neonatal Edition*, **85**: F100–4.

NHS Antenatal and Newborn Screening Programme (2011) An introduction to physical examination of newborn babies and those aged six to eight weeks. Screening tests for you and your baby (www.screening.nhs.uk).

NHS Quality Improvement Scotland (2008) Best Practice Statement – May 2008. Routine examination of the newborn.

NICE Clinical guideline 37 – postnatal care (www.nice.org.uk/nicemedia/pdf/CG37NICEguideline.pdf).

Townsend, J, Wolke, D, Hayes, J, *et al.* (2004) Routine examination of the newborn: the EMREN study. Evaluation of an extension of the midwife role including a randomized controlled trial of appropriately trained midwives and paediatric senior house officers. *Health Technology Assessment*, **8**(14): 1–10.

Wolke, D, Dave, S, Hayes, J, *et al.* (2002) Routine examination of the newborn and maternal satisfaction: a randomized controlled trial. *Archives of Disease in Childhood. Fetal and Neonatal Edition*, **86**: F155–60.

▨ Web link

http://newbornphysical.screening.nhs.uk

9

Congenital anomalies and common postnatal problems

Key points
- Isolated minor anomalies are common and many are of no clinical significance.
- Neonatologists have a golden opportunity to be the first to identify important problems.
- It is vital to consider gender, race, family history and number of minor abnormalities before investigating.
- Some apparently minor abnormalities can be the clue to underlying serious disease.

An anomaly is a structural defect which deviates from normal. Congenital refers to something which is present at birth; it does not necessarily imply either that there is a known cause or that there is an underlying genetic diagnosis. Isolated minor anomalies are common and are usually incidental findings (as long as they are truly isolated). Common minor anomalies are shown in Table 9.1.

However, there are some minor anomalies that do need further attention:

- more than three café au lait spots in Caucasians, or more than five in black African babies;
- multiple haemangiomas, or strawberry naevi in specific places, e.g. midline over the spine or on the face in the region supplied by the maxillary division of the facial nerve – associated with Sturge–Weber syndrome;
- oedema of feet associated with Turner syndrome;
- asymmetric crying facies (congenital heart disease);
- microcephaly/macrocephaly;
- micrognathia;
- midline skin defects over the spine.

Table 9.1 Common minor anomalies

Folded-over ears	Umbilical hernia, especially in African Caribbean babies
Hyperextensible thumbs	Hydrocele
Syndactyly of second and and third toes	Undescended testes in newborn period
Single palmar crease	Accessory nipples
Polydactyly especially if familial	Capillary haemangioma
Fifth finger clinodactyly	Simple dimple above the natal cleft
Third fontanelle	Single café au lait spot (up to 3 in Caucasian babies, 5 in African Caribbean babies)
Ear pits and tags (if hearing normal)	

Fifteen to twenty per cent of babies have one minor anomaly, and this carries a 3% risk of an associated major anomaly; 0.8% of babies have two minor anomalies, which is associated with a 10% risk of a major anomaly; 0.5% of babies have three minor anomalies, which has a 20% risk of a major anomaly. The prevalence of the more common major congenital anomalies is shown in Table 9.2.

■ Common findings in day-to-day practice

To aid the busy neonatal resident on the front line of the postnatal ward we provide our approach to some of the common findings and conundrums encountered in day-to-day practice. The list is not exhaustive and other conditions will be detailed in other chapters of the book but this approach has proved valuable to our residents. On encountering multiple minor or a major congenital anomaly you should examine the baby thoroughly and record all features. Do not give parents a diagnosis unless you are absolutely sure; always involve a senior member of the medical staff to help make the diagnosis and inform the parents. Once parents are informed of the diagnosis, support their relationship with the baby; review the baby frequently and offer information leaflets if appropriate.

Accessory auricles/ear pits/ear tags

Ear tags are common with isolated tags occurring in up to 1.7 per 1000 births, 6% of theses are bilateral. Isolated ear pits affect 1–5% of babies. These can be autosomal dominant in inheritance. With the advent of universal neonatal hearing screening in the UK no additional management is required (in areas without neonatal hearing screening the hearing should be tested in both ears). The previous practice of referral for renal scans is not indicated. If there are cosmetic concerns a referral to a plastic surgeon may (rarely) be indicated.

Accessory digits

These are a common finding and are often autosomal dominant. The previous practice of tying a suture around the pedicle of a loosely attached nubbin of an accessory digit is no longer acceptable practice. All accessory digits should be referred to a plastic surgeon for further management.

Table 9.2 Common major anomalies (Source: Office for National Statistics)

	Prevalence (per 1000 live births)
Congenital heart disease	6–8
Developmental dysplasia of the hip	1.5
Talipes	1.5
Down syndrome	1.5
Cleft lip/palate	1.2
Urogenital anomalies (e.g. hypospadias)	1.2
Spina bifida/anencephaly	0.5

Cleft lip and palate

All infants must have their entire palate inspected visually using a light and tongue depressor as part of the routine examination of the newborn. Otherwise it is easy to miss a cleft of the soft palate, which presents later on with feeding difficulties. Immediate referral to the local cleft lip and palate team is essential. In our region a clinical nurse specialist will usually come on day 1 to see the baby. We always attempt to keep baby with mother on the postnatal ward to help establish breast feeding, which is often achievable with support. Early involvement of speech and language therapists either in house or from the regional cleft team may help facilitate this. They can advise on and provide special feeding bottles where appropriate.

Developmental dysplasia of the hip

See p. 344. All babies should be examined using the Ortolani and Barlow tests postnatally and at 6 weeks. Babies with risk factors should be referred for an ultrasound scan (USS). Babies who have suspected developmental dysplasia of the hip should be referred for an urgent opinion from the orthopaedic surgeons.

Down syndrome

Babies with suspected Down syndrome should be examined by a senior member of medical staff. As a general rule if the diagnosis has been considered a karyotype should be sent to confirm or refute the clinical suspicion. A rapid fluorescent in-situ hybridization test can often confirm a diagnosis within a few days.

In addition to genetic diagnostic tests, remember:

- to test thyroid function at around a week of age;
- to check full blood count (including platelets) and serum bilirubin before discharge;
- that an echocardiogram should be performed as soon as possible after birth to look for associated congenital heart disease;
- that inpatient support is often helpful from a breast-feeding support/speech and language therapist; support from a counsellor or clinical psychologist may also be appropriate and excellent leaflets are available;
- that outpatient referrals should be made for ophthalmology review, hearing screening including brainstem responses (automated auditory brainstem response), and a hip ultrasound scan;
- to ensure that letters are sent to the GP, health visitor and child development centre, and that Down syndrome growth charts and inserts are placed in the parent-held records.

Brachial plexus palsy, including Erb's palsy

Erb's palsy results from an injury to the brachial plexus nerve roots, and has an incidence of around 1 in every 2000 births in the UK (unchanged for over 40 years) (Evans-Jones *et al.* 2003). The injury can involve the whole plexus, occasionally including the phrenic nerve (with diaphragmatic palsy) and resulting in a flail arm. More commonly the roots of C5–7 are involved, resulting in the characteristic posture of the upper limb which is internally rotated with flexion at the wrist (waiter's tip position). Klumpke's palsy (C8–T1) can occur but is rare in the newborn. Typically, there is a history of shoulder dystocia in a macrosomic baby. On examination an incomplete or absent Moro reflex is seen on the affected side. The baby should be carefully examined for the co-existence of a fractured clavicle (with X-ray if suspected or uncertain). There can be an associated Horner syndrome. Babies benefit from assessment from and follow-up with an experienced physiotherapist. Many cases are due to neuropraxia and in general the prognosis for recovery is good although only about 50% of babies had fully recovered by 6 months in the recent UK survey. Refer for specialist orthopaedic opinion at 2–3 months if there is no recovery of biceps function, because the best results are obtained with early nerve grafting in appropriately selected cases.

Extracranial haemorrhage

Extracranial bleeding is uncommon and is often associated with Ventouse extraction. The important distinction is between the common and harmless condition of cephalohaematoma and the potentially serious and occasionally life-threatening subgaleal (sometimes termed subaponeurotic) haemorrhage. The features are shown in Table 9.3. If the neonatologist is concerned that there may be a subgaleal bleed the baby needs careful assessment and monitoring (on a neonatal unit (NNU)). Measure the head at hourly intervals and watch for signs of significant blood loss; especially take note of tachycardia which may be the only initial sign. This may herald cardiovascular collapse if not managed appropriately.

Facial nerve palsy

This affects around 0.3% of births and is usually recognized with asymmetrical crying. In severe cases the baby may present feeding problems. Be careful to exclude hypoplasia of the depressor anguli oris muscle which is not facial palsy, in which case there is a high incidence of associated problems, e.g. 22q11 deletion. Most unilateral facial nerve palsies are due to neuropraxia associated with delivery and resolve within the first few weeks of life. Spontaneous recovery is to be expected in these babies, and occurs within 4 weeks in 90%. In bilateral cases think of Mobius syndrome, and in unilateral cases remember hemifacial microsomia and CHARGE (coloboma, heart defects, atresia of choanae, retardation of growth and/or development, genital/urinary abnormalities and ear abnormalities) syndrome. Adequate eye care, taping the eyelid shut in sleep if necessary and using artificial tears, is important while awaiting recovery because of the risk of exposure keratitis.

Gastrointestinal problems

The most common cause of vomiting in a well baby is posseting, with/without gastro-oesophageal reflux. Bilious vomiting is always abnormal and requires prompt

Table 9.3 Comparison of extracranial haemorrhage

	Cephalohaematoma	Subgaleal haematoma
Location	Usually the parietal bones Does not cross sutures	Beneath epicranial aponeurosis
Characteristic findings	Distinct margins Initially firm; more fluctuant after 48 hours	Firm to fluctuant; ill-defined borders, often 'boggy' swelling Crepitus or fluid waves
Timing	Increases after birth for 12–24 hours; resolution over 2–3 weeks	Progressive after birth Resolution over 2–3 weeks
Volume of blood	Not significant	May be massive

investigation. The baby should be admitted to the NNU, abdominal X-ray done and surgical opinion considered. The most important diagnosis not to miss is a malrotation, which can lead to volvulus and loss of bowel. Signs of abdominal problems which require senior assessment include:

- excessive vomiting;
- bile-stained vomiting;
- excessive weight loss (>10%);
- abdominal distension and/or discoloration;
- abdominal tenderness;
- delayed passage of meconium (>48 hours);
- passage of blood per rectum;
- pale stools.

Hydrocele

See p. 321.

Hypoglycaemia

See pp. 237–239.

Hypospadias

See p. 321.

Imperforate anus

See p. 278.

Inguinal hernia

Inguinal hernias are not common in term infants. They can normally be reduced back through the superficial inguinal ring. They should be distinguished clinically from a hydrocele. If freely reducible they should be referred as an outpatient to the paediatric surgeons. If not reducible (incarcerated) this is a surgical emergency; the baby requires immediate transfer for urgent surgery.

Jaundice

See p. 259.

Jitteriness

Jitteriness is a common neonatal finding. It is often due to either excessive startle response or benign myoclonic jerks. It is important to differentiate jitteriness from convulsions. If jitteriness is severe and accompanied by hypertonia it may have an underlying cause, e.g. hypoglycaemia, hypocalcaemia, drug withdrawal, polycythaemia or encephalopathy.

Maternal illegal drug use

See pp. 347–349.

Maternal medication and breast feeding

Most maternal medications are safe in the context of breast feeding (although most manufacturers advise avoidance). In general the benefits of breast feeding normally outweigh minor possible effects on the baby. There are a number of excellent reference texts which present the known data on individual drugs; we find our pharmacist a particularly valuable resource where information is not clear. Encourage mother to express and save milk pending decision.

Maternal thyroid disease

Disorders of thyroid function affect approximately 1 in 3000 newborn term infants, and the risk is increased among infants born to mothers who have thyroid disease (of most aetiologies), irrespective of disease activity and treatment. The routine screening using a blood spot will identify the majority of these patients. Infants of mothers with Graves' disease are at risk of neonatal thyrotoxicosis due to transplacental transfer of stimulating autoantibodies. Only 1–3% of babies delivered to mothers with this past history develop symptoms but the disease can be life-threatening. Testing for the presence and concentration of thyroid-stimulating hormone receptor antibodies during the third trimester in women with a history of Graves' disease helps to predict the babies at risk (for management see pp. 257–258).

Micrognathia

This may be diagnosed antenatally or be identified after birth. It may be an isolated finding or part of a Pierre Robin sequence. Babies may exhibit varying degrees of airway obstruction and feeding difficulties depending on the degree of micrognathia.

Murmur in a well baby

Cardiac murmurs are very common in the neonatal period and are often due to either a patent ductus arteriosus or flow murmurs through a structurally normal heart. Innocent murmurs are characterized by the '5Ss': short, soft, systolic, sternal edge (left) and symptomless. If a murmur persists beyond 24 hours it is our practice to organize an echocardiogram to reassure parents and exclude structural anomalies. If this is not available then four-limb blood pressure (although the value of this is very debatable) and a post-ductal oxygen saturation measurement should be organized prior to discharge with an outpatient echocardiogram arranged at a suitable centre. Parents should be advised to seek urgent medical help if their baby develops breathlessness, poor feeding, colour changes particularly cyanosis or other concerns about their baby's behaviour.

Petechiae

Petechiae are a common finding in neonates following delivery; however, they can also be an indicator of sepsis, disseminated intravascular coagulation, congenital viral infections or thrombocytopenia. It is often prudent to perform a full blood count (and to check the mother's platelet count) and manage accordingly.

Poor feeding

Experience will help you differentiate between the sleepy or poorly latching baby and one who has pathological cause for poor feeding. In general reassess for cleft palate and ask an experienced feeding support worker to assess as well. Possible causes include neurological, e.g. hypotonia or asphyxia, infection or other systemic illness – if in doubt, ask for a senior colleague's opinion. Beware the baby who was previously feeding well whose feeding behaviour changes.

Renal problems

1. Failure to pass urine in the first 24 hours: causes include intrapartum hypoxic ischaemia, poor fluid intake, renal anomalies, outflow obstruction, voiding in the delivery room (8% may not void again for 24 hours). Consider USS of the bladder to look for a large distended bladder and discuss with urology if appropriate.
2. Haematuria:
   - uncommon;
   - most common cause of pink staining on nappies is urate crystals (benign);
   - exclude vaginal bleeding in girl;
   - urine microscopy if concerned;
   - confirm vitamin K given at birth (see Haemorrhagic disease of the newborn – see p. 318).
3. Urinary tract infection – see p. 204.
4. Renal pelvic dilation – see pp. 326–327.

Respiratory distress

Infants with respiratory distress commonly present on the postnatal ward with varying degrees of tachypnoea (>60 breaths/min), cyanosis, expiratory grunting, sternal and subcostal recession, head bobbing and the use of accessory muscles of respiration. Common causes include:

- surfactant deficiency associated with preterm birth, perinatal asphyxia, maternal diabetes, hypothermia;
- congenital pneumonia – e.g. group B *Streptococcus*; may be associated with prolonged rupture of membranes, maternal fever, positive high vaginal swabs;
- meconium aspiration – usually term infants;
- transient tachypnoea of the newborn – delayed clearance of lung liquid, associated with caesarean section without preceding labour; this is often a retrospective diagnosis as the condition is self-limiting lasting 24–48 hours;
- pneumothorax, not an uncommon finding; it is estimated that this affects up to 1% of babies but the majority are minor and require no treatment;
- congenital malformations – e.g. hypoplastic lung, diaphragmatic hernia, cystic adenomatoid malformation;
- metabolic disorders;
- congenital heart disease causing heart failure.

All babies with significant respiratory distress (or mild respiratory distress that persists for more than 2 hours) should be admitted to the NNU for assessment, an infection screen and antibiotics, a chest X-ray and a blood gas. See p. 133 for further management.

Sacral dimples/clefts

- A simple sacral dimple is defined as one that is < 5 mm in size, in the midline, within 2.5 cm of the anus and is not associated with any other cutaneous stigmata. Simple dimples do not indicate spinal dysraphism, unless they occur in combination with other lesions and therefore no further evaluation is required.
- Approximately 50% of children with spinal dysraphism have overlying cutaneous markers including haemangiomas, hairy patch, mass or cutis aplasia. The presence of cutaneous markers with a spinal dimple or pit is highly suspicious.
- All midline lesions that are not simple sacral dimples are suspicious and the baby should have an ultrasound of the spine as a minimum investigation.

Seizures

Seizures are sometimes recognized on the postnatal ward. Initial management is resuscitation and stabilization if necessary and blood sugar measurement (hypoglycaemia is one of the most common causes on the postnatal ward and is devastating if not recognized and managed appropriately). All babies with seizures require admission to the NNU for further assessment and management (see pp. 217–220).

Single umbilical artery

This is a common finding and if an isolated anomaly no further management is required.

Skin rashes and birth marks

See Chapter 26.

Small for gestational age and clinically wasted babies

Small for gestational age is defined as birth weight <2nd centile (Table 9.4) but watch out for clinically wasted babies with higher birth weights. Associated problems include hypoglycaemia, hypothermia, polycythaemia and poor feeding. Ensure early and frequent feeds with maximal feeding support. Suggest expressing if the baby is not latching and sucking well. Encourage kangaroo care to help thermal stability; heated cots/incubators may be required to maintain the baby's temperature.

Table 9.4 Birth weights that are small for gestational age

Gestation	Birth weight	
	Boy	Girl
34 weeks	1550	1500
35 weeks	1750	1700
36 weeks	1950	1800
37 weeks	2100	2000
38 weeks	2250	2200
39 weeks	2500	2300
≥40 weeks	2600	2500

Sticky eyes

See p. 189.

Talipes equinovarus

See p. 343.

Tongue tie

Tongue tie or ankyloglossia is a congenital anomaly characterized by a short lingual frenulum, which may restrict mobility of the tongue. The severity of this condition is very variable from mild to severe with limitation of movement of the tongue resulting in a heart-shaped tongue on protrusion. Severe forms may result in difficulties with latching and breast feeding. The evidence for surgical intervention (division of tongue tie) is limited to one randomized trial and three case series, all of which used a subjective outcome measure. Although reported early adverse events are few, there are no studies looking at long-term complications or rates of breast feeding weeks after intervention. The National Institute for Health and Clinical Excellence has approved division of tongue tie as a service to be provided by the NHS (see Web link). On the basis of the current evidence we feel this procedure should only be offered to babies with significant limitation of tongue movement affecting latching and preventing breast feeding despite maximal breast-feeding support.

Umbilical discharge and flares

Periumbilical redness is not uncommon and may often be a result of pressure from the umbilical clamp. True periumbilical infection presents with redness and local discharge; it is usually due to staphylococci or *Escherichia coli*. Systemic antibiotics are indicated if the discharge is copious or oedema and inflammation are spreading onto the abdominal wall. A blood culture and swab of the discharge should be sent prior to commencing antibiotics.

Undescended testes

See also p. 330. Present in 5% of babies at birth; on examination they may be:

- normal – midpoint of the testis is at or below the midpoint of the scrotum;
- retractile – can be pulled into a normal position and will stay there for a time;
- high scrotal/suprascrotal/inguinal – can only be brought down to correct the position (if at all) temporarily and with discomfort owing to tension on the cord;
- non-palpable.

■ Reference

Evans-Jones, G, Kay, SPJ, Weindling, AM, *et al.* (2003) Congenital brachial palsy: incidence, causes and outcome in the United Kingdom and Republic of Ireland. *Archives of Disease in Childhood. Fetal and Neonatal Edition*, **88**: f185–9.

■ Further reading

Cartlidge, P, Shah, DK, Rennie, JM (2012) Care of the normal term newborn baby. In Rennie, JM (ed.) *Rennie & Roberton's Textbook of Neonatology*, 5th edition. Edinburgh: Elsevier, pp. 361–374.

Graham, JM (2007) *Smith's Recognizable Patterns of Human Deformation*, 3rd edition. Philadelphia: Elsevier.

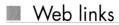 ## Web links

nice.org.uk
www.nice.org.uk/nicemedia/pdf/ip/ IPG149guidance.pdf

PART 3
Nutrition and fluid balance

10

Fluid and electrolyte balance

Key points
- Newborn babies, particularly those of very low birth weight (VLBW), can only regulate fluid and electrolytes within narrow limits.
- VLBW infants easily become dehydrated owing to large transepidermal fluid losses and an inability to concentrate urine.
- A postnatal diuresis and natriuresis is normal, and sodium should not be added to the intravenous fluids until this has occurred.
- Weight and serum sodium are the keys to correct management of fluid balance in the newborn.

Renal function in the neonate is limited. In essence, the neonate, and in particular the preterm neonate, can only regulate fluid and electrolyte homeostasis within narrow limits. The basic principles of management are standard and consist of providing maintenance fluid and electrolyte requirements and providing for ongoing losses. In neonatal medicine, the rapid changes which are seen make this a challenging aspect of intensive care requiring meticulous attention to detail.

Neonatal renal function and physiology

Human glomerulogenesis and nephrogenesis are complete by 34–35 weeks' gestation, though at term the glomeruli are still much smaller than in the adult. The tubules are not fully grown even at term, and only those of the juxtamedullary glomeruli extend deep into the medulla. These factors contribute to the low glomerular filtration rate (GFR) of the neonate, and his inability to concentrate urine. Expressing GFR per unit of surface area is inappropriate in the neonate, and GFR should be expressed per kilogram. When this is done the preterm neonate has a GFR of 0.5 mL/kg/min and the term neonate a GFR of 1.5 mL/kg/min compared with an adult value of 2 mL/kg/min. In clinical practice the serum creatinine concentration is the best guide to GFR. Urea is not helpful.

The renal blood supply arises from the aorta between T12 and L2; umbilical artery catheters must be positioned to end above or below this region (see Fig. 7.1). Renal blood flow is around $100 \, mL/min/1.73 \, m^2$ at term, and is lower in preterm babies or when a baby is ill.

Although well babies excrete the majority of a water load adequately, being able to reduce urine osmolality to <100 mOsmol/kg, when they are ill they are less able to do this, in part because of the lower GFR. Babies can only concentrate urine to a maximal osmolality of 600–800 mosmol/kg until they establish an adequate medullary osmotic gradient. This occurs much later in the neonatal period; by adult life a urine concentration of 1500 mosmol/kg can be achieved. Urinary sodium losses are high in the early neonatal period with up to 5% of the filtered sodium being excreted in the urine in the first few days, yet the natriuretic response to salt overload is also defective.

Plasma levels of mineralocorticoids and antidiuretic hormone (ADH) in neonates are within, or just above, the normal adult range, though the distal tubule, particularly in very low birth weight (VLBW) babies, responds poorly to the mineralocorticoids. Atrial natriuretic peptide (ANP) levels are high in the early neonatal period and, although the kidney may be relatively insensitive, high ANP may contribute to the high sodium excretion.

■ Water

At term, 75% of the baby's body weight is water and this percentage is higher in preterm babies. Part of the normal adaptation to extra-uterine life is a marked reduction in body water, especially from the extracellular fluid (ECF). Reduction in the ECF accounts for the early fall in body weight, and there is a change in the ratio of ECF to intracellular fluid from the 2:1 seen in fetal life to the 1:1 ratio which is normal for the neonate. After an initial period of 12–24 hours without diuresis the baby enters a diuretic phase (which is also a natriuresis) and then, after postnatal homeostasis is achieved, has normal sodium and water balance (Lorenz *et al.* 1995; Fig. 10.1). In ill preterm babies, characteristically those with respiratory distress syndrome (RDS), the onset of the diuretic and natriuretic phase is delayed.

The key to the management of fluid balance in the ill baby lies in recognizing and adapting to these phases of water and sodium balance, and in such babies fluid overload and dehydration readily occur.

Insensible water loss

Transepidermal and respiratory tract loss

The main route of insensible water loss is transepidermal water loss, which is particularly high in preterm infants (Table 10.1). Insensible loss also occurs via the respiratory tract. Respiratory tract water loss varies from 4 mg/kg/min when a term baby is asleep to 10 mg/kg/min when he is crying furiously (Riesenfeld *et al.* 1987). This corresponds to a loss of about 6–9 mL/kg/24 h, meaning that respiratory tract loss accounts for about half of the daily insensible loss in a term infant. Respiratory losses are eliminated when a baby is artificially ventilated with humidified gas. Transepidermal water loss is increased by overhead heaters, draughts and phototherapy lamps, and can be significantly reduced by high ambient humidity and covering the baby. Evaporation of water from the skin causes the baby to lose heat; reducing transepidermal water loss is an important component of thermoregulation. When calculating water replacement, an estimate of the insensible water loss needs to be added to the urine volume and any other losses (remember gut losses in babies who have undergone surgery).

Obligatory urine water loss

This arises from the volume of water needed to excrete the urea and other waste products generated from the baby's diet. Obligatory urine water depends on the renal solute load of the diet, which in turn varies according to the type of milk or other feed the baby is receiving. The renal solute load of breast milk is much lower than that of formula milks. The obligatory urine water is approximately 2–4 mL/kg/h.

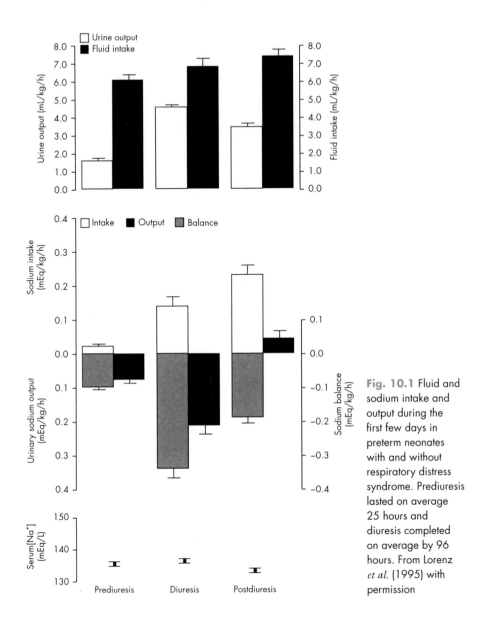

Fig. 10.1 Fluid and sodium intake and output during the first few days in preterm neonates with and without respiratory distress syndrome. Prediuresis lasted on average 25 hours and diuresis completed on average by 96 hours. From Lorenz *et al.* (1995) with permission

Table 10.1 Transepidermal water loss (g/kg/24 h) at an ambient humidity of 50% (from Hammarlund *et al.* 1983)

Gestational age	Postnatal age			
	0–1	3	7	14
25–27	129 ± 39	71 ± 9	43 ± 9	32 ±10
28–30	42 ± 13	32 ± 9	24 ± 7	18 ± 6
31–36	12 ± 5	12 ± 4	12 ± 4	9 ± 3
37–41	7 ± 2	6 ± 1	6 ± 1	6 ± 1

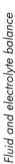

Stool water

In babies the water lost in stool is approximately 7 mL/kg/day (Patrick and Pittard 1988), although clearly the water loss varies with the number of stools and the fat content of the stool.

Fluid overload

In the first week of life, particularly in ill VLBW neonates, the first indication of fluid overload or retention is a weight loss of less than 1% per day, or weight gain. After the first week fluid retention results in a weight gain of more than 20 g/kg/24 h. The signs of fluid overload include oedema, which is often hidden around the back and flank of a baby who is nursed supine. The causes of fluid overload can be divided into causes of excessive intake, and fluid retention (Table 10.2).

Effects of excess fluid (overload or retention)

1. Heart failure, including massive pulmonary haemorrhage (pp. 161–162).
2. Pulmonary oedema – in lung disease this exacerbates the hypoxaemia.
3. In babies recovering from RDS, an increased incidence of patent ductus arteriosus (p. 296) and perhaps chronic lung disease (CLD) (Chapter 14).
4. Hyponatraemia, hypokalaemia.

Table 10.2 Causes of fluid overload

Excessive fluid intake
1. Excessive maintenance intravenous fluid including sodium, particularly when the normal postnatal diuresis and natriuresis has not yet occurred (see above)
2. Large boluses of bicarbonate, dextrose or blood products being given to sick babies without making allowances in the maintenance fluid intake
3. Excessive infusion through arterial catheters (umbilical or peripheral)
4. Human error or mechanical failure in the pumps controlling the IV fluid

Fluid retention
1. Renal failure, e.g. caused by asphyxia, hypotension, acidaemia
2. Congestive cardiac failure, e.g. with a patent ductus
3. Central nervous system damage (e.g. asphyxia, meningitis) causing inappropriate ADH secretion
4. Leaky capillaries owing to severe RDS, asphyxia, endotoxaemia, sepsis
5. A rise in central venous pressure owing to continuous positive airways pressure or intermittent positive pressure ventilation.
6. A combination of (4) and (5) – commonly seen in babies with RDS who, in addition, may be paralysed with pancuronium which eliminates the action of muscle activity on venous and lymphatic drainage
7. Extravasation of fluid into the extracellular space owing to hypoalbuminaemia
8. Indometacin or ibuprofen used to treat patent ductus arteriosus

ADH, antidiuretic hormone; RDS, respiratory distress syndrome.

5. Oedema of kidneys, liver and gut, making these organs (respectively) less effective at excreting urine, conjugating drugs and bilirubin, and more prone to necrotizing enterocolitis (NEC) (pp. 278–283).
6. Cerebral oedema, especially if there is co-existing asphyxial brain damage.
7. Sclerema.

Treatment

Treatment is tailored to the individual situation dependent on the underlying cause. The key to successful fluid management is careful assessment of the baby's fluid balance considering all sources of fluid intake and losses. In sick and very preterm babies this assessment may need to be done several times in a 24-hour period. Common clinical situations with fluid overload include:

1. Oedema due to fluid overload: restrict fluids to 30–40 mL/kg/24 h. This may be all that is necessary, but, if symptoms are present, consider furosemide 1–2 mg/kg IV.
2. In a seriously ill neonate oedema is often accompanied by hypoalbuminaemia and leaky capillaries. This is very common in the early stages of RDS or with sepsis, and recovery from the underlying disease is heralded by diuresis and clearing of the subcutaneous oedema (Fig. 10.1). However, while the baby is oedematous with weight gain, or no weight loss, fluid intake should be restricted to the minimum consistent with maintaining blood pressure and replacing transepidermal loss and urine water. For an average baby this corresponds to about 40–60 mL/kg/24 h.
3. Oedema due to inappropriate ADH secretion. The presence of an abnormally low serum osmolality combined with a urinary osmolality above 300 mosmol/kg H_2O establishes the diagnosis. The treatment is that of the underlying condition, plus fluid restriction to 30–40 mL/kg/24 h IV of an electrolyte solution containing the daily electrolyte requirements.
4. The baby with heart disease who develops heart failure (treatment p. 296).
5. After surgery. Perhaps due to a combination of replacement fluids leaking out, paralysis and some pre-renal renal impairment, fluid retention is commonly seen in the post-operative neonate who should have his fluids restricted as in (3) above.
6. Oedema following indometacin treatment. This will usually clear spontaneously on stopping treatment. If indometacin results in significant renal impairment the course may have to be stopped.
7. Hydrops fetalis (p. 312).

If, in any of these situations, on clinical or radiological grounds it is felt that oedema is significantly adding to the neonate's lung problem, exacerbating hypoxaemia, furosemide 1–2 mg/kg IV should be tried, with repeated doses given as necessary. If oedema is severe or progressive with a poor urinary output, dialysis or haemofiltration can be considered.

Dehydration

In the first week in neonates this is a weight loss of ≥3% per 24 hours. Thereafter the standard criteria for dehydration apply. A weight loss >2.5% is clinically significant, >5% moderate, and >10% severe. There is some evidence that the incidence of hypernatraemic dehydration is rising (Laing and Wong 2002).

Signs of dehydration

In addition to weight loss the dehydrated baby develops decreased skin turgor, sunken eyes, a depressed fontanelle and a reduced urinary output. Dehydration readily develops in neonates and is likely to occur with:

1. A high insensible transepidermal water loss (see above).
2. An osmotic diuresis due to glycosuria in VLBW babies receiving ≥10% glucose.
3. Gut fluid loss in diarrhoea and vomiting.
4. Inadequate intake – tissued IV line, fluid deliberately withheld to avoid overload, and in term babies due to failure to establish breast feeding (Chapter 11).
5. Overvigorous use of diuretics.
6. Pyrexia.
7. Rarely, due to diabetes insipidus associated with massive intraventricular haemorrhage or congenital diabetes insipidus.

The effects of the fluid loss include a progressive reduction of the plasma volume leading to hypoxia and acidaemia, gut underperfusion predisposing to NEC, pre-renal uraemia, and ultimately to shock; jaundice (Chapter 20); and electrolyte problems, in particular hypernatraemia.

Treatment

In a baby who is clinically dehydrated his fluid intake should:

1. Consist of a maintenance of 120–150 mL/kg/24 h.
2. Replace fluid losses. In acute dehydration the fluid lost is approximately equal to the weight loss in grams.
   - In well term babies this is often best given enterally as milk by either mouth or nasogastric (NG) tube.
   - Sick or preterm neonates will need IV replacement. If shocked a fluid bolus (10 mL/kg of 0.9% saline) may be required, otherwise replacement IV over 24–48 hours is preferable. The choice of fluid will depend on the duration and severity of associated hypernatraemia. It is essential not to bring high sodium down rapidly as this may result in cerebral oedema. In severe hypernatraemic dehydration with serum Na 150–169 mmol/L, 0.45% saline with 5% or 10% dextrose should be used to prevent a rapid drop in serum Na. In babies with a serum Na of ≥170 mmol/L, 0.9% saline with 5% or 10% dextrose should be used until Na levels fall below 170 mmol/L. Hypo-osmolar salt-poor fluids should not be used in this situation.
3. Allow for insensible loss from overhead radiant heaters (an extra 50–75 mL/kg/24 h).
4. Keep up with ongoing losses in diarrhoea, NG aspirate, cerebrospinal fluid (CSF) leak, etc.
5. Allow for pyrexia (an increased intake of 10 mL H_2O/kg/24 h for each 1°C above 37°C).

Overall, this may mean an intake of 250–300 mL/kg/24 h. Such babies require meticulous reassessment of their fluid requirements every 8–12 hours.

If there are signs of circulatory compromise the following regimen should be used: administer an initial resuscitation volume of 20–30 mL/kg of normal (0.9%) saline over 30–60 minutes. Then use the following steps to calculate the initial infusion rate:

1. Estimate daily maintenance fluid volume in mL (M).
2. Estimate the total deficit in mL (D); if the serum sodium is 149–169 mmol/L, aim to administer the deficit over 2 days (T=2); if the serum sodium is 170 mmol/L or above, aim to administer the deficit over 3 days or more (T=3 or more).
3. Calculate the initial infusion rate in mL/h as $[M + D/T]/24$.

Check serum electrolytes and blood glucose 1 hour after starting therapy and then 4 hourly for 12 hours. If the serum sodium is falling at a rate greater than 0.5 mmol/L/h, reduce the rate of infusion. Aim to reduce the serum sodium at a rate not exceeding 12 mmol/L/day (see above). Too rapid correction of hypernatraemia can cause cerebral oedema, convulsions and permanent brain injury. Extremely severe hypernatraemia (serum sodium greater than 200 mmol/L) requires correction by peritoneal dialysis.

■ Sodium

The normal serum sodium is 130–145 mmol/L. Values between 125 and 150 mmol/L are well tolerated but outside this range urgent treatment is required. The normal requirement for sodium in the neonate is 2–3 mmol/kg/24 h, and it is usually possible to calculate an electrolyte input which keeps healthy neonates in balance. However, in sick babies many factors are present which severely disrupt sodium homeostasis. Extreme preterm infants often require around 6 mmol/kg/24 h at the end of the first week of life.

Hyponatraemic babies (serum sodium <125 mmol/L) become listless, develop an ileus and may become hypotensive and convulse. With hypernatraemia (>150 mmol/L) the major hazard is the risk of cerebral venous sinus thrombosis, or seizures associated with rapid shifts in osmolarity. Avoid correcting the serum sodium too fast.

Hyponatraemia

Hyponatraemia is relatively rare in the first 48–72 hours. It is vital to understand that low serum sodium either can reflect low body sodium or can result from dilution (i.e. water overload) because the management of the two situations is quite different.

■ Water excess (dilutional hyponatraemia)

1. In babies born to hyponatraemic mothers, usually due to excess intravenous infusion of salt-free fluids during labour, or excessive water drinking during labour. This is the only common cause of first-day hyponatraemia.
2. With CNS injury causing inappropriate ADH production.
3. In renal failure or with reduced urine output secondary to indometacin or ibuprofen therapy.

■ Sodium depletion

1. In very small premature babies with poor renal conservation of sodium.
2. In preterm babies on a low sodium intake (e.g. just breast milk, or plain 10% dextrose IV).
3. Following furosemide, both acutely and in babies with CLD on 'maintenance' diuretics.
4. With diarrhoea or vomiting owing to excessive sodium losses. Similar losses may occur through an ileostomy.

5. 'Sequestered' sodium loss into the gut or into damaged cells (e.g. NEC – a low serum sodium is common in early NEC – or associated with sepsis).
6. Following external drainage of CSF for the treatment of hydrocephalus.
7. Salt-losing forms of congenital adrenal hyperplasia (CAH) (p. 255).

Treatment of hyponatraemia

Treatment depends on the cause; leaving aside the baby with gastrointestinal tract loss, CSF loss and CAH there are three common clinical situations:

1. Hyponatraemia in the ill neonate. This requires careful assessment. Examination of the intravenous fluid charts, urine output records and the baby's weight trend should help. The baby who is total body sodium depleted needs more sodium, whereas one who is retaining fluid does not need more sodium, just fluid restriction. Alternatively the hyponatraemia may be a marker of intravascular volume depletion, to which there has been an appropriate release of ADH resulting in water retention and a dilutional hyponatraemia. This requires volume replacement with a sodium-containing fluid.
2. Hyponatraemia, usually after the first week in an otherwise well baby who may be growing poorly. All this baby requires is an increased sodium intake, to as much as 10 mmol/kg/day or more, plus regular monitoring of his serum sodium.
3. True inappropriate ADH secretion. Usually as a result of brain (hypothalamic) injury excess ADH is produced despite normovolaemia, normal blood pressure and normal renal function. There is hyponatraemia and a low plasma osmolarity with inappropriately high urinary sodium and osmolarity. As well as treating the primary CNS disorder, treatment is fluid restriction (40–50 mL/kg/day) with judicious sodium supplementation, at least the normal daily requirement.

Acute severe hyponatraemia

In acute severe hyponatraemia (serum sodium <120 mmol/L), particularly if associated with neurological signs, the intravenous infusion of 3% sodium chloride may be justified. The rate of correction should not exceed 1 mmol/L/h and the infusion of 3% sodium chloride should be stopped before a normal serum sodium is reached. As 3% sodium chloride contains approximately 0.5 mmol/mL, the infusion of 1 mL/kg will raise the serum sodium by 1 mmol/L (if ECF volume is 50% of body weight; in extremely preterm babies ECF volume may be higher). Hence the rate of infusion of 3% sodium chloride should never exceed 1 mL/kg/h.

Hypernatraemia

Hypernatraemia develops if water losses exceed sodium losses or if too much sodium is given. It is primarily seen in ill extremely low birth weight (ELBW) neonates in the first 24–72 hours of life. Causes include:

1. an inadequate fluid intake for any reason;
2. small ill premature babies with a marked transepidermal water loss; more marked in those nursed under overhead radiant heaters; this is the most common cause of early hypernatraemia;
3. phototherapy, which has a similar effect to radiant heaters and also causes diarrhoea;

4. hyperglycaemia in premature babies receiving excessive dextrose causing an osmotic water loss;
5. diarrhea;
6. too much sodium as bicarbonate or from other sources such as drugs.

Treatment of hypernatraemia

Ideally hypernatraemia should be avoided by careful control of the baby's microenvironment, avoiding excess sodium intake (bicarbonate, blood and blood products, drugs and saline catheter flushes) and by maintaining appropriate fluid balance. However, if the serum sodium is above 150 mmol/L:

1. Minimize transepidermal water loss (humidify incubator, wrap baby in clothes or plastic).
2. Exclude osmotic diuresis.
3. Stop added sodium.
4. If the weight loss has been more than 3% per day, the baby is likely to be volume depleted. Increase fluid intake (sodium-free) accordingly. If the weight loss has been 1–3%, be careful to avoid fluid overload with its attendant hazards.

Potassium

The normal serum potassium is 3.5–5.5 mmol/L. Neonates tolerate levels of 3–6.5 mmol/L extremely well, but outside this range treatment is required. The normal neonate needs 1–3 mmol/kg/24 h of potassium, and disorders of potassium homeostasis are rare. Hypokalaemia is usually the result of poor control of intravenous fluid prescriptions and is readily treated by increasing the potassium intake. Hyperkalaemia is seen in ill VLBW babies who have been hypotensive and are in renal failure. The emergency treatment of hyperkalaemia is discussed with the management of renal failure on pp. 323–326.

Hydrogen ions and bicarbonate

See Table 13.3, p. 122, for normal values.

There are five important reasons for a neonate having a metabolic acidaemia – that is, a base deficit greater than 8–10 mmol/L. They are:

1. accumulation of lactic or other acids with asphyxia, hypotension, sepsis, hypoxia, or various inborn errors of metabolism (see Chapter 18);
2. the hydrogen ion load resulting from growth and the metabolism of high protein milks;
3. defective urinary acidification due to the low GFR, reduced urinary phosphate production, and reduced capacity of the neonatal kidney to make ammonia;
4. tubular bicarbonate leak; the bicarbonate threshold in a preterm baby may be as low as 12 mmol/L;
5. total parenteral nutrition (TPN) with hyperchloraemic metabolic acidosis (see Chapter 12).

Nothing can or should be done for factors (3) and (4), although occasionally a full-blown Fanconi tubular defect is seen after severe neonatal illness and needs bicarbonate replacement (2). The treatment of the causes of acidaemia listed under (1) and (5) is dealt with elsewhere.

▪ Calcium and phosphate

The normal serum calcium is in the range 2.2–2.6 mmol/L (1–1.4 mmol/L ionized calcium). Serum phosphate levels vary from between 2 and 2.6 mmol/L at birth to 1.5–2.9 mmol/L after the first week. Calcium and phosphate levels are higher in cord blood than in maternal plasma. Calcium is actively transported from the mother into the fetus, and the fetal phosphate rises owing to hypoparathyroidism induced by the high calcium.

Postnatally neonatal plasma phosphate may rise further owing to the low GFR and the higher phosphate intake in bottle-fed babies. Parathormone rises slowly in small sick babies, and will therefore have little phosphaturic effect on the neonatal renal tubule. However, neonatal vitamin D metabolism is probably normal.

Hypocalcaemia

Hypocalcaemia is common in the neonatal period, but allowance must be made for co-existent hypoalbuminaemia. On average, the serum calcium falls by 0.1 mmol/L for each 4 g by which the serum albumin falls below the mean for the baby's gestation.

Serum calcium levels above 1.75 mmol/L rarely cause any problem, but symptoms (see below) may develop if the serum calcium falls below 1.5 mmol/L. This happens:

1. during the first 24–48 hours in severely ill babies. This accounts for 95% of neonatal hypocalcaemia; the babies have a subnormal parathormone response to the low calcium, but high circulating levels of hormones such as glucocorticoids and calcitonin which depress plasma calcium;
2. in babies of diabetic mothers;
3. during an exchange transfusion with citrated blood; the citrate chelates the calcium causing a rapid drop in the plasma level.

Other rare causes of neonatal hypocalcaemia which should be sought if the problems listed above are not present include:

1. maternal and fetal hypovitaminosis D; this may be particularly common in babies from ethnic groups at risk from rickets;
2. babies fed on high-phosphate milks (e.g. unadulterated cow's milk): formerly common, now very rare;
3. renal failure;
4. primary hypoparathyroidism including DiGeorge syndrome;
5. maternal hypercalcaemia including that due to hyperparathyroidism, causing prolonged neonatal parathyroid depression.

The symptoms of hypocalcaemia depend on the age at presentation. In babies less than 72 hours old convulsions are rare; but these babies, particularly if on intermittent positive pressure ventilation, may be jittery. Hypocalcaemia developing during an exchange transfusion may cause convulsions, cardiac arrhythmias or tetany with a positive Chvostek sign (the facial nerve is tapped at the angle of the jaw, causing the ipsilateral facial muscles to contract momentarily). At the end of the first week in an otherwise well baby hypocalcaemia causes clonic fits. Hypocalcaemia may cause heart failure and apnoea at any time in the neonatal period.

Hypocalcaemia should be avoided by adequate treatment of the illnesses which predispose to it. Convulsions should be controlled pharmacologically (see Chapter 17) while investigating the cause of the hypocalcaemia, and the plasma calcium raised with oral or intravenous calcium supplements.

To prevent early hypocalcaemia in ill neonates, appropriate intravenous supplements of 10% calcium gluconate should be given. In general, 5–10 mL of 10% calcium gluconate (1.125–2.25 mmol of calcium) IV each 24 hours is all that is usually necessary.

Depending on the aetiology, specific therapy may be with phosphate restriction, calcium supplements, or treatment with vitamin D. In general, use the standard vitamin D preparations rather than the newer much more potent vitamin D metabolites such as 1-α-vitamin D or 1,25-vitamin D.

The dose of calcium for tetany or hypocalcaemic arrhythmias during an exchange transfusion is 1 mL of 10% calcium gluconate (equivalent to 0.225 mmol calcium) infused over 2 minutes under ECG control.

Hypercalcaemia

Neonatal hypercalcaemia is rare and usually iatrogenic. Occasionally, hypercalcaemia of 3.0–3.5 mmol/L may develop in the ELBW baby (<1.0 kg) who has become profoundly hypophosphataemic (<0.5 mmol/L). Treatment is with phosphate supplements, giving 2–3 mmol/kg/24 h of neutral phosphate. Rare cases of neonatal hyperparathyroidism have been described.

Hypophosphataemia

Hypophosphataemia is now being seen with increasing frequency in VLBW babies on TPN or in those receiving low-phosphate milks. In enterally fed babies this can be prevented by adding phosphate to breast milk. When severe it causes hypercalcaemia (see above).

▓ Magnesium

Abnormalities of magnesium homeostasis are now rare with the withdrawal of the high-phosphate milks. Magnesium sulphate is used for treating maternal pre-eclampsia and can give rise to high levels of magnesium in the neonate. He is usually asymptomatic but hypermagnesaemia can cause floppiness. Hypomagnesaemia may occasionally occur during parenteral nutrition. It can be treated by giving 0.2 mL/kg of a 50% solution of $MgSO_4$ intramuscularly.

▓ Practical fluid and electrolyte management

The single most useful measurement in assessing a baby's fluid requirement is his weight. In the first week of life the very premature baby should lose about 1–3% of his body weight per day. If he is not doing this he is being overhydrated; if he is losing more than this he needs more IV fluids. It is, therefore, essential that sick VLBW neonates are weighed at least daily, and in some cases twice daily as part of their intensive care.

A careful calculation of the exact fluid and glucose and electrolyte intake should be performed at least twice a day in sick or very preterm babies while on intensive care. The information required for assessing fluid requirements other than weight is: urinary output, packed cell volume, blood pressure, serum sodium and creatinine estimations and a clinical assessment of the baby's state of hydration and perfusion. Weighing the nappies is the easiest way of measuring urine output and should be standard practice while babies are requiring intensive care. Controlling the fluid intake by aiming to achieve some set biochemical goal such as a normal urinary osmolality or a specific urinary output without taking note of the clinical state and weight of

Table 10.3 Outline of fluid therapy in the newborn

Indicator	Frequency of estimation during intensive care	Response
Weight	Daily or twice daily	Aim for a weight loss of 1–2% per day for 5 days. Adjust volume of maintenance fluid accordingly
Urine output	Continuous, using nappy weights, or urine collection system. Review results 8 hourly	Aim for a urine output of at least 0.5 mL/kg/24 h on the first day, and 2–7 mL/kg/h thereafter. Adjust maintenance fluid, blood pressure support to achieve this. Urine output below 1 mL/kg/24 h for more than 8 hours requires renal failure management
Sodium	Daily or twice daily	**Omit** added sodium (a) until urine output is established and (b) if plasma Na > 145 mmol/L **Increase** input if low Na (<125 mmol/L) considered to be due to sodium depletion – otherwise restrict fluid
Glucose	At least 6 hourly during intensive care	Maintain level between 2.6 and 9 mmol/L by adjusting glucose concentration of fluid. Usual requirement 8–12 mmol/kg/min
Potassium	Daily or twice daily	**Omit** (a) on day 1 (b) if K >5.5 mmol/L (c) renal failure developing **Increase** (a) if K <2.5 mmol/L
Calcium	Daily	Give 5 mL 10% calcium gluconate/kg/24 h if serum calcium <1.75 mmol/L Give 10 mL/kg/24 h if Ca <1.5 mmol/L

the baby is ill-advised, and frequently results in serious overhydration. Nevertheless since the changes in the electrolyte concentrations in ill neonates are to some extent unpredictable all such babies should have measurement of their plasma electrolytes, urea and creatinine at least daily while they are in intensive care. Table 10.3 summarizes our approach to the interpretation of results. We start with a maintenance fluid of 10% dextrose and vary the concentration to keep the blood glucose between 2.6 and 9 mmol/L.

■ References

Hammarlund, K, Sedin, G, Stromberg, B (1983) Transepidermal water loss in the newborn VIII. Relation to gestational age and postnatal age in appropriate and small for gestational age infants. *Acta Paediatrica Scandinavica*, **72**: 721–8.

Laing, IA, Wong, CM (2002) Hypernatraemia in the first few days: is the incidence rising? *Archives of Disease in Childhood. Fetal and Neonatal Edition*, **87**: F158–62.

Lorenz, JM, Kleinman, LI, Ahmed, G, Markarian, K (1995) Phases of fluid and electrolyte homeostasis in the extremely low birthweight baby. *Pediatrics*, **96**: 484–9.

Patrick, CH, Pittard, WB (1988) Stool water loss in very low birthweight neonates. *Clinical Pediatrics*, **27**: 144–6.

Riesenfeld, K, Hammarlund, K, Sedin, G (1987) Respiratory water loss in relation to activity in fullterm infants on their first day after birth. *Acta Paediatrica Scandinavica*, **76**: 889–93.

Further reading

Modi, N (2012) Renal function, fluid and electrolyte balance and neonatal renal disease. In Rennie, JM (ed.) *Rennie & Roberton's Textbook of Neonatology*, 5th edition. Edinburgh: Elsevier, pp.331–344.

11

Neonatal enteral nutrition

Key points

■ Breast milk is the ideal food for babies of all weights and all gestations (supplements will be required for preterm babies).

■ When starting enteral nutrition in very low birth weight babies, breast milk is better tolerated than formula.

■ Breast milk has important anti-infective properties which are difficult to mimic.

■ Minimal enteral feeding should be started early and stopped only if there is clear evidence of gastrointestinal disease.

In order to grow and develop normally babies must have enough energy and a balance of carbohydrate, fat and protein with vitamins and minerals. Enteral feeding is the best way in which to deliver nutrition – stopping minimal enteral feeding should be seen as the last resort. Early nutrition also has biological effects ('programming') with important implications for later health, for example on cognitive function and cardiovascular disease risk. The aim of all nutritional support is to achieve as near to intra-uterine growth as possible. This translates to a rate of weight gain of 15–18 g/kg/day (Ehrenkranz *et al.*, 1999) while maintaining a normal body composition. Provision of nutrition by the enteral route is safer and easier than parenteral nutrition (Chapter 12). Human milk has important anti-infective properties and there are benefits of early feeding in establishing appropriate gut flora, which help to protect the preterm baby against necrotizing enterocolitis (NEC). For a full discussion of this enormous subject the reader to referred to Tsang *et al.* (2005) and Fewtrell and Chomtho (2012).

■ Infant nutrient requirements

The basic nutritional requirements for preterm infants as recommended by the European Society for Paediatric Gastroenterology, Hepatology and Nutrition (ESPGHAN) (Agostoni *et al.* 2010) and Tsang (2005) are given in Table 11.1.

Fluid

For routine feeding, volumes of 150–180 mL/kg/day of preterm infant formula or fortified breast milk fed to preterm babies are likely to achieve fluid and nutrient requirements.

Energy

A well preterm baby who is in a thermoneutral environment needs about 50 kcal/kg just to maintain essential body functions; if he is to grow he requires another

Table 11.1 Basic nutritional requirements for preterm infants

	ESPGHAN (Agostoni *et al.* 2010) requirements per kg per day	Tsang *et al.* (2005) requirements per kg per day
Fluid, mL	135–200	150–200
Energy, kcal	110–135	ELBW: 130–150 VLBW: 110–130
Protein, g	4–4.5 (<1 kg) 3.5–4 (1–1.8 kg)	26–30 weeks: 3.8–4.2 30–36 weeks: 3.4–3.6 36–40 weeks: 2.8–3.2
Fat, g (MCT <40%)	4.8–6.6	5.3–7.2
Carbohydrate, g	11.6–13.2	3.4–4.2
Sodium, mg	69–115	69–115
Potassium, mg	66–132	78–117
Calcium, mg	120–140	100–220
Phosphate, mg	60–90	60–140
Iron, mg	2–3	2–4
Vitamin, C mg	11–46	18–24
Folate, µg	35–100	25–50
Vitamin A, IU/kg	1332–3330	699–1498
Vitamin D, IU/day	800–1000/day	400
Vitamin K, µg	4.4–28	8–10

ELBW, extremely low birth weight; MCT, medium chain triglycerides; VLBW, very low birth weight.

5 kcal for every gram of weight gain. Energy requirements are dependent on the postconceptional age and birth weight of the preterm infant, with the smaller and sicker infants having higher requirements. At least 100 kcal/kg/day are needed. Sick babies need more, and although some babies grow well on 90–120 kcal/kg/day, particularly if the fat in their diet is well absorbed, many need 135 kcal/kg/day or even more. Enough calories need to be provided so that the baby uses all the protein in his diet for cell-building in order to achieve a positive nitrogen balance and does not break down protein for energy. This is the reason why the protein/non-protein calorie ratio is important.

Fat

Fat is the main energy source for babies and dietary fat should constitute at least 30% of the total caloric intake per day, but not more than 54%. Brain grey matter and the cells of the retina are rich in long-chain polyunsaturated fatty acids, and the availability of these in the diet has implications for cell membrane function. Fat can be stored in large quantities, as opposed to carbohydrate and protein, for which the storage capacity of the body is limited. For the newborn, using fat for energy marks a big change from fetal life during which the main energy source was glucose. Assuming a daily fat deposition of 3 g/kg, a 10–40% loss from malabsorption and 15% loss from unavoidable oxidation, the minimum fat intake is estimated at 3.8–4.8 g/kg/day (Table 11.1).

There are four major lipid types: glycerides, phospholipids, sterols and fatty acids. The fat globules in human milk consist mainly of triglyceride, with some cholesterol, phospholipid and fatty acids. Formula milks have only traces of cholesterol and few long-chain fatty acids. The amount of fat in breast milk changes with gestation and the phase of feeding. Fat in formula milk is constant and is derived from cow's milk and/or vegetable oils such as corn oil. These fats are less well digested and absorbed than fat from breast milk. Artificially fed premature babies may lose up to 50% of ingested long-chain fat in their stools. Clinical trials in preterm infants fed formulas containing both arachidonic acid and docosahexaenoic acid have shown beneficial effects on the developing visual system and cognition in the first year of life. ESPGHAN has published recommended intakes of both these nutrients.

Protein

The growing preterm baby requires a higher protein intake than the term baby, with the latest evidence suggesting up to 4.5 g/kg/day in extremely low birth weight (ELBW) infants, an intake that is often higher than it is possible to achieve using breast milk. Protein accretion in fetal life has been estimated as 1.7 g/kg/day; a preterm baby probably has obligatory protein losses of 0.7 g/kg/day. ESPGHAN and other authorities recommend that preterm babies should have a protein intake of at least 3 g/kg/day, and intra-uterine weight gain can be mimicked with protein intake of 3–3.5 g/kg/day and a high energy intake, although body fat percentage at term equivalent will be much higher than in an equivalent fetus. This protein intake can be achieved by adding fortifiers to breast milk. We monitor the growth velocity (World Health Organization Neonatal and Infant Close Monitoring chart; see Appendix 1) as well as urea, and the albumin level, aiming to keep the urea above 1.6 mmol/L.

Babies born at term require about 2.1 g/kg/day of protein. No more than 7–12% of the daily calorie intake should be derived from protein. In addition to the amino acids which are essential for adults, histidine, cysteine and tyrosine may be essential for newborn babies. The protein/non-protein calorie ratio is equally important in enteral and parenteral nutrition. Very high protein intakes should be avoided, particularly if casein-predominant formulas are used, as these may cause problems such as hyperaminoacidaemia and metabolic acidaemia.

Carbohydrate

The main carbohydrate in human milk and term formulas is lactose, whereas in preterm formulas it is a mixture of lactose and glucose polymers. Lactose is split up into the monosaccharides glucose and galactose by β-galactosidase (lactase), a brush border enzyme in the gut. Glucose is the principal circulating carbohydrate and is the primary source of energy for the brain (Chapter 18).

Minerals

Sodium

On formulas with a very low sodium content or unfortified breast milk, babies smaller than 1.50 kg may become hyponatraemic (Na <125 mmol/L) since they lose much more salt in their urine than full-term babies. Hyponatraemia is much less likely with preterm formulas or if fortifier is added to breast milk. We aim to keep the serum sodium >133 mmol/L in a preterm baby, using supplements or fortifier if necessary.

Calcium and phosphorus

Calcium is the most abundant mineral in the body, 99% of it being in bone. Babies born prematurely suffer an interruption of supply at a time of rapid accretion (about 2.5 mmol/kg/day or 120 mg/kg/day for calcium, and 2.2 mmol/kg/day or 70 mg/kg/day for phosphorus). Consequently preterm babies require much more calcium and phosphorus than can be provided by breast milk or standard infant formula. Metabolic bone disease of prematurity (p. 345) is mainly due to this dietary deficiency. Hypocalcaemia is discussed on p. 89.

Preterm babies require 60–100 mg of calcium and 40–70 mg of phosphorus/100 mL milk – values which are achieved only using preterm formulas or breast milk fortification or even additional supplementation. The present ESPGHAN recommendation is for a calcium–phosphate ratio close to 2:1. The reason for this is in part that the absorption of phosphate is close to 90%, but calcium is less (~50%) well absorbed. Babies less than 1.2 kg who are fed on breast milk without fortifier should receive an extra 0.5 mmol of phosphate per 100 mL feed given as a neutral phosphate solution (a mixture of Na_2HPO_4 + NaH_2PO_4). If their phosphate is still <1.25 mmol/L, an extra 0.5 mmol phosphate and 1 mmol calcium/100 mL should be put in their feeds, the phosphate being added first to avoid precipitation.

Iron

Iron is essential for brain development and many studies have shown an association between toddler iron deficiency anaemia and poor neurodevelopment. Commercial formulas have iron added to them, whereas all forms of breast milk are very low in iron, although the iron is in a form which is more readily absorbed than the iron in formulas. Iron is also a pro-oxidant, and non-protein-bound iron may cause the release of oxygen free radicals. Hence it is important to maintain a balance between avoiding iron deficiency and causing iron overload. Iron intakes of <2 mg/kg/day are likely to result in iron deficiency, particularly in babies of birth weight <1800 g, and ESPGHAN recommends an intake of 2–3 mg/kg/day. Prophylactic supplementation should be started at 2–6 weeks of age and continued after discharge, until 12 months of age.

Babies of 32–34 weeks' gestation or less are born before their body iron stores are laid down by transplacental transfer. Preterm babies need iron supplements after 2–6 weeks; where there have been multiple blood transfusions during the preterm period, the timing of supplementation may be directed by measuring the serum ferritin level. Iron supplementation is not then required if babies are fed on an iron-supplemented preterm formula. However, preterm babies who are fed on breast milk should receive 2.5 mg/kg/day of iron up to a maximum of 15 mg/day (5 mg/kg/day) and stay on this treatment until they are taking an adequate mixed diet. Iron supplementation in this way does not prevent the physiological anaemia of prematurity (p. 310), but it does prevent later iron deficiency.

Trace minerals

Humans require zinc, copper, selenium, chromium, molybdenum, manganese and iodine in addition to iron. Copper and zinc deficiency do occur rarely in ELBW neonates at 2–4 months of age, usually only in those who have been given prolonged total parenteral nutrition (TPN), or suboptimal enteral nutrition with inadequate trace mineral supplementation. Manganese toxicity has been reported with long-term TPN. Aluminium is not an essential trace mineral, but can accumulate during TPN.

Vitamins

Vitamins A, D, K and E are fat soluble; the B vitamins, folic acid and vitamin C are water soluble. Unsupplemented breast milk is short of some vitamins, and we routinely supplement all premature babies with multivitamin preparations such as Abidec or Dalavit (vitamins A_1 B_1 B_2 B_6 C and D). While still in the neonatal unit very low birth weight (VLBW) babies who are not being fed on supplemented breast milk or a preterm formula should receive additional vitamin D to achieve the recommended 800–1000 IU/day (not per kg). Vitamin D affects the calcium absorption rates and there has been a general consensus that the target value of circulating 1,25-dihydroxyvitamin D should be >80 nmol/L. We have noticed an improvement in osteopenia of prematurity since we increased our vitamin D supplementation to a total of 1000 IU/day from all sources of vitamin D.

Vitamin K deficiency bleeding (see Chapter 23) is much more common in breast-fed babies. To prevent it, all babies should receive 0.5–1.0 mg of vitamin K intramuscularly at birth.

Folic acid deficiency may reduce growth and may rarely cause a megaloblastic anaemia in both babies less than 2 kg at birth and survivors of haemolytic disease. We give babies on non-fortified breast milk 50 mg/kg/day of folic acid weekly until discharge.

Prebiotics and probiotics

Human milk contains more than 130 different oligosaccharides, the precise composition of which is genetically determined and varies in the population. GosFos is a mixture of short-chain galacto-oligosaccharides and long-chain fructo-oligosaccharides which can be added to preterm formula. Further work is needed to determine the hypothesis that GosFos supplementation of formula milk will reduce NEC, improve immunological function and reduce hospital-acquired infection. However, the majority of the preterm formulas used in the UK have prebiotic oligosaccharides added. There is also current widespread interest in the role of probiotics in the prevention of NEC and further trials are in progress.

■ Which milk to give?

For the healthy term baby all paediatricians will recommend breast feeding as the method of choice. Fresh human milk from the baby's own mother given along with the appropriate supplements is also undoubtedly the feed of choice for preterm babies.

For preterm babies there are several milk preparations available. They are, in order of choice:

1. 'Mother's own' fresh expressed breast milk (EBM) or, second, frozen breast milk, supplemented when required.
2. Banked breast milk.
3. Specially formulated 'preterm' formulas.

Colostrum should be given as soon as it is available and in the order of it being expressed.

'Mother's own' expressed breast milk

EBM is the best option, but more suitable as a sole food for a very preterm baby when supplemented. The huge advantages of immune protection, improved bonding and protection against NEC mean that every effort should be made to encourage mothers to produce milk for their own baby, even if their initial intention was not to breast feed. The protein, calorie and vitamin intake can be adjusted with supplementation when required. Exclusive EBM feeding can be given only if sufficient volume is produced, and long-term expression presents formidable challenges. Helpful advice is given by Lang (2002) and Jones and King (2005).

Breast milk supplements

All babies of birth weight <1500 g should be considered for fortification/ supplementation when they have begun to tolerate 150–180 mL/kg/day of EBM, usually after a period of 2 weeks. We start with half-strength fortification, increasing to full strength after 24 hours, using a multicomponent breast milk fortifier. Follow the manufacturer's instructions regarding the storage time and storage conditions for fortified breast milk. The majority of the UK multicomponent breast milk fortifiers have a 24-hour storage period when added to breast milk.

An alternative to multicomponent breast milk fortification is to fortify with individual macro- and micronutrients such as energy, protein, sodium, phosphate, calcium and vitamins and trace elements. There is, however, a risk of zinc deficiency if zinc is not added. None of the breast milk fortifiers in the UK contains iron, with the result that iron supplementation is needed.

Banked breast milk

Expressed breast milk from women who have delivered at term, and who have been lactating for some weeks or months, contains less protein and minerals than preterm EBM. The milk in breast milk banks is usually expressed milk which is superfluous to requirements or collected from the contralateral breast during suckling (drip breast milk), and is low in energy content. It is pasteurized, which affects the absorption of fat from banked milk, due to denaturation of the bile salt-stimulated lipase enzyme, and therefore has a lower energy content. Pasteurization reduces the viral load of cytomegalovirus, for example.

Preterm formula

For a newborn preterm baby to grow and accumulate sufficient nutrients and minerals to parallel intra-uterine growth, he requires a higher protein and mineral intake than would be provided by a standard infant formula or unfortified human breast milk. Special preterm formulas have therefore been produced with higher protein and mineral contents, in line with the ESPGHAN (Agostoni *et al.* 2010) and Tsang *et al.* (2005) guidelines (see Table 11.2). The composition of EBM can vary between expression and between mothers (~25% variance).

■ Anti-infection agents

There are many anti-infection agents in breast milk. These include lysozymes, lactoferrin, immunoglobulins and complement. Most of these anti-infection factors are reduced even by gentle pasteurization. If there are any benefits to the baby on the neonatal unit from these anti-infection factors, they will be available only if he receives fresh EBM from his own mother.

Table 11.2 Composition of mature human milk and nutritional criteria for the composition of infant formula for full-term infants per 100 mL (EC Directive, 2006/141/EC)

	Mean values for pooled samples of expressed mature human milk	Guidelines for infant formulas	
		Minimum	Maximum
Energy			
kJ	293	250	295
kcal	70	60	71
Protein (g)	1.3	1.1	2.1
Lactose (g)	7	2.8	NS
Total carbohydrate (g)		5.5	10.0
Fat (g)	4.2	2.6	4.1
Vitamins (mg)			
A	60	35	127
D	0.01	0.63	1.92
E*	0.35	0.5**	1.2**
K	0.21	2.4	NS
Thiamin	16	35	212
Riboflavin	30	48	212
Nicotinic acid	230	150	NS
Pyridoxine	6	22.5	124
B_{12}	0.01	0.06	NS
Folic acid	5.2	6.25	35
Biotin	0.76	1.0	5.3
C	3.8	6.25	22.1
Minerals			
Sodium (mg)	15	12.5	41.3
Potassium (mg)	60	37.5	112
Chloride (mg)	43	30	112
Calcium (mg)	35	30	97
Phosphorus (mg)	15	15	65
Magnesium (mg)	2.3	3.0	10.6
Iron (mg)	0.76	0.18	0.89
Iodine (mcg)	7	6.25	35
Zinc (mg)	0.295	0.3	1.1
Copper (μg)	39	21	74

NS, not specified.

* mg tocopherol equivalents.

** Minimum 0.5/g polyunsaturated fatty acids (PUFA); maximum 1.2/g PUFA.

Infection

Various viruses such as cytomegalovirus, herpes, hepatitis B, human T-cell lymphotropic virus 1 (HTLV-1) and HIV can be transmitted in breast milk, of which the most important are HIV and HTLV-1. It is for this reason that breast-milk banks should use only milk which has been pasteurized and obtained from women who have been tested and are known to be HIV and hepatitis B and C negative.

Drugs

These may get into breast milk if they are not protein bound. However, it is very unusual for drugs taken by the mother to have any serious implications for the breast-fed baby. Table 11.3 lists those which do and which should therefore be avoided. It is important to treat each mother individually and assess the specific medication needed and its effects on breast milk. Consult a pharmacist regarding alternative medications, when necessary, in order to preserve and use any available EBM as far as possible.

Tolerance

There is a wealth of clinical experience which says that, when starting enteral feeds in low birth weight babies who have been ill or had bowel problems, breast milk is better tolerated than formula. This is supported by scientific research which shows that breast milk passes though the stomach faster, releases gut hormones into the circulation and increases gut motility. Time to achieve full feeds is significantly shorter when breast milk is used.

Special milks

A wide variety of other formulas has been designed for situations such as allergy, malabsorption and inborn errors of metabolism. None of these was designed to meet the preterm infant's requirements and when they are used (for example, Neocate LCP for short gut after NEC) extra nutritional monitoring and adaptation are required. Many of these milks have a very high renal solute load, which can cause problems if the total fluid intake has to be restricted.

Table 11.3 Drugs which are contraindicated in breast-feeding mothers

Amiodarone
Ergot alkaloids
Etretinate (vitamin A derivative)
Gold salts
Immunosupressive drugs, cytotoxic drugs, e.g. ciclosporin, cyclophosphamide, methotrexate
Lithium
Morphine, methadone heroin and other drugs of addiction when used by addicts
Oral contraceptives
Phenindione
Radiopharmaceuticals
Tetracycline

Conclusions

The ideal starting diet for a term or preterm baby is fresh, unpasteurized breast milk from his own mother, and for a term baby this diet will suffice for many months. If 'mother's own' is unavailable, the next best starting diet for a preterm baby is pasteurized donor breast milk thawed from a breast milk bank. Once a preterm baby is established on enteral feeds, we would prefer to continue with 'mother's own' EBM, unpasteurized, supplemented for babies of birth weight <1500g or in bigger babies whose growth is suboptimal. We do not wait for bacteriological culture results before starting to give a mother's own milk to her baby. Freeze-thawing mother's own breast milk has to be done at times to bridge gaps in supply. If 'mother's own' EBM is not available, we would not continue with donor breast milk after using it to establish feeds, but would feed the baby on one of the preterm formulas.

When to start enteral feeds and when to increase the volume

Babies less than 34 weeks cannot usually sustain coordinated sucking and swallowing and require tube feeding. Healthy low birth weight babies should have an orogastric or nasogastric (NG) tube passed within 1–2 hours of delivery, and feeding with breast milk or formula milk can be started at once. Ideally some form of breast milk (see above) should be used to minimize the risk of NEC (see Chapter 21) and because it is better tolerated. Great care should be taken when starting feeds to aspirate the stomach 4–6 hourly to prevent pooling of milk and secretions in the stomach, and to assess the volume and nature of 'gastric residuals' and stool frequency, which are helpful in judging when to increase feed volume.

Minimal enteral feeding (trophic feeding)

Giving small, nutritionally insignificant, volumes of milk encourages the secretion of gut hormones, improves gut motility, helps in the earlier achievement of full enteral feeds and reduces the hazards of TPN. The presence of an umbilical artery catheter or a putative risk of NEC are not contraindications to trying enteral feeds so long as sensible precautions are observed. We start small bolus feeds of 1.0 mL every 4 hours as soon as possible and when mother's own milk is available (Table 11.4).

In babies at high risk of NEC we increase the feed volume slowly, at 20 mL/kg/24 h, whereas in babies at low risk we increase at a rate of at least 30 mL/kg/24 h. We monitor gastric residuals and as a rule of thumb do not become concerned about milky residuals of <25% of the feed volume. A residual of 3.5 mL is quite large for a preterm baby (Cobb *et al.* 2004). Aspirates of 2–3 mL in a <1000 g baby are not a sign of feed intolerance if the baby is clinically well. Assessment of suspected bile-stained aspirates should take into account the baby's overall clinical picture.

■ Healthy low birth weight babies

The volumes listed in Table 11.4 are a guide. It is particularly important to feed these volumes to babies who are small for dates and at risk from hypoglycaemia (see Chapter 18).

If the baby is unable to suck, then appropriate volumes of milk should be given hourly through an indwelling orogastric or NG tube. Low birth weight asymptomatic

Table 11.4 Initiating feeds in preterm infants

	Day 1	Day 2	Day 3	Day 4 and onwards
<27 weeks or <1000g or high risk*	1 mL 4 hourly	1 mL 2 hourly	1 mL hourly	Increase by 20mL/kg/day Aim to reach hourly feeds of 180mL/kg/day EBM or DEBM
Standard risk 27–31+6 or 1000–1500g	1 mL hourly	Hourly feeds Increase by 30mL/kg/day	Hourly feeds Increase by 30mL/kg/day	Aim to reach 180mL/kg/day EBM/DEBM Or 150mL/kg/day formula is tolerated
Standard risk >32 weeks	2–3-hourly feeds as tolerated Start at 60mL/kg/day	2–3-hourly feeds as tolerated Increase by 30mL/kg/day until 180mL/kg/day EBM Or 150mL/kg/day formula is tolerated	2–3-hourly feeds as tolerated Increase by 30mL/kg/day until 180mL/kg/day EBM Or 150mL/kg/day formula is tolerated	2–3-hourly feeds as tolerated Until 180mL/kg/day EBM Or 150mL/kg/day formula is tolerated

DEBM, donor-expressed breast milk (banked milk); EBM, expressed breast milk.

*High risk – preterm infants:

Intra-uterine growth restriction with reverse end-diastolic flow

Haemodynamically unstable on inotropes

Post-complex resuscitation

babies can be fed 2 hourly when they weigh about 1.30 kg and 3 hourly when they reach 1.50 kg. Well babies weighing more than 2 kg at birth usually tolerate 2–3-hourly feeds in the first 24 hours of life. Whenever NG feeding is started, the position of the NG tube should be checked radiologically by injecting air while listening over the stomach, or by aspirating acid stomach contents.

Sustained nipple feeding (breast or bottle) is rarely possible in babies of less than 34 weeks, but putting a much less mature baby to the breast, even briefly, will boost the mother's morale enormously. Non-nutritive sucking from a dummy helps weight gain in all preterm babies and should be offered during tube feeds when the baby is awake and well enough.

■ Sick low birth weight babies

Certain important generalizations govern the feeding of these babies:

1. The baby less than 32 weeks' gestation has caloric reserves for only 4–5 days' extra-uterine existence and enough glycogen for only a few hours.
2. An adequate caloric intake is necessary to prevent hypoglycaemia and jaundice, and may be one of the factors limiting neurological handicap in survivors.
3. The sooner a baby puts on weight and ceases to be catabolic, the sooner he recovers from serious neonatal illness.
4. If oral feeds are not tolerated or are contraindicated, intravenous feeding should be started as early as possible, within the first 24–48 hours.
5. Although milk is good for premature babies it can also do harm (Table 11.5). However, maintain minimal enteral feeds of small volume (e.g. 1 mL every 4 hours) whenever possible. This will maintain gut flora and assist later increase of feed volume.
6. The stomach contents must be aspirated every 4–6 hours once feeding is commenced.
7. Even when enteral feeding is established, electrolyte disturbances such as hyponatraemia and hypophosphataemia may still occur. Serum chemistry should be checked at least weekly and, if necessary, appropriate supplements given.
8. Enteral feeds should be stopped:
   - when the gastric aspirate every 3–4 hours is consistently larger than 50% of the volume of milk given (except with minimal enteral feeding) or the aspirate is 'dirty', e.g. blood or bile stained; 3.5 mL of residual is a large absolute volume for a very preterm baby;
   - if there are signs of intestinal obstruction;
   - if feeding triggers apnoeic attacks;
   - for 4–6 hours post extubation;
   - in babies suspected of inborn errors of metabolism;
   - during exchange transfusion.

If NG tube feeding is not being tolerated, the following can be tried.

Posture

Babies' stomachs empty better if they lie on their right side or are lying prone.

Table 11.5 Dangers of milk feeding in premature babies

Danger	Complication
Pooling in stomach	Regurgitation and aspiration
Compromised respiratory function (due partly to gastric distension and partly to nasal obstruction)	Recurrent apnoea ↓ PaO_2 ↓ Functional residual capacity
Introduction of infection (?due to indwelling tube)	Gastroenteritis Necrotizing enterocolitis
Electrolyte imbalance	Hyponatraemia Acidaemia Hypophosphataemia
Milk bolus obstruction	Gut perforation

Continuous infusion of milk through a nasogastric tube

Although a randomized controlled trial showed no benefit from continuous NG feeds, a wide body of clinical experience suggests that this method can be tried when establishing feeds remains a persistent problem or when no other treatment for gastro-oesophageal reflux disease has been successful. The most common technique is to use a syringe pump to infuse the milk down the NG tube. The use of a syringe pump is not ideal, however, and puts the baby at risk of infusing an enteral fluid parenterally. If giving continuous feeds, a certified enteral feeding pump should be used. A new supply of milk should be started every 2 hours in preterm infants and every 4 hours in a term infant. A significant amount of fat in the milk may adhere to the side of the tubes, thereby reducing the caloric intake. It is recommended not to use continuous feeding EBM at a volume of $\leq 4\,mL/h$ as the fat loss is too great.

Nasojejunal tube feeding

There is no point in using nasojejeunal feeding routinely since not only is it more difficult to set up, but it aggravates the steatorrhoea of prematurity (see above) and may also increase the risk of gut infection and NEC (pp. 278–283). It should therefore be used only if NG tube feeding results in persistent regurgitation and/or apnoea. Silastic tubes should be used. To get them through the stomach into the duodenum, either use an introducer or wait until the tube is carried through the pylorus by peristalsis. The position of the tube should be confirmed radiologically and the milk given as a continuous infusion using a syringe pump. An NG tube should be left in situ to detect regurgitation of milk back through the pylorus.

Intravenous glucose electrolyte solutions (Chapter 18)

In the short term (the first 2 days) this is the usual way of hydrating a >34-week baby and providing fluid during the acute phase of any neonatal illness. Intravenous glucose electrolyte solutions should be used for as short a period as possible as they do not nearly meet any macronutrient requirements in the preterm infant.

Intravenous feeding

This technique can be life-saving for the baby in whom enteral feeding is going to be impossible for a period longer than 2 days. It is described fully in Chapter 12.

■ References

Agostoni, C, Buonocore, G, Carnielli, VP, *et al.* (2010) Enteral nutrient supply for preterm infants: commentary from European Society for Paediatric Gastroenterology, Hepatology and Nutrition Committee on Nutrition. *Journal of Pediatric Gastroenterology and Nutrition*, **50**: 1–9.

Cobb, BA, Carlo, WA, Ambalavanan, N (2004) Gastric residuals and their relationship to necrotising enterocolitis. *Pediatrics*, **113**: 50–3.

Ehrenkranz, RA, Younes, N, Lemons, JA, *et al.* (1999) Longitudinal growth of hospitalised very low birth weight infants. *Pediatrics*, **104**: 280–9.

Fewtrell, M, Chomtho, S (2012) Infant feeding. In Rennie, JM (ed.) *Rennie & Roberton's Textbook of Neonatology*, 5th edition. Edinburgh: Elsevier, pp. 278–296.

Jones, E, King, C (2005) *Feeding and Nutrition in the Preterm Infant*. Amsterdam: Elsevier.

Lang, S (2002) *Breastfeeding Special Care Babies*, 2nd edition. Oxford: Balliere Tindall.

Tsang, RC, Uauy, R, Koletzko, B, Zlotkin, SH (2005) *Nutrition of the Preterm Infant: Scientific Basis and Practical Guidelines*, 2nd edition. Digital Educational Publishing.

■ Further reading

Deshpande, G, Rao, S, Patole, S, Bulsara, M (2010) Updated meta-analysis of probiotics for preventing necrotising enterocolitis in preterm neonates. *Pediatrics*, **125**: 921.

Lucas, A, Cole, TJ (1990) Breast milk and neonatal necrotizing enterocolitis. *Lancet*, **336**: 1519–23.

■ Web link

http://espghan.med.up.pt/position_papers/Enteral_Nutrient_Supply_for_Preterm_Infants.pdf

Parenteral nutrition

- Parenteral nutrition (PN) is an essential part of good neonatal intensive care, but requires careful monitoring, is associated with complications and is always second best to enteral nutrition.
- PN should be considered soon after birth in very premature babies, particularly those who are unlikely to tolerate enteral feeds.
- PN should only be administered with the help of a multidisciplinary nutrition team, including dietetic and pharmacy support, sterile manufacture and biochemical monitoring.

The caloric reserves of the neonate weighing 1.00 kg will sustain him for only 4–5 days in the absence of feeding. Giving 10% glucose (40 kcal/100 mL) will prolong survival to some extent, but neonates who, for any reason, are expected to be unable to tolerate enteral feeds by 3–4 days of age require some source of nitrogen and additional calories. This is the most common indication for parenteral nutrition (PN) on neonatal units, 'bridging the gap' until full enteral feeds are tolerated – usually a period of less than 3 weeks. Full PN – that is, providing all the fat, protein, carbohydrate, vitamins, minerals and calories to support normal growth – is life-saving in babies who have major gastrointestinal disease or chylothorax which preclude enteral feeding for weeks or months (Chapters 21 and 13, respectively).

Undertaking any form of intravenous nutrition demands the support of skilled personnel in pharmacy, dietetics and biochemistry, as well as the appropriate technical experience and equipment on the neonatal unit to maintain long lines and infuse small quantities accurately over prolonged periods of time. Appropriate vascular access is essential to the success of PN and requires a high level of skill because devastating complications can occur. The National Confidential Enquiry into Patient Outcome and Death (2010) report showed that neonatal PN was often delayed, inadequate, and associated with metabolic and line complications. Best practice recommendations were for multidisciplinary teams.

Composition of parenteral nutrition solutions

Although this topic can be made extremely complicated, it can be broken down to very simple basic rules.

Carbohydrate

Most neonates need at least 4–6 mg glucose/kg/min ($\cong$ 58–86 mL of 10% glucose/kg/24 h), but larger volumes or more concentrated solutions can be used if tolerated (i.e. blood glucose <6–7 mmol/L; no glycosuria) to increase the caloric intake. Many babies will tolerate 12 mg/kg/min ($\cong$ 130 mL of 12.5% glucose/kg/24 h) or more if the infusion rate is built up slowly over a period of days.

Protein

The protein solutions now used are mixtures of pure L-isomers of amino acids (Table 12.1). Various solutions are available. These solutions are certainly well tolerated although the ideal amino acid solution for preterm babies has yet to be found, but amino acid solutions designed for paediatric patients have been shown to result in a more favourable plasma aminogram, higher nitrogen retention and better weight gain in preterm infants. Trophamine, available in the USA and Europe, also has an acceptable composition. Vaminolact and Primene are electrolyte-free, which makes it easier to tailor the electrolyte requirements to the individual baby.

It is not usually advisable to give more than 3.0–3.5 g protein/kg/24 h because of the risks of hyperammonaemia, acidaemia and hyperaminoacidaemia. Optimal protein requirements for growth are in the range of 3.5–4 g/kg/day. Preterm infants require not only more amino acids than term infants but also qualitatively different amino acids. Cysteine, taurine, tyrosine and histidine have been considered as semi-essential amino acids in preterm infants.

Table 12.1 Composition (per litre of fluid) of amino acid solutions available for use in the newborn

Content per litre	Vamin 9 glucose (Pharmacia)	Primene 10% (Baxter Healthcare)	Vaminolact (Pharmacia)
Nitrogen (g)	9.4 (= 57.5 g first-class protein)	15	9.3
Energy (kcal/MJ)	650/2.7	250/1.05	240
Sodium (mmol)	50	0	0
Potassium (mmol)	20	0	0
Magnesium (mmol)	1.5	0	0
Calcium (mmol)	2.5	0	0
Acetate (mmol)	0	25	0
Chloride (mmol)	50	15.6	0
Glucose (g)	100	0	
Osmolarity (mOsmol/L)	1350	780	510
Isoleucine (g)	3.9	6.7	3.1
Leucine (g)	5.3	10.0	7
Alanine (g)	3.0	8.0	6.3
Arginine (g)	3.3	8.4	4.1
Aspartic acid (g)	4.1	6.0	4.1
Glutamic acid (g)	9.0	10.0	7.1
Glycine (g)	2.1	4.0	2.1
Lysine (g)	3.9	11.0	5.6

(continued)

Table 12.1 (Continued)

Content per litre	Vamin 9 glucose (Pharmacia)	Primene 10% (Baxter Healthcare)	Vaminolact (Pharmacia)
Phenylalanine (g)	5.5	4.2	2.7
Proline (g)	8.1	3.0	5.6
Serine (g)	7.5	4.0	3.8
Methionine (g)	1.9	2.4	1.3
Threonine (g)	3.0	3.7	3.6
Tyrosine (g)	0.5	0.45	0.5
Histidine (g)	2.4	3.8	2.1
Tryptophan (g)	1.0	2.0	1.4
Valine (g)	4.3	7.6	3.6
Cysteine (g)	1.4	1.89	1.0
Taurine (g)		0.6	0.3

Fat

Providing fat is essential if an adequate caloric intake is to be achieved in total parenteral nutrition (TPN), and non-nitrogen energy is vital in order that amino acids can be utilized effectively. Lipids are also required in order to prevent fatty acid deficiency. Previous concerns about the early use of lipid have largely been alleviated by the results of randomized controlled trials in which fat supplementation commenced on the day of birth. A 20% lipid emulsion should be started at 1 g/kg/24 h and increased daily by 1 g/kg to 3g/kg/24 h as tolerated.

Intralipid is made from soybean oil and does not have the optimum balance of linoleic–linolenic acid for the newborn brain but it is the only product readily available at present; 20% Intralipid is better tolerated than the 10% preparation. Monitoring of tolerance should be done with serum triglyceride levels as plasma turbidity is a poor indicator of triglyceride concentration. The infusion rate should probably be reduced if the plasma triglyceride concentration exceeds 1.8 mmol/L, and certainly if it is higher than 3 mmol/L.

Protein calorie/non-protein calorie ratio

This should be kept in the range of 1:8–1:10. Values less than 1:6 are likely to result in hyperaminoacidaemia and aminoaciduria.

Vitamins and trace elements

If some enteral feeding is tolerated, i.e. supplemental parenteral nutrition is being given, the neonate will receive adequate trace minerals orally and can be given a standard oral vitamin supplement (e.g. Abidec). Trace elements (zinc, selenium, copper and manganese) should be routinely added to the aqueous component of PN; Vitalipid should be added to the lipid component. Iron supplementation is not required as preterm neonates receive frequent top-up transfusions. Copper and manganese should be withheld when biliary stasis is present. We use Peditrace (Table 12.2); the older Pedel contained too much manganese for preterm babies.

Table 12.2 Contents of one 10 mL vial of Peditrace

Mineral	Amount in micrograms	Amount in μmoles
Zinc	2500	38.2
Copper	200	3.15
Manganese	10	182
Selenium	20	253
Iodine	570	30

Solivito and Vitlipid are used to provide water- and fat-soluble vitamins, respectively (see Tables 12.3 and 12.4 for composition). The dose of Solivito is 0.5 mL/kg/day to a maximum of 5 mL in 24 hours, and Vitlipid 1mL/kg/day to a maximum of 10 mL in 24 hours. A lot of vitamin D and E is lost by adherence to the plastic of the tubing. These vitamins should be added as soon as PN is begun.

Electrolytes

These are prescribed on a daily basis according to the guidelines outlined in Chapter 10. Sodium and potassium are added often as chlorides; this results in a hyperchloraemia when large amounts of sodium are given to replace losses in very preterm babies. More recent formulations provide some of the sodium as acetate, which reduces the incidence and severity of hyperchloraemia. If a baby does become hyperchloraemic, a metabolic acidosis ensues.

Table 12.3 Composition of 1 mL of Solivito (water-soluble vitamins)

Vitamin	Amount
Vitamin B_1	3 mg
Vitamin B_2	3.6 mg
Nicotinamide	40 mg
Pantothenic acid	15 mg
Vitamin B_6	4 mg
Vitamin C	100 mg
Biotin	60 μg
Folic acid	0.4 mg
Vitamin B_{12}	5 μg

Table 12.4 Composition of 1 mL of Vitlipid

Vitamin	Amount
Vitamin A	230 units
Vitamin D_2	1 μg
Vitamin E	0.64 mg
Vitamin K	20 μg
+ emulsifying agents	

Calcium and phosphate pose major problems since their solubility product is readily exceeded and they precipitate out. Their solubility depends on the acidity of the solution, and thus mainly on the concentration of the protein solution; the higher the concentration of Vamin/Vaminolact/Primene, the more calcium and phosphate that can be given. A range of 1.5–2.2 mmol/kg/24 hours of both calcium and phosphorus should be given in IV feeding solutions, starting with the lower dose and building up by 10% per day. If TPN is provided in glass containers the calcium should be given as calcium chloride to avoid the potentially neurotoxic concentrations of aluminium found as a contaminant in calcium gluconate preparations (Bishop *et al.* 1997); this is not, however, a problem with TPN supplied in plastic.

Hypophosphataemia often develops in very low birth weight babies receiving PN. If the phosphate remains below 0.8 mmol/L, the only practical solution is to give an infusion of IV phosphate using one of the formulations below (dissolved in 10% dextrose) and to stop the PN for a few hours. Recommendations regarding infusion are a maximum rate of potassium phosphate 0.5 mmol K/kg/h and aim to give about 0.5–1 mmol PO_4/kg in 12 hours. Formulas currently available are: potassium phosphate 17.42%, 1 mL contains 2 mmol K and 1 mmol PO_4; potassium acid phosphate 13.6%, 1 mL contains 1 mmol PO_4 and 1 mmol K; sodium glycerophosphate, 1 mL contains 1 mmol PO_4 and 2 mmol Na.

Intravenous feeding solutions

We use Vaminolact, and give fat as 20% Intralipid. The Vaminolact is added to a glucose electrolyte solution by our pharmacy. The amount of Vaminolact and concentration of glucose and electrolytes are decided daily on the basis of the age of the baby, his tolerance of IV glucose, and in particular the desired caloric intake for the next 24 hours. Intralipid is included after the first day or so of PN, bearing in mind the caveats outlined above. Water- and fat-soluble vitamins, and trace elements, are added as discussed above.

Route of infusion

All the fluids used in intravenous feeding can be given through a peripheral vein. However, the fluids are very irritant and frequently thrombose the vessels. If extravasation occurs, permanent scarring may result. Thus, this route has limited application and should only be used for the short term, when it is not possible to insert a central venous catheter and PN is indicated. For long-term feeding, use a long line sited in a major central vessel. Because of the risk of introducing infection through an intravenous feeding line, it should never be used for anything other than the intravenous feeding solution.

Monitoring of intravenous feeding

Daily or twice daily:

- Weight.
- Urinary glucose, blood glucose.
- Electrolytes.
- Haematocrit.

Weekly:

- Magnesium.
- Calcium and phosphorus (daily in the first week).

- Bilirubin.
- Protein, albumin (daily in the first week).
- Liver enzymes; transaminases, alkaline phosphatase.
- Triglycerides.
- Blood gases.
- Haemoglobin, white count and platelets, C-reactive protein (CRP).

Complications of parenteral nutrition

Catheter related

Central lines are a potent cause of thrombosis in newborns, in whom venous obstruction is otherwise rare. If extravasated subcutaneously from a peripheral line, irritant PN solutions can cause unsightly scarring. Extravasation from central lines into all sorts of spaces has been described.

Metabolic

Hyperglycaemia is common, although tolerance to the high glucose infusion rates required to achieve an adequate calorie input can be achieved if the concentration is built up slowly. Sometimes insulin has to be used. Hyperammonaemia also occurs, and urea should be monitored and kept below 6 mmol/L. Hyperchloraemic metabolic acidosis has already been mentioned. High phenylalanine levels have been detected in babies receiving amino acid solutions, but so far no adverse effect on outcome has been demonstrated.

Cholestatic jaundice

About a third of preterm babies who receive PN for more than 2 weeks develop jaundice (see Chapter 20) and this figure rises to 80% after 2 months of PN. Biliary sludging and calculi may develop. In most cases the jaundice resolves once enteral feeding is established, but in some it progresses to cirrhosis and liver failure. Factors increasing the incidence of this complication are prematurity, duration of PN, sepsis and surgery.

Infection

This is the major complication of PN, and can lead to removal of precious central lines. The risk of infection can be minimized by a meticulously aseptic insertion technique, and rigorous adherence to the rule about not using the line for anything other than PN. We use antifungal prophylaxis in preterm babies with central venous lines.

Infection may be suspected on the basis of the routine weekly blood tests, or it may present with an insidious deterioration in the baby's condition, often accompanied by a low-grade pyrexia, changes in the white blood cell count, a falling platelet count and a rise in CRP. Occasionally the baby develops a full-blown septicaemic illness.

The usual pathogen isolated when there is a gradual deterioration is coagulase-negative staphylococci (CONS). If use of the long line is not essential, the safest course of action is to remove it, and to treat the baby with flucloxacillin, vancomycin or teicoplanin. If the line is crucial, and CONS is grown, it is well worth trying the effect of parenteral antibiotics given through the line or as 'locks'. For more pathogenic bacteria, or with fungal infections arising from the line, there is probably no alternative but to remove it, in addition to vigorous treatment of the infection.

Acknowledgement

Thanks to Fiona McGuire, our fantastic pharmacist, for her help with this chapter.

References

Bishop, NJ, Morley, R, Day, JP, Lucas, A (1997) Aluminum necrotoxicity in preterm infants receiving intravenous-feeding solutions. *New England Journal of Medicine*, **29**: 1 557–61.

National Confidential Enquiry into Patient Outcome and Death (NCEPOD) (2010) A mixed bag – an enquiry into the care of patients receiving parenteral nutrition. www.ncepod.org.uk.

Further reading

Ehrenkrantz, RA (2007) Early, aggressive nutritional management for very low birthweight infants: what is the evidence? *Seminars in Perinatology*, **31**: 48–55.

Koletko, B, Goulet, O, Hunt J, *et al.* (2005) Guidelines on paediatric parenteral nutrition of the European Society of Paediatric Gastroenterology, Hepatology and Nutrition (ESPGHAN). *Journal of Pediatric Gastroenterology and Nutrition*, **41** (suppl 2): S1–87.

PART 4

Diseases and their management

114

13

Acute disorders of
the respiratory tract

Key points

- Fetal lung liquid fills the airways and must be cleared rapidly from the lungs at birth for normal gas exchange to start.
- The lung of a normal term baby has only a fifth of the final number of alveoli and very preterm babies have no alveoli at all.
- By 15 minutes of age major changes in blood gases, lung mechanics and pulmonary perfusion have already taken place, and by 60 minutes lung function is close to normal.
- Right-to-left shunts are common in the neonate; the true shunt is estimated from the pre-ductal PaO_2 after breathing 100% oxygen for 15 minutes.
- Surfactant is a complex mixture of phospholipids, neutral lipids and protein. Surfactant appears in the lung during the third trimester of pregnancy.
- The oxygen affinity of fetal and early neonatal blood (P_{50}) is increased, in part owing to a reduced effect of 2,3-diphosphatidylglycerol in red cells when fetal haemoglobin is present.

Respiratory physiology

Lung growth and development

The term baby has 50 million alveoli, a number which increases to 250 million by adult life. Most of this increase occurs during the first 18 months, the surface area of the lung rising from 3 m² to 70 m². This growth potential is important during the treatment of babies with chronic lung disease (Chapter 14). The growth factors involved are still under study. The canalicular stage of lung development occurs between 17 and 27 weeks of gestation. During this phase capillaries begin to appear and gas exchange can occur when the capillaries approximate to the air spaces. This enables gas exchange to occur and determines extra-uterine survival. During the canalicular stage bronchioles terminate in acinar units, not alveoli. Alveoli begin to appear as shallow indentations at about 32 weeks' gestation, but many alveoli form after birth. During fetal life the lung is filled with lung liquid which has a completely different composition to amniotic fluid and plasma. It is produced by active transport mechanisms, the dominant one being the transfer of chloride from plasma into the lung fluid. In human fetuses lung fluid first appears during the second trimester, and by full term alveoli contain approximately 30 mL/kg.

The onset of respiration

The following are all important in initiating breathing:

1. *Physical stimuli.* In newborn animals delivered into a bath of warm saline or onto a warm bench beside the mother, physical stimuli such as cold or touching the fetus can initiate respiration. If, however, the newborn is kept warm and has an intact umbilical circulation, breathing is rarely sustained. Newborn babies are suddenly exposed to light, gravity, sound and cold – an immense sensory input.
2. *Chemoreceptors.* An important factor in the initiation of breathing is stimulation of the central chemoreceptors by the changes in blood gas concentrations which follow cord clamping. The role of the peripheral chemoreceptors remains controversial, since, if they are denervated, respiration still starts after the cord is clamped.
3. *Central nervous system (CNS) activity.* Respiratory centre activity may also be involved in the onset of respiration. In animals, this area becomes much less electrically active if the sensory input to the CNS is removed.

When aerating the lungs at birth the neonate generates an opening pressure of at least 20 cmH$_2$O to overcome the viscosity of the fluid in the airway, the surface tension within the fluid-filled lung, and the elastic recoil and resistance of the tissues of the chest wall, lungs and airways. Large positive end expiratory pressures above 30 cmH$_2$O are also generated, which help to squeeze the liquid out of the lungs. By the time of delivery, the lungs contain about 30 mL/kg of fluid. Shortly before the onset of labour the production of fetal lung liquid is reduced by β-adrenergic stimulation, which may also serve to activate the epithelial sodium ion pumps. Lung epithelial cells change from chloride-secreting to sodium-absorbing at birth, a function which they then retain throughout life. Activation of sodium absorption across the alveolar epithelium at birth moves alveolar liquid into the lung interstitium from where it is removed rapidly via the lymphatics and the pulmonary capillaries. The lungs appear lucent on X-rays within two or three breaths, and a normal functional residual capacity (FRC) is established within 60 minutes (Fig. 13.1).

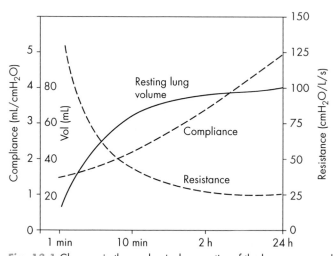

Fig. 13.1 Changes in the mechanical properties of the lungs expressed on a logarithmic scale during the first day of life. From Godfrey (1981)

Pulmonary perfusion

All the factors involved in the onset of respiration – lung expansion, the fall in $PaCO_2$ and the rise in PaO_2 – have an independent effect to increase pulmonary blood flow immediately after delivery (Fig. 13.2). Thereafter, pulmonary vasodilatation is maintained by powerful endothelium-derived vasodilators, including endothelin 1, prostacyclin and nitric oxide, the release of which is stimulated by the expansion and ventilation of the lung (Ziegler *et al.* 1995).

Mechanics of respiration in the newborn

See Table 13.1.

Rate

The normal newborn baby breathes 30–50 times per minute when asleep at all gestations. This is the respiratory rate at which the calculated work of breathing is minimal. When awake the normal respiratory rate is up to 60 breaths/min. The normal newborn breathes irregularly with apnoeic pauses of up to 10 seconds.

Functional residual capacity and thoracic gas volume

Normally these two measurements of resting lung volume are similar, but, in the newborn, the thoracic gas volume (TGV) may be 30–35 mL/kg compared with an FRC of only 20–25 mL/kg. Whether this represents genuine air trapping or is a methodological artefact remains uncertain.

Dead space (V_D), tidal volume (V_T), minute volume (V_E) and vital capacity (V_C)

These are similar in premature and full-term babies, when expressed per kilogram of body weight.

Lung compliance (C_l)

This is the change in volume in millilitres, for unit change in pressure in cmH_2O. Compliance measured in the spontaneously breathing baby is the dynamic compliance

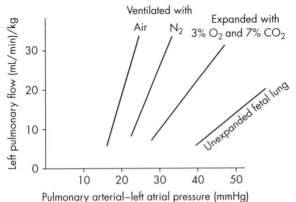

Fig. 13.2 Effect of expansion of lung with 3% O_2 and 7% CO_2 in nitrogen (equivalent to ventilation without change in blood gases), ventilation with nitrogen (equivalent to blowing off CO_2), and ventilation with air on pulmonary vascular resistance in mature fetal lambs. From Dawes (1966)

and is inversely proportional to the respiratory rate. Static compliance is measured (in adults) by the subject voluntarily holding his breath at different points during inspiration and expiration, an experiment which it is difficult to reproduce in babies. To compare compliance at different lung volumes, specific compliance is used, which is the compliance divided by the FRC. During the first few days of life, compliance increases up to the normal value of 5 mL/cmH$_2$O (Fig. 13.1).

Airways resistance (R$_{AW}$)

Pulmonary resistance (R$_L$) is calculated by measuring inspiratory and expiratory flow (in L/s) using a pneumotachograph and dividing this into the pressure difference between the mouth and the oesophagus (equivalent to the intrapleural pressure). To measure airways resistance (R$_{AW}$) the alveolar pressure has to be estimated and this can be done only with a plethysmograph. Alveolar pressure can then be substituted for oesophageal pressure in the calculations. If the flow measurements are made using a

Table 13.1 Lung function in the newborn

Measurement	Full term	Preterm (if different from term)	Adult
Thoracic gas volume (TGV) (mL/kg)	30–35	35–45	30
Functional residual capacity (FRC) (mL/kg)	27–30	20–25	30
Total lung capacity (mL/kg)	55–70		80–85
Vital capacity (V$_C$) (mL/kg)	35–40		60
Tidal volume (V$_T$) (mL/kg)	4–7		7
Alveolar volume (V$_A$) (mL/kg)	3.8–5.8		4.8
Dead space (V$_D$) (mL/kg)	2.0–2.5		2.2
V$_D$/V$_T$	0.3		0.3
Alveolar ventilation (V$_A$) (mL/kg/min)	100–150		60
Minute ventilation (V$_E$) (mL/kg/min)	200–260		90
Lung compliance (C$_L$) (mL/cmH$_2$O)	5–6	0.5–3.0	200
Specific compliance (C$_L$/FRC) (mL/cmH$_2$O/ml)	0.04–0.06	0.012–0.05	0.04–0.07
Total pulmonary resistance (R$_L$) (cmH$_2$O/L/s)	40–45		1.7–2.6
Airway resistance (nose breathing) (R$_{AW}$) (cmH$_2$O/L/s)	25–30	60–80	3.5
Airway resistance (mouth breathing) (R$_{AW}$) (cmH$_2$O/L/s)	15	25–30	1.3
Specific conductance (nose breathing) (SG$_{AW}$) (cmH$_2$O/L/s/mL FRC)	0.31	0.35–0.5	0.1
Work of breathing (g.cm/min)	1500	500	16,000–50,000
Diffusion capacity for CO (DL$_{CO}$) (mL/CO/min/mmHg)	0.8–3.0	0.3	15–25

face mask rather than a mouthpiece or endotracheal tube (ETT), the nasal resistance will be included in the measurement. Half of the airways resistance in the neonate is in the nose.

The reciprocal of the resistance is conductance, which can be expressed as specific conductance (SG_{AW}), i.e. conductance per millilitre of FRC. Normal values are given in Table 13.1, and the rapid postnatal fall is shown in Fig. 13.1. The abnormal stiffness of the lung in respiratory distress syndrome (RDS) results in a change of the pressure–volume curve. Normally air is retained until low volumes are reached (hysteresis). In RDS, large pressure changes are needed to achieve a small increase in volume and during deflation the lung volume follows a similar track to the inflationary curve (Fig. 13.3).

Work of breathing

This can be derived from the formula $W = 0.6PV$, where P is the pressure swing during respiration in cmH_2O and V is minute volume in mL. A wide range of normal values has been obtained in the newborn, averaging around 1500 g.cm/min. This represents about 1% of the total metabolism of the full-term baby.

Pulmonary gas exchange

Ideally the ratio of alveolar ventilation (V_A) in mL/min to pulmonary capillary blood flow (Q_C) in mL/min – the ventilation–perfusion ratio – is 1. In the normal adult lung the value is 0.8–0.9, and in the normal newborn the value is lower, particularly during the first few hours of life.

A right-to-left shunt occurs when blood returns to the left side of the heart without being oxygenated. There are four shunt sites in the newborn:

1. Cardiac veins draining into the left side of the heart and anastomoses between the bronchial and pulmonary circulations.
2. The foramen ovale and ductus arteriosus during postnatal circulatory adaptation.

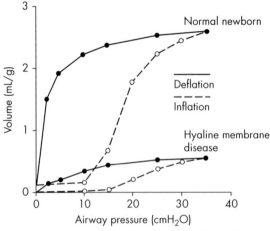

Fig. 13.3 Pressure–volume loops in excised lung of neonates dying with and without respiratory distress syndrome (RDS). In RDS the deflation curve follows the inflation curve and little air is retained at zero pressure. In normal lungs much more air is retained on the deflation limb of the loop (the phenomenon of hysteresis). Reproduced with permission from Gribetz *et al.* (1959)

3. Intrapulmonary shunting owing to pulmonary arterial blood going through the lung without passing a ventilated alveolus – this is a true intrapulmonary shunt with a V_A/Q_C of 0.
4. Intrapulmonary shunting owing to partially ventilated alveoli having a lower PaO_2 than elsewhere in the lungs. These cause V_A/Q_C ratios less than normal, but greater than 0. This component of the shunt can be eliminated by breathing pure oxygen for 15–20 minutes, which eventually washes all the nitrogen out of even poorly ventilated alveoli and equalizes the PaO_2 throughout the lung. This procedure is known as the hyperoxia test. If the PO_2 does not exceed 20 kPa (150 mmHg) in 100% oxygen there is a right-to-left shunt due to congenital heart disease (CHD) (Chapter 22), very severe respiratory disease, or persistent pulmonary hypertension of the newborn (PPHN) (p. 162).

These four shunts constitute the total venous admixture, but if the fourth site is eliminated by inhaling pure oxygen, what is left is the true right-to-left shunt. A measurement of the size of the shunt is the A–aDO$_2$ (alveolar–arterial oxygen difference in mmHg). This is normally less than 2 kPa (<15 mmHg). When breathing pure oxygen, the A–aDO$_2$ indicates the true right-to-left shunt.

Regulation of respiration

The central neural control of respiration is modulated by the chemoreceptors and mechanoreceptors.

Central control

The 'respiratory centre' sited in the dorsal and ventral respiratory group of neurones within the medulla generates the central respiratory rhythm. Afferents from many parts of the brain, in addition to those from chemoreceptors and mechanoreceptors, act on these neurones. Excitatory neurotransmitters in this region include glutamate, serotonin, substance P and catecholamines; inhibitory agents include GABA, glycine, endorphins, adenosine and the E prostaglandins.

Chemoreceptor function

Central chemoreceptors on the ventral surface of the medulla and the peripheral chemoreceptors in the carotid and aortic bodies modulate respiratory control in the neonate. The latter are relatively unimportant in the early neonatal period, as they are in the onset of respiration at birth.

Oxygen chemosensitivity

When a baby is in a cool environment his responses to hypoxaemia are different from those obtained when he is in the neutral thermal environment (Fig. 13.4) and are different from those of older babies and adults. In a thermoneutral environment, hypoxia (10–12% oxygen) causes hyperventilation for 1–2 minutes. The baby then hypoventilates, and premature babies in particular develop periodic breathing or even apnoea. In a cool environment, respiratory depression is the only response to hypoxaemia (Fig 13.4). The reason for this unusual response to hypoxia is not understood, but by 5–7 days of age hypoxia causes a sustained increase in minute and tidal volumes. Breathing 100% oxygen for 30–60 seconds decreases ventilation by 10–15% in all neonates; in premature babies this may cause apnoea.

Carbon dioxide chemosensitivity

Both premature and full-term babies have a lower $PaCO_2$ than adults. The reason for this is uncertain.

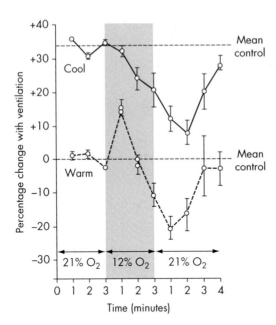

Fig. 13.4 Percentage change in ventilation while breathing air and 12% oxygen in normal term babies in cool and warm temperatures. From Ceruti (1966)

At term the central chemoreceptors are functional at the low $PaCO_2$, and the CO_2 response curve is left-shifted compared with the adult's. Premature babies, however, when they are having apnoeic attacks, have a flattened CO_2 response curve, and the response curve may be right-shifted (i.e. they are less sensitive to increases in $PaCO_2$). Well-oxygenated premature babies have a steeper CO_2 response curve. Raising the $FICO_2$ in preterm and term babies stimulates respiration.

Mechanoreceptors

Vagal afferents from the lung, as well as mechanoreceptors in the muscles of respiration, are stimulated by the distortion of respiratory movement, and the more the distortion, the more they act to inhibit the drive to inspiration. During rapid eye movement sleep, when resting muscle tone is minimal, the distortion of the rib cage caused by diaphragmatic activity results in major activation of this feedback loop, with a shortening of the inspiratory time, irregular breathing and even apnoea. This is probably a manifestation of the Hering–Breuer inflation reflex (cessation of the inspiratory drive with lung inflation). The reflex is also active in term babies. Head's paradoxical reflex or the inspiratory augmenting reflex in which lung inflation provokes a further major inspiratory effort is also present in the neonate. It may be important at birth in helping to expand the lung and establish an FRC.

Surfactant

The lungs of all animals are lined with a layer of lipoprotein which keeps the pressure constant within the alveoli irrespective of their diameter. Lipoproteins which lower surface tension in vitro to less than 10–15 dyn/cm are known as surfactants. Surfactant is synthesized in the type II or granular pneumonocytes of the alveolar epithelium and is stored in the lamellar bodies of these cells. It is released by fusion of the lamellar body membrane with the cell wall. Surfactant is 90% lipid and 10% protein (Table 13.2).

There are four main surfactant proteins: SP-A, SP-B, SP-C and SP-D. SP-A is the largest and most abundant and is involved in the regulation of surfactant metabolism.

Table 13.2 Surfactant data: percentage composition of lipids

	Babies with respiratory distress syndrome	Mature babies
Phosphatidylcholine	61.7	80.9
Sphingomyelin	11.0	2.0
Phosphatidylglycerol	0.9	3.7
Phosphatidylethanolamine	11.7	4.5
Phosphatidylinositol	4.9	–
Phosphatidylserine	5.3	–
Lysophosphatidylcholine	2.0	–
Neutral lipid	Approx. 10%	Approx. 10%

SP-B and SP-C play an important role in the surface tension-lowering activities of the surfactant complex. SP-D interacts with SP-A and has anti-infection properties.

About 85% of the lipid is phospholipid, the remainder being neutral lipid, cholesterol and sphingomyelin. The major phospholipids of surfactant are phosphatidylcholine (lecithin), phosphatidylglycerol and phosphatidylinositol. The phosphatidylcholine from alveolar surfactant is primarily dipalmitoylphosphatidylcholine (dipalmitoyl lecithin (DPL)), which constitutes 50–60% of all surfactant phospholipid. DPL alone does not reduce surface tension, and phosphatidylinositol or phosphatidylglycerol must be present. These appear one after the other in the neonatal lung, and until at least one of them has appeared the lungs remain unstable.

Surfactant and type II pneumocytes appear in the human lung at about 20 weeks' gestation. The amount present increases slowly until, following a surge at about 30–34 weeks, the lungs are mature, and the baby should not develop RDS when delivered. Many agents increase the amount of surfactant in neonates' lungs. These include drugs which have been used therapeutically, such as steroids (pp. 129–130), agents of theoretical interest but which have raised little practical interest such as aminophylline, oestrogens, β-mimetics and bromhexine, and addictive drugs including heroin and cocaine. Babies born to mothers abusing these two agents have a lower incidence of RDS than gestation-matched controls.

At birth, surfactant is released from the pneumocytes. The most important factor in this seems to be distension and ventilation of the lungs, though adrenergic agents and prostaglandins may well play a part. Postnatally, surfactant synthesis is sensitive to cold, hypoxaemia and acidaemia. Postnatal exposure to temperatures less than 35°C, and pH less than 7.25, causes a rapid fall in the amount of surfactant in pharyngeal aspirates. Surfactant, once released, has a half-life of about 10 hours. Some is washed up the bronchial tree with normal fluid movement, some is ingested by alveolar macrophages which contain phospholipases, and some is broken down by tissue phospholipases. However, the majority, probably 90%, is taken up by the type II pneumocytes and recycled into the alveolus as fresh surfactant. The rate of breakdown is increased when breathing pure oxygen, and by overventilation.

Blood gases

Table 13.3 gives average blood gas values for normal full-term and premature babies during the first month of life and includes values obtained from babies less than 1 hour old in whom particular care was taken to avoid asphyxia and early neonatal hypothermia.

Table 13.3 'Normal' blood gas values in the newborn

	PaO_2				$PaCO_2$				H^+			
	kPa	mmHg	kPa	mmHg	kPa	mmHg	kPa	mmHg	nmol/L	pH	nmol/L	pH
15 minutes	11.6	87			3.7	28			48	7.32		
30 minutes	11.4	86			4.3	32			43	7.37		
60 minutes	10.8	81			4.1	31			40	7.40		
1–6 hours	8.0–10.6	60–80	8.0–9.3	60–70	4.7–6	35–45	4.7–6	35–45	46–49	7.31–7.34	42–48	7.32–7.38
6–24 hours	9.3–10.0	70–75	8.0–9.3	60–70	4.4–4.8	33–36	3.6–5.3	27–40	37–43	7.37–7.43	35–45	7.36–7.45
48 hours–1 week	9.3–11.3	70–85	10.0–10.6	75–80	4.4–4.8	33–36	4.3–4.5	32–36	42–44	7.36–7.38	40–48	7.32–7.40
2 weeks					4.8–5.2	36–39	5.1	38	43	7.37	48	7.32
3 weeks					5.3	40	5.1	38	42	7.38	49	7.31
1 month					5.2	39	4.9	37	41	7.39	49	7.31

The values at 15, 30 and 60 minutes are from our own unpublished observations on full-term babies. Data from 1 hour to 1 week are drawn from the literature on arterial samples. Data beyond 1 week are for full-term babies. Values in italics are those for premature babies; those not in italics are for full-term babies.

Measurement of SpO_2 in term babies shows that this is usually >95% by 10 minutes of age with a range from 87% to 99% (Dawson *et al.* 2010).

Oxygen transport

The position of the oxyhaemoglobin dissociation curve is controlled by pH, temperature, the intracellular concentration of 2,3-diphosphatidylglycerol (2,3-DPG), and the interaction between these three factors and the haemoglobin present in the red cells. A decrease in pH and a rise in temperature and 2,3-DPG move the curve to the right, decreasing the affinity for oxygen (more oxygen given up at the same PaO_2). A rise in pH or a fall in body temperature and 2,3-DPG have the reverse effect.

The blood of the neonate has a left-shifted oxyhaemoglobin dissociation curve, owing to the fact that within the cell fetal haemoglobin reacts poorly with 2,3-DPG. The position of the oxyhaemoglobin dissociation curve, and thus the oxygen affinity of whole blood, is expressed as the P_{50}. This is the partial pressure of oxygen at which the haemoglobin molecule is 50% saturated. For adult blood the P_{50} is 27 mmHg, and for fetal blood it is 19.5 mmHg. The fact that the newborn baby's blood has a high affinity for haemoglobin (low P_{50}) makes it more difficult to assess hypoxaemia clinically, since cyanosis occurs at a lower PaO_2 than in the adult. Furthermore, since high-affinity fetal blood is reluctant to release oxygen to the tissues, in pulmonary diseases with hypoxaemia, tissue oxygenation may be more effective if the circulating blood is of adult (i.e. transfusion) origin.

■ Differential diagnosis of neonatal respiratory disease

Respiratory illness starting within 4 hours

Almost all the lung diseases which affect the neonate can develop within the first 4 hours of life; indeed, the development of symptoms before 4 hours of age is an essential diagnostic prerequisite for surfactant-deficient RDS. Differentiating this condition from all the other causes of early neonatal dyspnoea is usually easily done on the basis of a history, simple clinical examination, chest X-ray (CXR) and the fact that most of the other problems usually occur in mature babies (Table 13.4).

The most difficult diagnostic problem at all gestations is differentiating RDS from congenital or intrapartum pneumonia. Furthermore, since these types of pneumonia and surfactant-deficient RDS can co-exist, it is impossible to exclude pulmonary infection as a component of the respiratory distress in any given baby – hence the need to put all breathless neonates on antibiotics. However, the following features greatly increase the likelihood that infection is responsible for some, if not all, the baby's respiratory illness:

- prolonged rupture of the membranes;
- maternal fever;
- positive culture on high vaginal swabs before delivery;
- purulent vaginal discharge;
- offensive liquor.

Clinical signs in the baby suggesting pneumonia rather than RDS are pyrexia or persisting hypothermia, unusual hypotonia, jaundice before 12 hours of age, profound hypoxaemia without hypercapnia, early onset of apnoeic attacks, and persisting hypotension.

Table 13.4 Differential diagnosis of respiratory symptoms and signs in the newborn

Condition	Gestation	History	Examination[a]	Gases[b]	Presentation[c]		Chest X-ray	Comments
					<6 hours	>6 hours		
Respiratory distress syndrome	Preterm				+++	Never	Usually diagnostic, see Fig. 13.6 and 13.7	Working diagnosis in all preterm neonates unless CXR suggests alternative. Always consider infection
Transient tachypnoea of the newborn	Term > preterm	Often CS delivery		Mild hypoxaemia rarely needing >40% FiO_2	+++	Rarely	Diagnostic but see pp. 154–155	Most common cause of breathlessness in term babies. By definition a mild disease
Meconium aspiration	Term[d]	Meconium liquor, post-maturity	Meconium-stained baby		+++	Never	Streaky	Diagnosis usually obvious on history. Infection may co-exist
Pneumothorax or pneumo-mediastinum	Term > preterm	Can be high pressures used at resuscitation			++	Rarely[f]	Diagnostic	
Massive pulmonary haemorrhage	Preterm > term	Asphyxia, heart failure, bleeding tendency. Artificial surfactant	Crepitations, pallor. Blood in endotracheal tube. Often associated with patent ductus		+	+++	Unhelpful; usually a whiteout	Diagnosis based on clinical findings
Post-perinatal hypoxia ischaemia	Term[e]	Birth depression, fetal distress	Other features of hypoxic ischaemic encephalopathy (pp. 220–223)	Metabolic acidaemia with respiratory correction	++	Never	Unhelpful	Respiratory correction of a metabolic acidaemia

Condition	Gestation	History	Examination[a]	Gases[b]	Presentation[c]		Chest X-ray	Comments
					<6 hours	>6 hours		
Infection (pneumonia)	Any	Maternal pyrexia, PROM	Rarely helpful	Often severe acidaemia and easy to reduce $PaCO_2$ without increasing PaO_2	++	+++	Unhelpful in most, may show patchy changes	Impossible to exclude in any baby with respiratory distress. Working diagnosis in the absence of specific chest X-ray findings in babies older than 6 hours
Congenital lung malformation	Term > preterm	Usually normal. May have antenatal USS diagnosis	Rarely helpful	May be profound hypoxaemia with raised CO_2	+++	+	Can be diagnostic	Diaphragmatic hernia, cysts, effusions, agenesis present this way. TOF should not present this way (p. 275)
Congenital heart disease	Term > preterm		Murmurs, heart size, signs of heart failure	CO_2 normal or reduced. In cyanotic CHD PaO_2 rarely > 13.5 kPa even in 100% oxygen with IPPV	Rarely	+++	May be helpful or diagnostic	The alternative common diagnosis in babies presenting after 6 hours of age, and particularly after 24 hours. Echocardiogram usually diagnostic
Pulmonary hypoplasia	Any	Prolonged rupture of membranes	Potter's facies Dwarfed	Profound hypoxaemia and hypercapnia	+++	Never	Diagnostic, very small lungs	Virtually always rapidly fatal
Persistent pulmonary hypertension	Term > preterm	May have had antenatal hypoxia	May hear murmur of tricuspid incompetence	Marked hypoxaemia with normal or reduced CO_2	+++	+	Usually normal or nearly normal	Can be difficult to exclude CHD unless echocardiogram available

(continued)

Table 13.4 *(Continued)*

Condition	Gestation	History	Examination[a]	Gases[b]	Presentation[c]		Chest X-ray	Comments
					<6 hours	>6 hours		
Inhalation of feed	Any	Usually obvious			Rarely	+++	Unhelpful	Should not happen; normal term babies rarely inhale, so seek alternative diagnosis such as infection
Inborn error of metabolism	Term > preterm	May be positive FH or FH of unexplained neonatal deaths	No evidence of lung disease. Tachypnoea driven by acidaemia	Severe metabolic acidaemia, with respiratory correction; low $PaCO_2$	Rarely	+++	Often normal	Diagnosis based on blood changes, plus ketonaemia in many cases
Primary neurological disease	Term > preterm	May be positive FH or FH of unexplained neonatal deaths. Polyhydramnios	Hypotonia. Areflexia, myopathic facies, deformities. No lung disease	Gases normal, unless apnoeic	++	++	Often normal	Usually easy to identify as a group
Upper airway obstruction	Term > preterm	May be typical in choanal atresia	Stridor. Problems resolve on intubation. Laryngoscopy may be diagnostic	Gases normal when intubated; $PaCO_2$ raised beforehand	++	++	Often normal	

CHD, congenital heart disease; CS, caesarean section; CXR, chest X-ray; FH, family history; IPPV, intermittent positive pressure ventilation; PROM, premature rupture of membranes; TOF, tracheo-oesophageal fistula; USS, ultrasound scan.

[a] Mentioning features other than cardinal features of respiratory disease (p. 130).

[b] Most conditions cause hypoxaemia and hypercarbia; only if the blood gas patterns differ from this is it noted here.

[c] Frequency of presentation graded + to +++; rarely and never.

[d] If preterm consider *Listeria*.

[e] Severely asphyxiated premature babies get respiratory distress syndrome.

[f] Usually a complication of preexisting severe lung disease, especially hyaline membrane disease.

A low white blood cell (WBC) count (total $<6 \times 10^9/l$) with neutrophils below $2 \times 10^9/L$ is very suggestive of infection within the first 24 hours. Other laboratory tests are rarely helpful. C-reactive protein (CRP) takes several hours to rise and gram stain of various secretions or gastric aspirate is a poor discriminator. Group B beta-haemolytic *Streptococcus* (GBS) antigen detection tests have a high false-positive rate.

Differentiating RDS from cyanotic CHD in the first few hours of life is less difficult now that echocardiography is readily available. The types of CHD presenting so early in life usually produce abnormal physical findings, an abnormal electrocardiogram, and a very large heart and either very oligaemic or hyperaemic lung fields on CXR. Differentiating PPHN from RDS is rarely a problem and may be purely semantic since pulmonary hypertension is common in babies with severe RDS. Differentiating isolated PPHN (p. 162) from cyanotic CHD or ascertaining whether a baby who undoubtedly has surfactant-deficient RDS also has co-existing CHD (cyanotic or otherwise) requires echocardiography.

Respiratory illness starting de novo after 4 hours

In essence there are only five possibilities:

1 pneumonia – bacterial and viral;
2 CHD with pulmonary oedema;
3 congenital malformation;
4 the dyspnoea of acidaemia due to underlying metabolic disease;
5 rare, late-onset lung disease of the very low birth weight (VLBW) baby (e.g. Wilson–Mikity, pp. 178–179; chronic pulmonary insufficiency of prematurity).

Differentiating these conditions rarely poses any problems, since typical clinical, radiological or electrocardiogram (ECG) changes are virtually always present.

■ Respiratory distress syndrome; hyaline membrane disease

Key points

- Respiratory distress syndrome (RDS) is due to surfactant deficiency as a result of prematurity and/or asphyxial lung damage.
- All women with threatened preterm delivery between 23 and 34 weeks of gestation should be considered for antenatal steroids, which reduce the risk of RDS.
- The treatment of RDS involves respiratory, surfactant and intensive care support.
- Preterm babies of less than 28 weeks' gestation should receive surfactant as soon as possible after birth (prophylaxis). Other babies should be given surfactant if they require ventilation and the diagnosis of RDS is confirmed (rescue treatment).
- The choice of surfactant preparation is largely a matter of individual preference. The rapid mode of action of natural surfactants means that good monitoring is essential, particularly to avoid hypocarbia.
- All babies at risk of RDS should be closely monitored for evidence of respiratory failure.
- Artificial ventilation should be instituted early if the blood gases deteriorate or the baby has persistent apnoeic attacks, and continued from birth in babies intubated for resuscitation.

- Randomized trials comparing different levels of blood gas control in RDS have not been done. There is general consensus that ventilation should be adjusted to maintain the following:
  - pH above 7.25;
  - PaO_2 in the range 6–10 kPa (45–75 mmHg);
  - $PaCO_2$ in the range 5–7.5 kPa (37.5–56.0 mmHg). Upper limit depends on pH.
- Successful treatment of RDS requires careful monitoring of blood gases, electrolyte levels and blood glucose concentrations in addition to monitoring of body weight, heart rate, respiration and blood pressure. Total parenteral nutrition is required in very preterm babies.
- Failure to respond to surfactant is rare, and advice from an experienced neonatologist should be sought if a baby remains in >60% oxygen and requires high peak ventilator pressures (>26 cmH$_2$O) after two doses of surfactant.
- Steroid therapy has been shown to reduce the duration of mechanical ventilation, but in view of possible adverse effects this treatment should be considered only for babies who remain ventilator dependent in significant amounts of oxygen after 2 weeks of age.

Aetiology

Four factors are important in the aetiology of surfactant-deficient RDS:

1 prematurity;
2 perinatal asphyxia;
3 maternal diabetes;
4 caesarean section.

Prematurity

Since surfactant does not appear in the lungs until the second trimester, and not in large amounts until the third trimester, gestational age is the major determinant of RDS (Fig. 13.5). However, not all premature babies will develop the disease and it can occur at term.

Perinatal asphyxia

Asphyxia predisposes to RDS in various ways. Hypoxaemia and acidaemia reduce surfactant synthesis, and the asphyxiated preterm baby may have such feeble respiratory efforts that he cannot release what surfactant he does possess from the pneumonocytes. Much more important, however, is the fact that asphyxia damages the pulmonary vasculature, allowing protein-rich fluid to leak out onto the alveolar surface where it inhibits surfactant activity. In term babies with surplus surfactant this is of no consequence, but in preterm babies with small surfactant reserves it results in lungs that are rapidly rendered surfactant deficient and thus non-compliant and atelectatic.

The association between asphyxia and RDS has major clinical implications. With premature babies every effort must be made to avoid asphyxia during labour, using cardiotocogram (CTG) and pH measurements, and delivering by caesarean section if there is evidence of fetal compromise. The prognosis for such babies is also improved if they are promptly and vigorously resuscitated after birth by intermittent positive pressure ventilation (IPPV) to establish FRC, release surfactant and control the baby's oxygenation and acid–base status, enabling the normal postnatal fall in pulmonary artery pressure to occur.

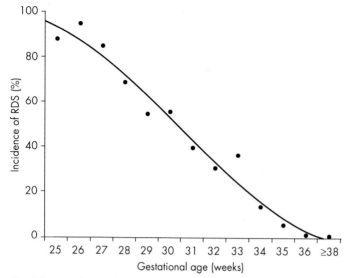

Fig. 13.5 Incidence of respiratory distress syndrome (RDS) at different gestations. From Stevens and Sinkin (2007). Reproduced with permission from the American College of Chest Physicians

Maternal diabetes

Maternal diabetes is associated with an increased incidence of RDS. In part, this is due to elective, prelabour delivery by caesarean section, but it is also due to delay in surfactant maturation, in particular the appearance of phosphatidylglycerol. In recent years, with first-class antenatal control of maternal diabetes allowing delivery to be delayed until 38–40 weeks' gestation, RDS is less often seen in this situation.

Caesarean section

Caesarean section carried out before labour in women beyond 32 weeks' gestation is associated with an increased incidence of both RDS and transient tachypnoea of the newborn (TTN) in the babies, presumably because they have been denied the β-adrenergic-mediated surfactant release and reduction in fetal lung liquid which occurs in the 24–48 hours before spontaneous labour. However, in babies of less than 32 weeks' gestation caesarean section has minimal effect on the incidence of RDS, and anxieties on this score should not influence the decision whether or not a very preterm baby should be delivered vaginally or by caesarean section.

Prevention of respiratory distress syndrome

Avoiding the four problems listed above will help to reduce the incidence of RDS, and of these the most important are the prevention of prematurity and asphyxia. However, there are other ways in which the incidence and the severity of neonatal RDS may be reduced: the administration of steroids antenatally to the mother, and the prophylactic administration of surfactant to the baby at resuscitation, and, ideally, both.

Antenatal steroids

It is now recognized that giving these drugs antenatally has many beneficial effects (Table 13.5) in addition to influencing surfactant synthesis.

Table 13.5 Benefits of antenatal steroids

Improved Apgar scores
Maturation of lung structure
Initiation of surfactant apoprotein synthesis
Improved nitric oxide-mediated pulmonary venous relaxation
Reduced pulmonary capillary leakiness
Interaction with postnatal exogenous surfactant therapy
Increased resistance to high oxygen exposure
Higher blood pressure in the neonatal period
Higher neonatal white cell counts
Less patent ductus arteriosus
Less germinal matrix–intraventricular haemorrhage
Less necrotizing enterocolitis
Less disability in the survivors

An overview of the results of 18 trials enrolling more than 3700 babies provides clear evidence that corticosteroids reduced the risk of RDS, with a typical odds ratio for RDS of 0.35 (95% confidence interval (CI) 0.26–0.45) and for death from RDS of 0.6 (95% CI 0.48–0.76) (Crowley 1997). The greatest benefit against RDS is seen when the time interval between the start of treatment and delivery is more than 48 hours and less than 7 days. The Royal College of Obstetricians and Gynaecologists in the UK recommended that two doses of betamethasone should be given 24 hours apart or four doses of dexamethasone 12 hours apart. Betamethasone is preferred as it has been associated with lower rates of periventricular leukomalacia (PVL). The value of repeated courses is doubtful. Antenatal betamethasone should be considered for all women who threaten to deliver at less than 34 weeks.

Prophylactic surfactant

See pp. 137–138.

Clinical signs of respiratory distress syndrome

RDS presents within 4 hours of birth with:

- sternal retraction, intercostal and subcostal recession;
- an expiratory grunt;
- tachypnoea above 60 breaths/min.

Babies with these signs are said to have respiratory distress. There are many other causes of respiratory distress presenting by 4 hours of age (Table 13.4), but these can usually be excluded comparatively easily on the basis of history, clinical signs and CXR (Figs 13.6 and 13.7). The baby can then be diagnosed as having 'respiratory distress syndrome', with the implication that the lungs are surfactant-depleted. If the lungs were examined histologically they would show hyaline membrane disease (HMD). If one is being semantic, the term HMD should be used only if there is histological proof of the diagnosis.

Since respiratory distress may be transient, the definition of RDS usually includes some statement about the duration of symptoms. However, common to all definitions of the disease is that the signs should be present *before* 4 hours of age, should still be there *at* 4 hours of age, and should persist for some period *beyond* 4 hours of age.

Without supplementary inspired oxygen, the baby is cyanosed (cyanosis is not a sign of RDS but a sign of a baby where the treatment of the RDS is out of control). Listening to the lungs reveals that the air entry is reduced and there may be a few crepitations. The baby is inactive, tends to lie in the frog position, and often has moderate generalized subcutaneous oedema owing to increased capillary leakiness and delayed onset of the normal postnatal diuresis. Babies with RDS pass only small amounts of urine, have an ileus, and may not pass meconium until the third or fourth day of life.

Natural history of respiratory distress syndrome

In uncomplicated RDS, surfactant begins to reappear in the lungs (and laryngeal aspirate) at about 36–48 hours of age. The illness therefore gradually gets worse over the first 24–36 hours as the baby tires. His condition then stabilizes for 24 hours and from 60–72 hours of age he steadily improves. By the end of the first week he has usually recovered.

Histopathology

The earliest histological changes in RDS are interstitial oedema and congestion of the alveolar walls leading to desquamation of the type II alveolar epithelial cells. The alveolar ducts dilate, but the alveoli become atelectatic because of the surfactant deficiency. There is exudation of plasma into the alveoli and airways, and this further compromises surfactant function. The proteins in this exudate coagulate to form the characteristic hyaline membranes which line the respiratory bronchioles and alveolar ducts.

Radiology

There is a reticulogranular pattern due to the atelectasis, and the air-filled major airways stand out as radiolucent areas – the so-called 'air bronchogram' (Fig. 13.6). In severe cases the lungs cannot be clearly separated from the cardiac border (Fig. 13.7). To some extent the severity of the X-ray changes reflects the severity of the disease; but if assisted ventilation or continuous positive airways pressure (CPAP) is being used or surfactant has been given, atelectasis is reduced and the CXR changes may look surprisingly mild.

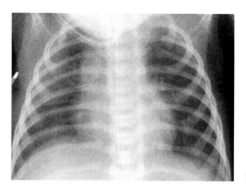

Fig. 13.6 Mild respiratory distress syndrome

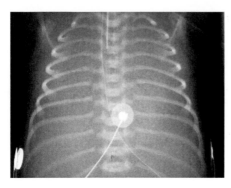

Fig. 13.7 Severe respiratory distress syndrome 'whiteout'

Pathophysiology of respiratory distress syndrome

Once the baby's lungs become depleted of surfactant, the alveoli collapse and the lungs become very stiff. This causes the following changes in pulmonary physiology (Table 13.6):

- lung compliance falls to about 25% of normal; there is a decreased FRC, TGV, crying V_C, and an increased dead space and dead-space/tidal-volume ratio, with a comparatively normal R_{AW};
- an increased work of breathing;
- increased intrapulmonary shunting (pp. 118–119) and severe hypoxaemia;
- hypoventilation, causing a respiratory acidaemia.

Many of the other features of RDS are secondary to hypoxaemia. They include:

- pulmonary artery and right heart pressure at or above fetal level (pulmonary hypertension), facilitating right-to-left shunts through the ductus arteriosus and the foramen ovale;
- vascular damage, causing transudation of fluid onto the alveolar surface (p. 115) and into the subcutaneous tissues;

Table 13.6 Respiratory function tests in babies with respiratory distress syndrome (RDS)

	Normal	RDS
Compliance (mL/cmH$_2$O)	5–6	<1.0
Airway resistance (cmH$_2$O/L/s)	40–45 (total)	55–95 (inspiratory) 140–200 (expiratory)
FRC (mL/kg)	30	5–20
V_T (mL/kg)	5–7	3–7
V_E (mL/kg/min)	200	250–350
V_A (mL/kg/min)	150	50–90
V_C (mL/kg)	35–40	20–25
V_D/V_T	0.3	0.55–0.6
Work of breathing (g.cm/kg/min)	500	2500–3500

FRC, functional residual capacity; V_A, alveolar ventilation per minute; V_D, dead space; V_E, minute volume; V_T, total volume.

- hypotension – the baby may have a low blood volume dating from the time of delivery and as a result of the capillary leak; in addition, hypoxaemia depresses the myocardium and prevents peripheral vascular responsiveness. Acidaemia has similar effects;
- severe metabolic acidaemia, partly the aftermath of birth asphyxia and also from lactic acid accumulation during the anaerobic glycolysis of hypoxaemia. The lactic acidaemia and hypoxaemia are also aggravated by the hypotension so that a vicious cycle develops which perpetuates surfactant deficiency pp. 133–138;
- decreased perfusion and/or oxygenation of other tissues, impairing their function, e.g.
  - the kidney – poor water and $(H)^+$ excretion;
  - the gut – ileus and mucosal injury with necrotizing enterocolitis (NEC) (pp. 278–283);
  - the CNS – intracranial haemorrhage (pp. 226–230).

Investigation of respiratory distress syndrome

Within an hour of admission basic investigations should be requested on all babies suspected of having RDS. This is both to confirm the diagnosis and to exclude other possibilities, as well as establishing baseline values for monitoring the progress of disease (Chapter 7). These investigations include:

- haemoglobin, WBC count and platelets (?need to transfuse or ?evidence for infection);
- electrolytes, creatinine, calcium (establishing baseline);
- blood gases (initiating treatment);
- group and crossmatch (in preparation for transfusion);
- deep ear and throat swabs (?infection);
- blood culture (?infection);
- CXR (diagnostic and noting the position of an umbilical artery catheter (UAC), ETT).

There is normally no need to do a lumbar puncture and babies with respiratory disease tolerate the procedure poorly (pp. 363–364). Subsequent investigation is described under monitoring.

■ Treatment of respiratory distress syndrome

The aim of treatment is to keep the baby alive and in good condition until he starts to synthesize his own surfactant 36–48 hours after birth. This means avoiding hypoxaemia, acidaemia and hypothermia, which inhibit surfactant synthesis, and achieving complete control of the baby's cardiorespiratory, electrolyte and renal homeostasis. In addition, the baby should receive synthetic surfactant to tide him over until endogenous synthesis is effective (pp. 137–138).

Monitoring

See Chapter 7 for more information on intensive care monitoring techniques. The following should be monitored continuously in all babies with RDS:

1. ECG.
2. PaO_2: we use intermittent arterial gases backed up by continuous transcutaneous oxygen tension ($TcPO_2$) and oximetry (SpO_2) (pp. 58–59). The last two are not suitable for monitoring of arterial oxygen tension alone because they cannot reliably detect hyperoxaemia.
3. Blood pressure, ideally from the arterial catheter.
4. Respiratory activity/apnoea monitor.

The following should be monitored 3–4 hourly and more frequently if necessary:

1. Temperature, pulse, respiratory rate.
2. $PaCO_2$, arterial pH and base deficit; glucose.

The following investigations should also be carried out routinely:

1. Packed cell volume (PCV)/full blood count, electrolytes, calcium and albumin daily or twice daily.
2. CXR daily or every other day in the acute phase.

Temperature control

Essentially, keep the baby in the environmental temperatures appropriate for his weight. If the baby stays cold, carry out the procedures suggested on pp. 52–53.

Acid–base homeostasis

It is important to keep the baby's H^+ below 65 nmol/L (pH >7.25), since surfactant synthesis is inhibited below this value. Furthermore, at somewhat lower pH values, body functions such as cardiac output are impaired. Acidaemia has an effect on the oxygen dissociation curve, too.

Metabolic acidaemia

A base deficit of more than 5 mmol/L indicates a metabolic acidaemia. There has been much argument about whether correction of metabolic acidaemia is more dangerous than the persisting acidaemia. There can be no doubt that overenthusiastic correction of metabolic acidaemia is harmful. Rapid infusions of hypertonic base cause big surges in the intravascular volume, which may lead to intracranial haemorrhage, and sodium bicarbonate can cause hypernatraemia. In general, it is better to find and treat the cause rather than to give base.

The most important reaction to the presence of a metabolic acidaemia is not how to treat it but to find out why it developed. Is it due to the baby developing some complication such as hypotension, hypoxaemia, sepsis, anaemia or a metabolic error? Babies given early total parenteral nutrition tend to develop a hyperchloraemic acidaemia, which can be reduced by replacing some of the sodium chloride with sodium acetate. The obvious solution to the arguments about whether or not to correct metabolic acidaemia is to prevent these complications occurring. If this is done, metabolic acidaemia will be rare except in the immediate post-birth asphyxia period, or following episodes of sudden collapse such as a blocked ETT or a tension pneumothorax.

Base therapy should be considered in all babies whose base deficit exceeds 10 mmol/L. If the baby is stable, well perfused, normotensive, mature and the degree of acidaemia is between 5 and 10 mmol/L, spontaneous correction is common, and it is reasonable to withhold therapy and measure the base deficit again after 2–3 hours. In sick babies, particularly those of less than 32 weeks' gestation, base deficits above 10 mmol/L should probably be corrected. Sodium bicarbonate should usually be used and the rate of infusion should never exceed 0.5 mmol bicarbonate/min:

$$\text{Dose in mmol of sodium bicarbonate} = \text{base deficit (mmol/L)} \times \text{body weight (kg)} \times 0.4$$

(8.4% sodium bicarbonate contains 1 mmol of bicarbonate/mL). This calculated dosage will always undercorrect the acidaemia, and the blood gases should always be checked within an hour, or sooner if the baby's condition does not improve. Despite the fact that many babies have a co-existing respiratory acidaemia, the infusion of bicarbonate to correct metabolic acidaemia rarely causes a rise in $PaCO_2$ of more than 0.6–1.3 kPa (5–10 mmHg).

Metabolic alkalaemia

This may be seen following excessive use of bicarbonate but is also seen in babies with severe chronic lung disease (CLD) who have CO_2 retention and chloride depletion due to vigorous diuretic therapy.

Respiratory acidaemia and alkalaemia

A respiratory alkalaemia, i.e. a $PaCO_2$ below 4 kPa (30 mmHg), may occur if hyperventilation is stimulated by acidaemia. However, it is commonly iatrogenic, due to overvigorous IPPV. It must be avoided, since preterm babies with $PaCO_2$ values below 3 kPa (approximately 20 mmHg) have an increased incidence of PVL (pp. 230–231). An induced hypocarbic alkalaemia was formerly often used in the treatment of term babies with PPHN (p. 162); now that nitric oxide has become more widely available, overventilation, with its attendant risks, is not necessary. Liberal administration of base should be used to keep the pH at normal levels in PPHN.

$PaCO_2$ is raised (respiratory acidaemia) in all but the mildest cases of RDS and may reach 13.3 kPa (100 mmHg) or more if untreated. Cerebral blood flow increases by about 10% for each rise of 1 kPa in $PaCO_2$. Because of the role of increased cerebral blood flow in the aetiology of germinal matrix–intraventricular haemorrhage (GMH-IVH) (pp. 226–230), it is prudent to keep the $PaCO_2$ below 7.0–7.5 kPa (52.5–56.0 mmHg) in very preterm babies at risk from this complication.

$PaCO_2$ measurements in RDS are of value in the following situations:

1. A steadily rising $PaCO_2$ at any stage in the disease is an indication that ventilatory assistance is likely to be needed or that the ventilator settings are not achieving adequate gas exchange.
2. A sudden rise in $PaCO_2$ may be an indication of acute changes in the baby's condition, e.g. pneumothorax, collapsed lobes, misplaced ETT.
3. A swift rise in $PaCO_2$ (often accompanied by hypoxaemia) during an attempt to wean a baby off IPPV or CPAP indicates that the time was not appropriate for that change in therapy.
4. A gradual rise in $PaCO_2$ at the end of the first week in a low birth weight baby on a ventilator who has previously been stable may herald the development of a patent ductus arteriosus (PDA) (p. 296) or CLD (Chapter 14).

Fluid and electrolyte balance

See also Chapter 10.

Great care must be taken to prevent excessive fluid administration in babies with RDS since:

■ in the presence of hypoalbuminaemia and increased capillary leakiness, excessive fluid intake may aggravate interstitial pulmonary oedema and worsen the hypoxaemia;
■ fluid overload predisposes the baby to complications of RDS, including PDA, NEC and CLD.

For these reasons use fluid restriction, aiming to give insensible losses plus urine output only, with no added sodium. A good starting point is to give 60 mL/kg/24 h in the first 24 hours, although extremely preterm babies will certainly need more than this owing to high insensible losses. Thereafter fluid intake should be guided by the principles laid down in Chapter 10. However, since fluid overload is damaging, be prepared to keep the intake to 50–60 mL/kg/24 h for several days if the baby is oedematous, oliguric and not losing weight. Muscle-relaxing agents often aggravate problems with oedema and fluid retention.

Sick babies are very prone to both hypernatraemia and hyperkalaemia in the first few days. Controlling sodium and potassium balance is described on pp. 86–88.

Hypocalcaemia is also common in the first 48 hours of life, with levels at or below 1.5 mmol/L. The baby's plasma calcium can be kept within the normal range by adding 5–10 mL of 10% calcium gluconate every 24 hours to the infusion fluid. This can usually be discontinued by 5–6 days of age.

Premature babies are often hypoalbuminaemic, since they have low levels at birth, and liver synthesis may be compromised if they are very ill. There is a poor correlation between serum albumin and oedema in babies. Evidence suggests that albumin may have detrimental effects when given to older children and adults in intensive care units; as yet there are very few data specific to the newborn but frequent infusions of albumin are best avoided. If hypovolaemia is suspected, saline will increase the circulating volume. Infusion of albumin to correct hypoalbuminaemia is not helpful when the baby still has leaky capillaries.

In the first 24–48 hours most babies with severe RDS are oliguric. Recovery from RDS is heralded by a spontaneous diuresis and resolution of subcutaneous and pulmonary oedema. Diuretic treatment has not been shown to hasten this process when used routinely in RDS. However, confronted by a profoundly hypoxaemic oedematous oliguric preterm baby with severe RDS, no harm can come from a trial of furosemide (2 mg/kg), which can be repeated if there is a diuresis and improvement in the baby's blood gases.

Blood volume and blood pressure

In ill babies, blood pressure (BP) is most easily and safely monitored with a direct recording of arterial BP from an indwelling cannula. Normal values are given in Appendix 3. Babies with severe RDS are often hypotensive in the first few hours of life. In some cases the hypotension is due to hypovolaemia, in others it is due to depression of cardiac and vascular function by severe metabolic disturbance and hypoxaemia. Whatever the cause, hypotension must be corrected as a matter of urgency in sick infants, particularly if there is reduced capillary filling, raised lactate and oliguria. There is no universally agreed definition of neonatal hypotension, which in any case relates to gestational age. A good general rule is to aim to keep the mean BP above the baby's gestational age in weeks, with the systolic pressure being at least 10 mmHg higher than this. If the hypotensive baby's PCV is less than 40%, he should be given a blood transfusion; but if his haematocrit is at least 45%, normal saline (0.9%) should be used, otherwise polycythaemia may develop.

Initially give 15 mL/kg of saline or blood; larger transfusions than this should be given only if there is clear evidence that the hypotension is hypovolaemic (i.e. no signs of heart failure, but persisting anaemia and low central venous pressure). If hypotension persists in the absence of signs of hypovolaemia, the correct treatment is to give inotropic support.

The two inotropes most widely used are dopamine and dobutamine. Dopamine at doses of <8–10 μg/kg/min has a direct inotropic β-adrenergic effect on the heart, while at the same time causing renal vasodilatation by dopaminergic mechanisms.

Because of its beneficial effect on renal blood flow, dopamine is widely used in the first 24–48 hours in babies with severe RDS, even in those whose hypotension is only borderline. Clear evidence that this is beneficial is lacking.

Dobutamine has primarily a β-adrenergic inotropic effect on the myocardium. It has few peripheral actions and no specific effects on the renal vasculature. If the BP is not adequate after volume replacement and dopamine up to 15 μg/kg/min, give dobutamine up to 20 μg/kg/min. If after volume replacement, dopamine and dobutamine a VLBW baby remains hypotensive, the prognosis is poor.

Other inotropes including isoprenaline and adrenaline (epinephrine) can be tried. In refractory hypotension hydrocortisone 2.5 mg/kg 6 hourly for 48 hours can be tried, the dose being tailed off subsequently. Remember to ask about maternal labetalol therapy; this can cause persistent neonatal hypotension.

Blood loss into the laboratory

Chronic iatrogenic hypovolaemia, anaemia and hypotension are caused by the frequent blood sampling of intensive care. Some neonatal units note all blood sampled (blood log) and transfuse when 10% of the blood volume has been removed. Others wait until the PCV is below 40% or the baby becomes hypotensive before transfusing. Whichever method is used, small sick babies may require several top-up transfusions of 10–15 mL/kg of blood. Donor exposure can be reduced by using blood prepared as pedi-packs, where a single unit is divided into up to eight small satellite bags. This system is now widely used, with no harm resulting from the use of older blood for top-up transfusions (see p. 311 for more detail regarding blood transfusions).

Drug therapy in respiratory distress syndrome

In general, the only drug of value in the management of RDS is exogenous surfactant. Other drugs may be used (Table 13.7) and antibiotic therapy is routine.

Surfactant therapy

Exogenous surfactant has made a dramatic impact on the incidence and severity of RDS. Surfactant is even more effective when combined with antenatal steroids; the treatments have synergistic effects. Surfactant reduces the neonatal mortality from RDS by about 40% and reduces air leaks by up to 60%, with beneficial effects on IVH (Morley 1997; Soll 2009).

Table 13.7 Drugs occasionally required in babies with respiratory distress syndrome

General indication	Drugs available
Analgesia for intubation, chest drains, infusions	Morphine, fentanyl, paracetamol
To assist intubation and ventilation	Pancuronium, vecuronium, atracurium; atracurium/suxamethoniunfor intubation
Treatment of patent ductus arteriosus	Indometacin
To assist extubation	Hydrocortisone, caffeine
To treat pulmonary hypertension	Nitric oxide, prostacyclin, magnesium sulphate, tolazoline
To treat hypotension	Dopamine, dobutamine, adrenaline, hydrocortisone
To correct acidaemia	Bicarbonate

Recent meta-analyses favour prophylactic natural surfactant. Our current practice is to give prophylactic natural surfactant to babies of less than 30 weeks' gestation who require intubation for resuscitation. In more mature babies, surfactant should be given as rescue therapy as soon as the baby is intubated. If, after prophylactic therapy in the labour ward, the baby continues to have significant RDS, we give a further dose at 12 hours. Two doses are better than a single dose and, if the baby remains very ill, further doses, up to a maximum of four, can be given.

Oxygen therapy

This is the most complex, important and difficult part of the treatment of RDS. In general, we aim to keep the PaO_2 in the range 6.0–10.0 kPa (45–75 mmHg). The lower limit is chosen to allow some leeway before the PaO_2 falls to the dangerously hypoxic levels at which acidaemia develops, the ductus arteriosus opens and surfactant synthesis decreases. The upper limit is chosen to minimize the risk of retinopathy of prematurity (ROP) (pp. 332–335). Although this aim appears simple, it is difficult to achieve because in addition to the severe lung disease there are clinical problems, most of which are unique to the neonate.

The different methods of oxygen monitoring and the target saturations are described in Chapter 7.

Oxygen administration by nasal cannulae

For babies on long-term oxygen, typically those with CLD, O_2 can be administered by nasal cannulae. These allow the baby to sit up, bottle feed and play while still receiving O_2. An estimate of the oxygen concentration received is given in Fig. 13.8.

High-flow nasal cannula (HFNC) oxygen using specifically designed systems that humidify the oxygen is now used in some centres as an alternative to CPAP. It has the potential to reduce nose trauma associated with CPAP. It is essential that such systems do not obstruct the nares, using appropriately sized nasal cannulae to prevent excessive pressure delivery to the infant's airway and lung overexpansion. The mechanisms of action are not completely understood but it has been suggested that such systems may either deliver low levels of CPAP or 'flush' the anatomical dead space with oxygen. Randomized trials with long-term outcomes are required to determine whether HFNC is more or less efficacious than CPAP.

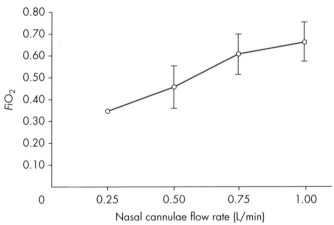

Fig. 13.8 Hypopharyngeal oxygen concentration (PhO_2) at different nasal cannulae oxygen flows. From Vain *et al.* (1989) with permission

Continuous positive airways pressure

Arguing teleologically, the grunt in RDS is a marker of the sudden opening of the glottis which had been held closed in an attempt to increase intrapulmonary pressure, blow open collapsed alveoli, reduce the atelectasis and the size of the right-to-left shunt, and thus improve oxygenation. CPAP attempts to mimic this effect on the baby's lungs by splinting the alveoli open with applied pressures of up to 8–10 cmH_2O. Furthermore, splinting the alveoli open and reducing the shearing forces in them helps to preserve alveolar surfactant.

Lung function

The effects of CPAP on lung function are surprising. The FRC increases, respiration becomes regular, though the rate may increase or decrease, and the airways resistance falls. However, compliance, minute volume and tidal volume all fall, and the work of breathing may actually increase owing to the effort required to overcome the resistance of the ETT or the nasal prongs used to administer CPAP. Despite this the A–aDO$_2$, V/Q ratio and right–left shunt all usually improve, and most important of all the PaO_2 usually rises. The $PaCO_2$ rarely rises unless pressures greater than 10 cmH_2O are used.

Cardiovascular effects

In normal babies, 50% of the applied CPAP reaches an oesophageal pressure balloon, whereas in babies with RDS, less than 30% of the pressure is transmitted. In babies with RDS, the central venous pressure rises by 10–20% during the application of CPAP and the pulse pressure falls slightly.

Techniques for giving continuous positive airways pressure

Although CPAP can be delivered by ETT, double nasal prongs are now the most widely used and safest technique for administering CPAP. Nasal masks are also in common use and may be valuable to provide a 'rest' for the nose from prongs. Various devices can be used to provide CPAP. The simplest is to use an underwater seal which provides a bubble CPAP system; most ventilators will have a CPAP mode. Commonly in the UK specifically designed CPAP devices are used which may produce either single or bi-level pressure. During bi-level CPAP two alternating levels of CPAP are delivered which can be syncronized with the baby's respiratory effort. Theoretically this may recruit unstable alveoli, and the delta pressure generates a tidal volume, potentially reducing respiratory work.

Complications of using prong CPAP include:

1. nasal trauma leading to nostril deformity;
2. feeding problems because the gas flow distends the stomach;
3. pneumothorax;
4. failure, with a need for IPPV.

Many of these complications can be avoided by careful nursing and by inserting an open-ended nasogastric tube to drain gas out of the stomach. CPAP should not be undertaken in units without facilities for the rapid recognition and treatment of pneumothorax, or the ability to give IPPV. A major drawback of CPAP is that, since the baby is not intubated, surfactant cannot be given. The proven benefits of prophylactic surfactant therapy place significant constraint on the early sole use of CPAP in babies with RDS.

Indications for using CPAP in babies include:

1. PaO_2 <8 kPa (60 mmHg) in >40% oxygen;
2. recurrent apnoea with or without RDS;
3. mild hypercapnia or mild hypoxaemia in infants who have recently been extubated.

CPAP is of no benefit in infection or meconium aspiration.

The earlier CPAP is started in babies with RDS, the more effective it is. Various groups have reported remarkable success with early CPAP and a 'mini-touch' technique. However, if CPAP is required within 1–2 hours after birth in a baby less than 27 weeks' gestation, such a baby should be treated with surfactant. This can be done using the INSURE technique (intubation–surfactant treatment–extubation). The evidence in favour of prophylactic surfactant is such that we strongly recommend elective intubation in the delivery suite for babies of 27 weeks or less, who should then be given surfactant and transported, still ventilated, to the neonatal unit for further assessment. Many larger babies tolerate CPAP badly, thrashing around in irritation when prongs are shoved up their noses. The main early indication for CPAP is to keep the lungs stable and expanded in babies with mild RDS or TTN who need >40% oxygen in the first 24 hours of life. Early CPAP (from the delivery room) aids recruitment of FRC and has been shown to be of benefit in the management of very preterm babies.

The management of babies on continuous positive airways pressure

Babies on CPAP require all the biochemical and physiological monitoring described in Chapter 7.

Initially 5–6 cmH_2O CPAP should be applied. It is very difficult to get CPAP pressures higher than 8 cmH_2O using nasal prongs. Once the baby's condition improves, CPAP should be weaned. There are theoretically three ways of weaning off CPAP. The first is to gradually reduce the CPAP pressure by 1–2 cmH_2O at a time. Second, CPAP can be stopped using trial periods (initially 1 hour) off CPAP twice a day. This time can then gradually be increased until the baby no longer requires CPAP. Finally, at a point where a baby is thought to no longer require CPAP, it can be stopped. This latter strategy has been shown to reduce the time on CPAP compared with weaning strategies.

■ Mechanical ventilation: intermittent positive pressure ventilation

The indications for starting IPPV in RDS are:

1. sudden deterioration with apnoea or irregular gasping respirations;
2. failure to establish satisfactory respiration after resuscitation in the labour ward (preterm babies who are intubated for resuscitation and given prophylactic surfactant are best continued on artificial ventilation from birth);
3. deteriorating blood gases.

The third category is the most difficult to define. The criteria outlined here are those for babies in the first 24–48 hours of life who are suffering from RDS and are usually deteriorating. For babies with CLD (Chapter 14), a relative hypoxaemia and quite

Acute disorders of the respiratory tract

marked hypercapnia are acceptable and safe prices to pay for not putting the baby back on the ventilator. The same blood gases would be an indication for starting ventilation in a baby with acute RDS.

Watching for a deteriorating trend is the key to avoiding a situation where the baby collapses with hypoxaemia, which is difficult to reverse. This means frequent blood gases taken from a reliable source, ideally an indwelling arterial line. Optimal care for a baby with RDS involves anticipating the need for artificial ventilation well before a disaster arises.

In general, PaO_2 values should be kept above 5.5–6.0 kPa (40–45 mmHg). If a VLBW baby cannot reliably maintain a PaO_2 above 5.5 kPa in 40–45% oxygen in the first few hours, he should be intubated and ventilated and given surfactant. In bigger and more mature babies, IPPV should be considered if more than 60% O_2 is needed to keep the PaO_2 >5.5 kPa (40 mmHg). Tight control of the $PaCO_2$ is also important. There is a clear link between hypercarbia and GMH-IVH, mediated via an increased cerebral blood flow. Low $PaCO_2$ has been associated with PVL, and levels below 3 kPa (20 mmHg) must be avoided. We aim to keep the $PaCO_2$ between 5 and 7.5 kPa (37–56 mmHg) in the first 48 hours in VLBW babies, and the $PaCO_2$ should not be allowed to rise above 8 kPa (60 mmHg) until these babies are more than 72 hours of age. In bigger babies, the rate of rise of $PaCO_2$ and the baby's overall condition should be considered before starting IPPV on the basis of a raised $PaCO_2$ alone. Hypercarbia associated with a pH <7.2 is an indication for ventilation.

Intubation (see pp. 358–359)

1. Awake intubation is painful and associated with a stress response which is detrimental to the baby. We use fentanyl 2–5 µg/kg, atropine 10 µg/kg and suxamethonium 1 mg/kg. Alternatives are 50–100 µg/kg of morphine and 0.5 mg/kg of atracurium. Fentanyl is a better choice of analgesic than morphine because the time to onset is quicker. We now use paralysis and analgesia for all intubations except those on the labour ward and in a dire emergency. The main difficulty is the time taken to obtain and draw up the drugs, particularly because fentanyl has to be kept in the controlled drugs cupboard.
2. The length of the ETT from the nostril or lips of babies of different weights is shown on p. 359.
3. Do not change tubes unnecessarily. Intubating babies never does them any good. Therefore only inflict reintubation on them if the tube is dislodged or blocked.
4. Immobilization of the tube at the nose or mouth is important to prevent it slipping out or traumatizing the larynx by sliding up and down. Various techniques are in routine use involving fixation either to a bonnet or to adhesive pads adhered to the baby's face.
5. Try to keep the baby's head in a constant degree of slight extension on his trunk. Flexing and extending his neck causes vast differences in ETT position and traumatizes the laryngeal mucosa.
6. Ensure that there is as small a dead space as possible between the ventilator circuit and the baby. However, we find that allowing an extra 2 cm of ETT is not a problem and we favour this arrangement since it considerably reduces nasal trauma and allows much greater mobility for the baby without using a complex head harness.
7. A good humidifier is essential, aiming to keep the inspiratory gas temperature at 37.0°C, to achieve 100% relative humidity.
8. RDS is not a disease in which airway secretions are increased. There is no need to suck out the ETT routinely in babies with RDS during the first 36–48 hours.

Sucking the baby out causes hypoxaemia, hypercapnia, hypertension and bradycardia, all of which are bad for him and predispose him to GMH-IVH (pp. 226–230). Suction should not be done for at least 4 hours after surfactant is given unless the ETT is blocked. After the first 48 hours the frequency should be tailored to the amount of secretions, usually sucking the tube out once or twice per day. The sucking out should be swift and efficient. If secretions are tenacious, 0.5 mL of normal saline can be instilled into the ETT prior to suction but should not be routine. The nurse needs to keep a very close watch on the baby; if he becomes cyanosed, if the reading of a continuous PaO_2 machine falls to 6.6 kPa (50 mmHg) or the saturation falls below 85%, she must stop. Suctioning time should be kept to 15 seconds and is ideally carried out with a system which allows continuous ventilation rather than requiring disconnection from the ventilator. If the baby is attached to an ECG monitor, suctioning should be stopped and IPPV restarted if the heart rate falls below 80 beats/min.

Choice of ventilator

Traditionally, neonatal ventilators have been designed as pressure-limited, time-cycled machines although improvements in technology have more recently allowed volume-limited ventilators to be developed. These are attractive because 'volutrauma' may be more important than 'barotrauma' in the genesis of CLD. Many modern neonatal ventilators offer high-frequency oscillation and the facility for continuous on-line monitoring of pressure, volume, flow and compliance. Patient-triggered ventilation is increasingly used, with the stimulus used for the trigger varying from an in-line flow or pressure sensor to an external respiration detector. Some ventilators can 'trigger' from the baby's efforts on both the inspiratory and expiratory phase.

■ Ventilation

Key points

- Effective ventilation is likely to be achieved only when the chest wall moves, ideally moving in phase with the ventilator.
- The PaO_2 is directly related to the mean airway pressure (MAP). MAP is dependent in turn on peak inspiratory pressure (PIP), positive end expiratory pressure (PEEP) and the duration of inspiration (see Fig. 13.9).
- Carbon dioxide tension is mainly affected by the minute ventilation (MV = tidal volume × rate). If ventilating well, the tidal volume is proportional to the tidal pressure, thus CO_2 elimination is altered by changing the rate and the difference between PIP and PEEP. Slow rates, short expiratory times and high levels of PEEP are more likely to cause CO_2 retention.
- The blood gases in a ventilated baby are likely to be better if he is breathing synchronously with the ventilator (or if he is making no spontaneous respiratory effort).
- In addition to achieving better blood gases and synchrony at fast rates, there is now clear evidence that the incidence of pulmonary interstitial emphysema and pneumothorax is less in babies ventilated at rates of 60–80 breaths/min with an inspiratory time of 0.3–0.5 seconds.
- $PaCO_2$ values below 3 kPa (approx 20 mmHg) must be avoided in preterm babies as this predisposes them to white matter injury (pp. 230–231).
- Artificial ventilation damages the lungs. Use the lowest settings compatible with achieving satisfactory blood gases. The most important determinants of lung injury

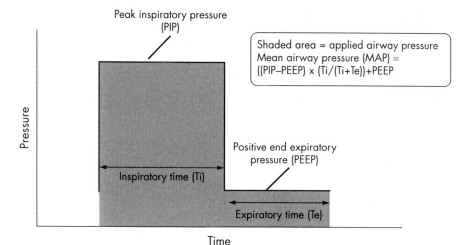

Peak inspiratory pressure (PIP)

Shaded area = applied airway pressure
Mean airway pressure (MAP) =
((PIP–PEEP) x (Ti/(Ti+Te))+PEEP

Pressure

Inspiratory time (Ti)

Positive end expiratory pressure (PEEP)

Expiratory time (Te)

Time

Fig. 13.9 Diagram to show relationship of ventilator settings to mean airway pressure

are the degree and the duration of PIP. Try whenever possible to reduce the PIP and avoid long inspiratory times. In particular, avoid an inspiratory (I) time which is longer than the expiratory (E) time (a reversed I:E ratio).

Modes of ventilation

One of the most confusing aspects of ventilator modes is that different terms are used by different ventilator manufacturers. We have tried to include as many synonymous terms as possible to aid the reader.

CMV (continuous mandatory ventilation)/IPPV (intermittent positive pressure ventilation)/IMV (intermittent mandatory ventilation)

In this mode the operator sets all parameters and the ventilator delivers the inspiratory breaths at regular intervals irrespective of the infant's own breathing. This can result in large pressure swings, asynchronous breathing and an increased risk of pulmonary leaks and long-term lung injury.

SIMV (synchronized intermittent mandatory ventilation)

In this mode the operator still sets all the parameters on the ventilator but the ventilator detects the baby's inspiratory flow during his own breathing and synchronizes the delivered breaths to the baby. The ventilator will still deliver a preset number of breaths, i.e. if the baby is breathing faster than the set rate, additional breaths are not supported; conversely, if the baby is breathing slower, additional non-synchronized breaths will be given.

SIPPV (synchronized intermittent positive pressure ventilation)/PTV (patient trigger ventilation)/ACV (assist control ventilation)

In this mode the operator sets a backup rate rather than an actual rate. The ventilator detects each inspiratory flow and supports each breath that the baby takes. If the baby breathes slower than the set ventilator rate, it will deliver additional breaths to make the baby's respiratory rate up to the set rate.

With trigger ventilation, short inspiratory times must be used (0.3–0.32 seconds). If a long inspiratory time is used there is a risk the baby will try to actively breathe out while the ventilator is still delivering a mechanical inflation. A Cochrane Review comparing SIPPV/SIMV with continuous mandatory ventilation showed SIPPV/SIMV was associated with a shorter duration of ventilation (weighted mean difference –34.8 hours, 95% CI –62.1, –7.4). During weaning there was a trend to a shorter duration of weaning using SIPPV (weighted mean difference –42.4 hours, 95% CI –94.4, 9.6), although this was not statistically significant.

VTV (volume-targeted ventilation)/VG (volume guarantee)

In VTV, rather than setting a peak inspiratory pressure (PIP) the operator sets a maximum inspiratory pressure. They additionally set a target volume (Vt), which is usually 4–6 mL/kg. The ventilator then uses the lowest inspiratory pressure to deliver the set volume of breath based on its 'experience' gained from the previous delivered breath. VTV does not work in babies with a large ETT leak calculated by (inspired volume/expired volume) × 100. If the leak is above 50%, VTV is unlikely to be successful. Often the most appropriate action is to consider the reason for the leak and act appropriately to reduce it.

In a meta-analysis of 12 randomized trials, VTV was shown to be significantly associated with reduced mortality and CLD compared with conventional pressure-limited ventilation. VTV reduced the combined outcome of death or bronchopulmonary dysplasia (BPD) (relative risk (RR) 0.73 (95% CI 0.57–0.93), (number needed to treat (NNT) 8 (95% CI 5–33)). VTV modes also resulted in reductions in pneumothorax (RR 0.46 (95% CI 0.25–0.84), NNT 17), days of ventilation (mean days (MD) –2.36 (95% CI –3.9 to –0.8)), hypocarbia (typical RR 0.56 (95% CI 0.33–0.96)) and the combined outcome of PVL or grade 3–4 intraventricular haemorrhage (typical RR 0.48 (95% CI 0.28–0.84), NNT 11). Although VTV can be used in conjunction with all modes of ventilation it is most logically used in conjunction with SIPPV.

Pressure support ventilation (PSV)

In PSV the inspiratory time is determined by the baby's own spontaneous respiration and not by the setting on the ventilator. In reality, preterm babies have been found to have too short an inspiratory time for this mode to work well and ventilation in this mode is therefore less efficient and relatively ineffective.

Initial ventilator settings using conventional pressure-limited time-cycled ventilation in respiratory distress syndrome

The settings which need to be considered include:

- flow rate of gases through the ventilator circuit;
- inspired oxygen concentration (FiO_2);
- peak inspiratory pressure;
- positive end expiratory pressure;
- duration of inspiration (T_I) and expiration (T_E), which determines the rate in breaths per minute.

As a general guide start VLBW babies on:

- flow of 8 L/min;
- oxygen concentration adjusted to achieve saturation ~88–92%;
- PIP of around 18 cmH$_2$O;

- positive end expiratory pressure (PEEP) of 5 cmH$_2$O;
- inspiratory time of 0.4 seconds, a rate of 60 breaths/min (T$_I$:T$_E$ = 1:1.2).

For larger babies born near term, start with a PIP of 18–25 cmH$_2$O. Watch for chest movement and synchrony between the baby's respiratory effort and the ventilator. Use the minimum level of PIP which is required to move the baby's chest. Check a blood gas 20 minutes after starting ventilation and adjust the settings accordingly.

Changing ventilator settings in respiratory distress syndrome

Aim to keep the blood gases in the range PaO$_2$ 6.0–10.0 kPa (45–75 mmHg) and PaCO$_2$ 5–7.5 kPa (37–56 mmHg) with a pH above 7.25. Vigorous high-pressure ventilation to keep the PaCO$_2$ in the normal range (Table 13.4) is not necessary and is associated with a higher incidence of chronic lung disease.

Solutions to unsatisfactory blood gases in respiratory distress syndrome

1. To improve oxygenation when the PaCO$_2$ is normal. In this situation, with the PaCO$_2$ 5–7.5 kPa (35–50 mmHg), there are three alternatives:
   - increasing the inspired oxygen concentration;
   - increasing the respirator rate;
   - increasing the mean airway pressure (MAP) without increasing the peak pressures (by increasing T$_I$ or the level of PEEP).
   Try increasing the FiO$_2$ first, then gradually increase the T$_I$ towards 0.5 seconds, but never let the T$_I$:T$_E$ ratio exceed 1. These manoeuvres increase the MAP. If they fail, increase the PIP and accept the lowish PaCO$_2$ as long as it is not below 3 kPa. Increasing the PEEP to above 7 cmH$_2$O is rarely of any benefit.
2. To improve oxygenation when the PaCO$_2$ is low <4.5 kPa (35 mmHg). Consider:
   - wrong diagnosis – the baby has compliant lungs, so there may be another cause for hypoxaemia (e.g. CHD, pneumonia, PPHN;
   - gross overventilation – overventilation prevents adequate pulmonary perfusion and reduces the PaO$_2$. The CXR in such babies shows lung fields which are black, with low, flat diaphragms and a small heart shadow.
   If none of these diagnoses applies, the baby probably has severe RDS. To improve oxygenation try to sustain the MAP but change other things in ways that might increase the PaCO$_2$ (e.g. increasing PEEP or decreasing the rate).
3. To lower a high carbon dioxide concentration (PaCO$_2$ >8–9 kPa (60–70 mmHg)) with an acceptable level of oxygen. There are several alternatives:
   - increasing the rate but to no more than 90 breaths/min;
   - reducing the PEEP, but not to below 3 cmH$_2$O, since PEEP preserves surfactant;
   - reducing the inspiratory time (but not to less than 0.2 seconds);
   - lengthening the expiratory time.

These options are summarized in Table 13.8.

Initial ventilator settings using volume-targeted ventilation in respiratory distress syndrome

- Set Vt. The normal range for Vt is 4–6 mL/kg and in general we would set initial Vt at 4.5—5 mL/kg for babies <1000 g and 4.0–4.5 mL/kg for babies >1000 g.

Table 13.8 Summary of adjustments to ventilator settings on the basis of blood gas results

Oxygen	Carbon dioxide	Action
Low PaO_2	High $PaCO_2$	Increase PIP – which will increase MAP. In spontaneously breathing babies an increased rate may work
Low PaO_2	Normal $PaCO_2$	Increase FiO_2; ↑ MAP but maintain PIP (i.e. ↑ PEEP or ↑ Ti)
Low PaO_2	Low $PaCO_2$	Consider alternative diagnoses to RDS; overventilation
Normal PaO_2	High $PaCO_2$	↓ PEEP; ↑ rate; keep MAP constant
Normal PaO_2	Normal $PaCO_2$	Sit tight! unless weaning
Normal PaO_2	Low $PaCO_2$	↓ Rate; maintain MAP
High PaO_2	High $PaCO_2$	Rare. Check for mechanical problems, e.g. blocked tube ↓ PEEP: ↓ Ti: ↑ rate
High PaO_2	Normal $PaCO_2$	↓ MAP (usually by ↓ PIP): ↓ FiO_2
High PaO_2	Low $PaCO_2$	Overventilated – ↓ pressure; ↓ rate; ↓ FiO_2

MAP, mean airway pressure; PEEP, positive end expiratory pressure; PIP, peak inspiratory pressure; RDS, respiratory distress syndrome; Ti, inspiratory time.

Note, the smaller the baby, the higher the initial Vt required. Do not set Vt too low, i.e. below 3.5 mL/kg.

■ Set the PIP. This needs to be set higher than you would set on pressure-limited time-cycled ventilation to allow for inter-breath fluctuations. Remember this is not the pressure that the baby will necessarily receive. We set the PIP 4 cmH$_2$O higher than we would use on conventional ventilation.

■ Set PEEP to start at 5 cmH$_2$O and alter as per lung inflation.

■ Set Ti 0.32 seconds – short inspiratory times help to achieve triggering and reduce lung injury.

■ Set backup rate at 40 breaths/min to enable the baby to trigger as many ventilations as possible (triggered breaths require less pressure to deliver the same Vt). However, if the infant is apnoeic or has poor respiratory drive, a backup rate of 50–60 breaths/min may be required to maintain minute ventilation.

■ Set FiO_2 to achieve saturation ~88–92%.

Adjusting ventilator settings using volume-targeted ventilation in respiratory distress syndrome

In VTV, weaning or increasing ventilation should be on the basis of volume. There is no point reducing the pressures without reducing the set Vt – all you will do is make the ventilator alarm. Increasing the Vt may require increasing the set PIP to achieve the new volume.

■ When the baby is overventilated, reduce the prescribed volume in 0.5 mL/kg increments to a minimum of 3.5–4.5 mL/kg. If the baby is underventilated or underoxygenated, increase the tidal volume in 0.5 mL/kg increments to a maximum of 6 mL/kg (unless there is BPD or the baby is >3 weeks old and ventilator dependent where higher Vt may be required).

■ Do not decrease Vt below 3.5 mL/kg as this is likely to be less than the baby's spontaneous tidal volume and therefore can result in the baby receiving continuous endotracheal CPAP. Most babies can be extubated from a Vt of 4–4.5 mL/kg.

■ Wean the backup rate to a rate well below the baby's natural respiratory rate and then allow the baby to self-wean. Usually a backup rate of 30–40 breaths/min is sufficient. There is no benefit to reducing the rate further if the baby is breathing above the ventilator on SIPPV as each breath is assisted.

Failure to respond to ventilator manipulations

Confronted with a baby who fails to respond to these manipulations and remains hypoxic in high FiO_2 with a high CO_2, always check the CXR and consider the following possibilities:

1. There are mechanical problems such as a blocked tube, a leak around the tube, ventilator failure. Check all machinery for leaks, try hand-ventilating with a bag and mask, insert a larger ETT.
2. The baby has only moderately severe HMD but has uncorrected acidaemia,* hypotension* or hypoglycaemia*. Check pH, blood pressure, PCV, glucose and treat accordingly.
3. Incorrect diagnosis or a complication of RDS has developed:
   (a) pneumothorax or pulmonary interstitial emphysema (PIE) (p. 159);
   (b) CHD* (mature > premature) (Chapter 14);
   (c) pulmonary haemorrhage (pp. 161–162);
   (d) pulmonary oedema/fluid overload/PDA (p. 296);
   (e) persistent pulmonary hypertension* (mature > premature) (p. 162);
   (f) overventilation* (see above);
   (g) pneumonia and septicaemia*; especially GBS sepsis (pp. 197–198);
   (h) intracranial haemorrhage* (pp. 226–230);
   (i) pulmonary hypoplasia (after very prolonged rupture of membranes with oligohydramnios).

   * These conditions will usually have a reduced or normal $PaCO_2$ whereas in the others it will be considerably raised.

High-frequency oscillatory ventilation

The strategy of high-frequency oscillatory ventilation (HFOV) is to inflate the lungs and recruit 'lung units' (immature babies do not yet have alveoli, p. 114) by applying a continuous distending pressure which keeps the lung at the optimal place on its hysteresis curve (Fig. 13.3). Oxygenation and carbon dioxide removal occurs via an oscillating pressure waveform superimposed on the MAP. High-frequency oscillators are essentially airway vibrators (a piston pump or vibrating diaphragm) that operate at frequencies of around 10 Hz (1 Hz = 1 cycle per second, 60 cycles per minute). During HFOV, inspiration and expiration are both active. A continuous flow of fresh gas rushes past the vibrating source that generates the oscillation and a controlled leak or low-pass filter allows gas to exit the system. Pressure oscillations within the airway produce a 'tidal volume' of 2–3 mL around a constant MAP, which maintains lung volume in a fashion equivalent to using very high levels of CPAP. The volume of gas moved in the 'tidal volume' is determined by the amplitude of the airway pressure oscillation (ΔP). The settings that need to be considered for oscillatory ventilation are:

■ flow rate of gases through the ventilator circuit (usually fixed around 6–8 L/min);
■ inspired oxygen concentration;
■ MAP;
■ oscillatory frequency;
■ oscillatory pressure amplitude – ΔP;
■ inspiratory–expiratory ratio or percentage of cycle as inspiratory time.

Oscillators are powerful tools, and in 'rescue' mode HFOV can save some babies with severe RDS who have failed to respond to conventional ventilation and surfactant. HFOV is particularly effective in the management of hypercarbia. What is less certain than rescue is the role of HFOV used as the primary mode of ventilation in RDS in today's population of very small babies who have received antenatal steroids and postnatal surfactant. The randomized controlled trials published to date have shown no benefit in reduced over conventional ventilation.

Indications for HFOV

- Failure of RDS to respond to surfactant and IPPV.
- Primary mode of ventilation for RDS (not proven and not our current practice).
- Meconium aspiration syndrome (MAS) with homogeneous disease, without pneumothorax.
- Pneumonia failing to respond to conventional ventilation.
- Severe bilateral uniform PIE with hypercarbia.

Relative contraindications for HFOV – use with care

- Hypotensive baby dependent on inotropic support.
- Inhomogeneous lung disease.
- Pre-existing pneumothorax – need to use a high FiO_2/low-volume strategy.

Starting oscillation from birth in preterm < 1000 g with RDS:

- FiO_2 40%.
- Frequency 15 Hz.
- Percentage of inspiratory time 33%. This is relevant only on the Sensor Medics as the I:E ratio is fixed or determined by the machine on the other oscillators.
- MAP 6–8 cm increase by 0.5–1 cm every 10–15 minutes until no further improvement in PaO_2 – at that point do a CXR to check the level of the diaphragms.
- Oscillatory amplitude – increase until the chest wall is just perceptibly 'bouncing', usually about 18 cm H_2O. Generally the oscillation is in the region of 2–3 times the MAP.

Changing to oscillatory ventilation from conventional ventilation

- Keep the FiO_2 the same as that which the baby is already receiving.
- Set the frequency to 10 Hz.
- Set the inspiratory fraction to 0.33%.
- Set the MAP as 2 cmH$_2$O above that used on IPPV, increase by 0.5–1 cmH$_2$O every 10–15 minutes until no further improvement in PaO_2. At that point do a CXR to check the level of the diaphragms.
- Amplitude (power, ΔP) – increase until the chest wall is bouncing, usually about 18 cmH$_2$O.

Ventilator changes during HFOV
Oxygenation is dependent primarily on:

- MAP;
- F_iO_2;
- blood pressure.

As mentioned above, increase MAP by 0.5–1 cmH$_2$O every 10–15 minutes until there is no further improvement in PaO_2. Aim for FiO_2 30–40%; if in lower FiO_2, reduce the MAP (but not lower than 6 cmH$_2$O). At that point do a CXR to check the level of the diaphragm; overventilation is present if the lung margin is below the ninth rib. If oxygenation decreases while on oscillation, assess whether the baby is hypovolaemic or hypotensive and perform a CXR.

Carbon dioxide elimination is mainly dependent on the amplitude; if the $PaCO_2$ increases, the amplitude should be increased. If hypercarbia is a significant problem despite a reasonable oscillatory amplitude, the frequency can be reduced – we use 15 Hz for small preterms, 10 Hz for larger babies and 8 Hz in those with significant hypercarbia, e.g. meconium aspiration. The effect of reducing the frequency is to increase the time for which the high and low pressures are acting and hence increase the tidal excursion of the chest and in turn improve CO_2 elimination.

Weaning from high-frequency oscillatory ventilation

The aim during weaning is to maintain optimum lung volume, therefore reduce FiO_2 before MAP. Once the FiO_2 is down to 30%, reduce MAP by 0.5–1 cmH$_2$O steps, monitoring the blood gases regularly. If during weaning the PaO_2 decreases, it is likely that you are reducing the MAP too slowly. Perform a CXR to check for overdistension.

Nitric oxide in respiratory distress syndrome

Nitric oxide has not been shown to be of benefit in preterm babies and has no place in the routine care of preterm neonates.

Other therapy

Antibiotics

We put all ventilated babies on antibiotics at birth for three reasons:

1. Severe early-onset sepsis can masquerade as RDS.
2. Sepsis can co-exist with surfactant-deficient RDS.
3. Once intubated the lung will be colonized with pathogens which can cause either pneumonia or septicaemia.

We use penicillin and amikacin until cultures are available at 48 hours. If the initial cultures are negative and the CRP is less than 10 mg/L at 48 hours, we stop antibiotics unless the secretions or the CXR suggest pneumonia is developing.

Analgesia/paralysis

Being on a ventilator is undoubtedly uncomfortable and stressful. High catecholamine levels have been found in such babies and there is a relationship between very high levels of stress hormones and adverse outcome. The aim is to achieve a settled baby on the ventilator in whom a reversal of the sedative effect can be rapidly achieved for weaning.

Paralysis with pancuronium or atracurium is a last resort but is still required from time to time. These drugs have undesirable side effects, but it is clear that they considerably reduce the number of pneumothoraces in babies breathing out of phase with the ventilator. Situations where muscle relaxants are indicated, apart from severe RDS with asynchrony, include PIE and pneumothorax (pp. 158–159), PPHN (p. 162), meconium aspiration (pp. 155–157), massive pulmonary haemorrhage (pp. 162–163) and diaphragmatic hernia (pp. 276–277). Babies who are given muscle relaxants because they are fighting the ventilator are frequently doing a lot of their own 'ventilation' and in such cases it will often be necessary to increase the ventilator pressures to achieve adequate blood gases after the drugs are given. The other main side effect is that the absence of spontaneous movements causes some peripheral oedema.

Paralysed babies must always be monitored carefully since they are unable to sustain even feeble respiratory efforts if they become disconnected from the ventilator or if their ETT blocks.

◼ Sudden deterioration on intermittent positive pressure ventilation

What to do when a baby's condition suddenly deteriorates when on IPPV is shown in Fig. 13.10. The important causes of deterioration are as follows.

- ◼ *Blocked ETT.* Check that the chest is moving. This is the key to assessing neonatal ventilation at all times, and a baby whose chest is not moving as well as it was earlier and whose blood gases are developing increasing hypercarbia is likely to have a blocked tube. On modern ventilators, looking at the flow graph and reviewing the resistance can also provide evidence of a blocked tube (poor flow and high resistance). If the problem does not resolve with suction, the ETT must be changed. If the chest still does not move, the baby has a blocked trachea, a bilateral pneumothorax or very stiff lungs. The only solution to a blocked trachea is direct suction below the cords using a large-bore suction catheter. This can be life-saving on occasion; a solid blood clot, or lump of meconium or vernix cannot be aspirated up an ETT with a small-bore suction catheter passed through it.
- ◼ *Pneumothorax* (p. 160). Pneumothorax can cause a catastrophic deterioration with hypoxaemia, hypercarbia and hypotension. If time permits, a CXR should be taken

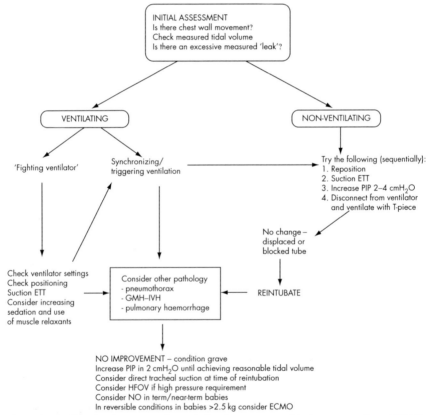

Fig. 13.10 Algorithm for action when a baby deteriorates suddenly on a ventilator. ECMO, extracorporeal membrane oxygenation; ETT, endotracheal tube; GMH-IVA, germinal matrix–intraventilator haemorrhage; HFOV, high-frequency oscillatory ventilation; NO, nitric oxide; PIP, peak inspiratory pressure.

to confirm the diagnosis. In the emergency situation, diagnosis can be confirmed by the clinical signs and by transillumination. Any pneumothorax which is associated with a deterioration in blood gases should be drained with a proper chest drain. A small pneumothorax which is found on a routine CXR in an unventilated baby can be observed because the air will absorb. However, if a baby with even a small pneumothorax requires artificial ventilation, the air leak is likely to enlarge and become a tension pneumothorax, so a drain should be inserted.

- *GMH-IVH* (pp. 226–230). A large GMH-IVH may be responsible whenever any baby weighing less than 1.5 kg suddenly deteriorates, whether or not he is receiving IPPV. The baby is difficult to resuscitate and remains hypoxic and acidaemic with a poor peripheral circulation; there is often a fall in haematocrit.
- *Pulmonary haemorrhage*. The clue to this diagnosis is a frothy pink endotracheal aspirate. Pulmonary haemorrhage is often associated with haemorrhagic pulmonary oedema because of a PDA (p. 296). There is usually a coagulopathy. The CXR shows widespread patchy infiltration. Pulmonary haemorrhage is difficult to treat but the best advice is to increase the ventilator settings, paralyse the baby and replace clotting factors with fresh frozen plasma, cryoprecipitate and platelets as indicated.

Gradual deterioration on intermittent positive pressure ventilation

There are six major diagnoses to consider if a baby's deterioration is more gradual:

1. Infection.
2. GMH-IVH.
3. PDA.
4. Partial blockage of the ETT.
5. Anaemia/hypotension.
6. Slow development of air leak.

Infection

With the exception of babies who present acutely ill with sepsis (usually GBS) within the first few hours, an infectious cause of deterioration is unusual in the first few days, since antibiotics will have been given to all babies on admission for the reasons given on p. 149. After this period, by far the most common cause of septicaemia is coagulase-negative staphylococci (CONS). CONS is particularly common in babies on long-term IPPV with central lines in situ to administer total parenteral nutrition. Any other organism can cause septicaemia (p. 188). Pneumonia may also cause problems in the following situations:

1. Secondary infection with an organism such as *Candida* or *Pseudomonas* not covered by penicillin and aminoglycoside.
2. Re-infection in a neonate on long-term IPPV some time after an initial course of antibiotics was completed.

Both septicaemia and pneumonia usually present over a period of hours rather than days, with some combination of the following signs:

- increasing lethargy, decreased peripheral perfusion, pallor;
- temperature instability;

- increasing jaundice;
- nasogastric feeds no longer tolerated, vomiting, abdominal distension;
- increased thick (purulent) secretions up the ETT and a positive culture of the aspirate;
- deteriorating lung function – PaO_2 falling, $PaCO_2$ rising;
- on auscultation, localized or generalized crepitations;
- CXR changes that are patchy (suggesting pneumonia).

With CONS septicaemia the only clinical features usually present are the first two, whereas more clinical features are present in those with pneumonia. Laboratory confirmation with a raised WBC count with a neutrophilia, a raised CRP and a fall in the platelet count is usually present.

Most of the above clinical findings are also compatible with deteriorating RDS in a small sick baby, with pulmonary oedema from a PDA or the development of CLD, but since they could also mean infection, one should start antibiotics or broaden or change the spectrum of cover. If CONS sepsis is a possibility, always include flucloxacillin, teicoplanin or vancomycin. If no organisms grow, this course of antibiotics can be discontinued after 5–10 days.

GMH-IVH (pp. 226–230)

As well as the acute deterioration (see above), there may be a more stuttering deterioration, with the baby becoming pale and unresponsive with deteriorating blood gases. The diagnosis can be confirmed by cerebral ultrasound.

Patent ductus arteriosus (p. 296)

This is a common cause of deterioration towards the end of the first week. The typical clinical and echocardiographic signs will usually be present.

Partial blockage of the ETT

The nurses may suspect this because of difficulties passing the endotracheal suction tube, increasing airways resistance, decreasing tidal volumes, or there may be conducted sounds audible on chest auscultation. The only way to confirm this diagnosis is to change the ETT.

Anaemia/hypotension

Hypotension may be due to sepsis or GMH-IVH, but can also be due to fluid or blood loss from any cause. Losses due to the blood removed for laboratory analysis must always be replaced by transfusion.

Other causes

Other conditions causing gradual deterioration are:

- infection in other sites, e.g. meningitis, NEC;
- development of any type of air leak;
- electrolyte imbalance, especially marked hyponatraemia, hypocalcaemia, hypo- or hyperkalaemia;
- hypoglycaemia;
- development of severe CLD with bronchial hypersecretion.

Weaning off intermittent positive pressure ventilation

Once a baby is stable on the ventilator, off muscle relaxants and with satisfactory blood gases for 12 hours or so, the weaning process can begin. Some babies who were intubated in the labour ward are soon found to have a normal CXR and minimal disease, and in such cases weaning can be rapid. However, in general, in babies with typical RDS, the temptation to wean them rapidly within the first 48 hours should be resisted since they often deteriorate if this is done and require vigorous ventilation for resuscitation. Remember that the natural history of RDS is that the disease worsens in the second 24-hour period, although this typical picture has altered with the advent of antenatal steroids and postnatal surfactant. The weaning process is as follows. This process may take several weeks, or may be achieved in 24 hours. Using a volume-guided form of ventilation can allow weaning to be performed 'automatically'.

Generally speaking, the smaller the baby, the slower the process. Following every change in the ventilator setting the blood gases should be checked within 1–2 hours to ensure that the PaO_2 and $PaCO_2$ are still satisfactory. If they are not, revert to the previous ventilator settings. In VLBW babies more than 72 hours old who are no longer at high risk of GMH-IVH, it is reasonable to allow the $PaCO_2$ to rise to 7–8 kPa during weaning, as long as the pH is >7.2.

Since more damage is done to the lungs by high pressures than by high oxygen concentrations, try to reduce the pressure first, but always preserve a PEEP to splint the alveoli open and preserve surfactant. In general, reduce the pressure by 2–3 cmH$_2$O at a time and the oxygen by 5–10% at a time. Bigger reductions can be made if the PaO_2 is much above 13.3 kPa (100 mmHg) or the CO_2 well below 5.6 kPa (40 mmHg).

Extubation

There are no 'absolute' values to define when to extubate a baby. Smaller babies may be able to generate less respiratory drive themselves than bigger babies. Once a baby has been weaned to a peak inspiratory pressure of 16 cmH$_2$O or less (or is using such pressures on volume-guided ventilation) and is showing sustained respiratory effort, extubation should be considered, although some babies will extubate from higher pressures. Preterm infants <32 weeks should be commenced on caffeine to improve respiratory drive and because this is associated with improved long-term motor outcomes, and indeed we start caffeine early in very preterm babies because of the evidence that neurodevelopmental outcome is improved. Most preterm infants have been traditionally extubated to CPAP, although biphasic CPAP and high-flow oxygen systems are being used increasingly. Whatever technique is used it is important to recognize that the recently extubated extreme preterm infant is among the most challenging infant to nurse (significantly more difficult than a baby with an ETT). The challenges include maintenance of a patent airway, appropriate positioning of the non-invasive ventilation often with the infant prone, performing appropriate chest physiotherapy and suction – all while maintaining minimal handling. We generally stop feeds around the extubation, although nutrition should not be compromised for more than a few hours. A gradual rise in $PaCO_2$ up to 8–8.5 kPa (60–65 mmHg), or a gradual fall in PaO_2, can be allowed so long as the baby is breathing well, looks clinically well and holds his pH above 7.25. These blood gas changes are often transient over the 6–12 hours after extubation and then improve.

Long-term difficulties with weaning and extubation

Repeated failure to wean a baby off IPPV may be due to the following:

1. Persisting problems with secretions. Leave an ETT in situ for 3–5 days, + IMV combined with a vigorous programme of chest physiotherapy, ETT suction and antibiotic therapy if appropriate before trying again.
2. Recurrent apnoea once extubated. The baby should be reintubated and the dose of caffeine increased. If apnoea persists off IMV, this may be a sign of a small GMH-IVH, sepsis, or gastro-oesophageal reflux.
3. PDA and/or pulmonary oedema. Babies in this situation are particularly likely to deteriorate if their PCV is less than 40%. Reintubate, control fluids, give furosemide if in pulmonary oedema. Treat PDA and try again.
4. Chronic lung disease. If this is severe it may take several months to wean the baby off both IMV and CPAP. Patience, minimal ventilator settings, steroids and diuretics are the treatment (Chapter 14).
5. Laryngeal oedema or stenosis. In the short term these can usually be circumvented by good humidification and some nasal CPAP. Occasionally, dexamethasone 0.5–1.0 mg 24–48 hours before extubation. If this fails, reinsert a nasal ETT (+ IMV) taking great care to immobilize it. Leave for 48–96 hours before reattempting extubation under dexamethasone cover. In some babies moderate degrees of subglottic stenosis can be controlled with long-term nasal CPAP until the baby grows and the stenosis resolves. A cricoid split operation can be tried but tracheostomy is a last resort in such babies, since if one is inserted it is very unlikely that decannulation will be possible in under 6 months.
6. Very small babies who repeatedly fail extubation should have their nutrition maximized by the enteral or intravenous route. Ten days and 250 g later, they will probably extubate easily.
7. Underlying neurological problems: GMH-IVH is considered above, but primary muscle disorders, e.g. dystrophia myotonica, may present this way.

■ Transient tachypnoea of the newborn

This condition affects mainly mature babies, but does occur in those born prematurely.

Aetiology

TTN is attributed to delayed clearing of the fetal lung liquid after the onset of respiration. It is more common in babies delivered by caesarean section before the onset of labour. In many cases there is a mild abnormality of surfactant.

Clinical signs

The baby, typically delivered in good condition at 38 weeks' gestation by elective caesarean section after an uneventful pregnancy, develops respiratory distress within an hour or two of delivery. He has mild grunting and little sternal, intercostal or subcostal recession, but the respiratory rate may be 100 breaths/min. On auscultation the chest sounds normal with good air entry, there are no râles. Cyanosis may be present in air but is relieved by putting the baby into 30–40% O_2.

Another group of babies who probably have the same disease show a different clinical picture. These babies have often dropped their body temperatures to around

35°C, breathe quite slowly, have varying degrees of recession but grunt loudly. When their body temperature rises to normal, they convert to the more typical clinical pattern of TTN.

The differential diagnosis is given in Table 13.4, but in the first few hours of life TTN cannot, with confidence, be distinguished from the early stages of GBS pneumonia or sepsis.

Radiology

The CXR shows 'wet lungs', with prominent vascular markings and fluid in the fissures.

Treatment

In mature babies not at risk from ROP, peripheral arterial samples and oximetry are adequate for the initial evaluation, which usually shows mild hypoxaemia with normal acid–base data. Arterial catheterization is rarely necessary, unless the baby requires more than 40% O_2, or if there is any doubt at all about the nature or severity of his disease. Because of the risk of GBS sepsis, after taking cultures we put all tachypnoeic neonates on penicillin and amikacin until the culture results are known to be negative. Although the disease is due to delayed clearing of pulmonary fluid, furosemide is of no benefit.

During the first 12–24 hours the baby should be hydrated with intravenous 10% dextrose, but oral feeds can often be started by 24 hours of age, if not before. Give 1–2 hourly feeds to start with and aspirate the nasogastric tube every 4–6 hours to ensure that the stomach is emptying. As soon as the baby has satisfactory blood gases when he is breathing air and is tolerating enteral feeds, he should be returned to his mother on the postnatal ward. Respiratory rates of 50–60 breaths/min may persist for several days, but this is no reason for keeping the baby on the neonatal unit.

Minimal respiratory disease

This title is given to those babies who have mild symptoms for 4–6 hours after birth, some grunting or a respiratory rate of 50–60 breaths/min and then recover. Careful observation, occasionally oxygen and taking care to exclude infection is all that is required.

■ Meconium aspiration

Key points

- Meconium aspiration syndrome (MAS) is a disease of postmature babies usually born through thick meconium.
- Vigorous suction of the airway at birth reduces the incidence and severity of MAS.
- Early treatment with intermittent positive pressure ventilation, paralysis, low levels of positive end expiratory pressure and surfactant can usually prevent progress to severe persistent pulmonary hypertension of the newborn requiring nitric oxide or even extracorporeal membrane oxygenation .

This condition is limited to mature babies, since premature babies virtually never pass meconium *in utero*. Meconium staining in preterm labour strongly suggests *Listeria* infection (p. 202). Passage of meconium occurs in 10% of all labours at term (15–20%

after 41 weeks). Meconium-stained liquor is a poor marker of fetal asphyxia unless there are co-existing changes in the CTG or fetal pH.

Aetiology

When meconium is present in the liquor and the upper airway before, during or immediately after delivery, it can be inhaled. Inhalation of meconium causes airway obstruction, air trapping and overdistension of the lungs, with a considerable risk of pneumomediastinum and pneumothorax. The irritant properties of meconium also cause a chemical pneumonitis, and the presence of inhaled organic material predisposes to bacterial infection and denatures surfactant on the alveolar surface.

Clinical signs

The baby's skin, nails and umbilical cord are often meconium stained. Respiratory distress appears quickly after birth and may be severe. Air trapping causes lung over-distension, anterior bowing of the sternum and an increased anteroposterior diameter to the chest. On auscultation there are widespread added sounds with rhonchi, and fine or sticky crepitations. Differential diagnosis is rarely a problem (Table 13.4), but other conditions may co-exist, particularly hypoxic ischaemic encephalopathy, pneumothorax and pneumonia.

Radiology

The lungs look overexpanded and contain multiple areas of streaky atelectasis. As the disease progresses the lungs become more diffusely opaque owing to chemical pneumonitis and/or bacterial superinfection.

Treatment

Every effort should be made to prevent this condition by meticulous intrapartum care, including the avoidance of fetal hypoxic ischaemia. It is now appreciated that meconium can be 'gasped' in before birth and the stimulus for fetal gasping is often hypoxia. MAS occurs in only 1% of deliveries in which the baby is born through meconium-stained liquor, and MAS is more likely if the meconium is thick (pea-soup meconium) because this occurs when there is oligohydramnios, which is linked to poor placental function and fetal hypoxia. Thin, watery, pale green liquor, merely tinged with meconium, is not usually followed by MAS. In practice, the difficulty in agreeing definitions of 'thick' and 'thin' means that paediatricians have to attend all deliveries where the liquor is meconium stained, although their presence at deliveries where the liquor is only faintly stained is often superfluous. If the newborn infant is vigorous, no attempt should be made to visualize the cords as this has not been shown to be effective. However, in a floppy apnoeic infant the upper airway should be cleared under direct vision using a laryngoscope as long as there is a heart rate >60 beats/min. If meconium is seen at or beyond the vocal cords, intubation and tracheal suction should be done. Remember that meconium can block the trachea.

Babies should be treated rapidly and aggressively to ensure adequate oxygenation and carbon dioxide elimination. Blood gas analysis should be carried out frequently, and a UAC or peripheral arterial line should be inserted into ventilated babies with MAS to both facilitate blood gases and measure blood pressure. The underlying reason for this approach is to minimize the risk of and treat any pulmonary hypertension that will arise if the baby remains hypoxic and hypercapnic. Most babies hyperventilate in an attempt to keep their $PaCO_2$ normal. A progressively rising $PaCO_2$ is an indication of severe disease with persistent plugging of the airways with meconium. The finding of a baby with significant respiratory distress often with a high oxygen requirement is an indication for early intubation and ventilation. Babies with MAS can be very difficult to ventilate; muscle relaxants such as pancuronium are virtually always necessary.

All babies should receive broad-spectrum antibiotic prophylaxis from the moment of birth. Give the usual broad-spectrum antibiotic cocktail in use on the unit, often penicillin and gentamicin or amikacin.

Surfactant is of value and should be given to ventilated babies with MAS. Large amounts may be needed. The risk of pneumothorax is very high and a chest drain set should be readily available.

The ventilator settings are different from those required in RDS, since these babies have gas trapping, an increased airways resistance and a chemical pneumonitis. Settings should include a long expiratory time and lower levels of PEEP. Many babies respond well to HFOV.

Many babies with severe MAS have pulmonary hypertension. Dopamine should be used to keep the systemic pressure above the pulmonary pressure (dobutamine should be avoided, with noradrenaline (norepinephrine) used as second-line inotrope). The mean arterial pressure should be maintained around 50 mmHg, and once this is achieved nitric oxide can be beneficial to lower the pulmonary pressure. Plasma magnesium levels should be measured and magnesium sulphate (which acts as a pulmonary vasodilator) should be given to keep plasma levels at the upper end of the normal range.

Our experience is that with adequate and vigorous early therapy the need to progress to extracorporeal membrane oxygenation (ECMO) is rare, but as these babies are usually >2 kg and >37 weeks' gestation if they remain profoundly hypoxic with an oxygenation index of 30–40, ECMO is an option. If babies with MAS are not responding to treatment by 12–24 hours, consider ECMO – do not wait for days.

The babies have often suffered from hypoxia–ischaemia *in utero* and if they have they are at risk from hypoxic ischaemic encephalopathy (HIE) and renal problems. Great care is therefore required to avoid fluid overload. Seizures may not be clinically apparent in paralysed babies and consideration should be given to electroencephalographic monitoring. Assessment of the CNS is particularly important if ECMO is being considered. While therapeutic hypothermia is now standard care for babies with moderate–severe HIE, it may also worsen pulmonary hypertension and is therefore contraindicated in severe PPHN.

Pulmonary interstitial emphysema, pneumothorax, pneumomediastinum

Key points

- The incidence of air leaks has been markedly reduced to about 10% of ventilated babies by antenatal steroids, postnatal surfactant and synchronous ventilation.
- Pulmonary interstitial emphysema (PIE) and pneumothorax can be asymptomatic in preterm babies on intermittent positive pressure ventilation (IPPV) with severe lung disease. To detect air leak, which will alter the type of IPPV applied, a chest X-ray should be done at least daily.
- All pneumothoraces should be drained if symptomatic or present in babies requiring IPPV and the drain attached to suction of 10–20 cmH_2O.
- Management of PIE is by 'gentle' IPPV with permissive hypercapnia using ventilator rates of 80–100 breaths/min. High-frequency oscillatory ventilation may be indicated.

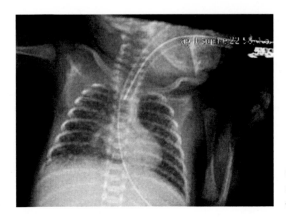

Fig. 13.11 Chest X-ray showing severe bilateral pulmonary interstitial emphysema

Pneumopericardium, pneumoperitoneum, subcutaneous emphysema

All these air-leak problems are serious complications of high-pressure ventilation. Air leak increases the mortality rate and the incidence of intracranial haemorrhage. This has occurred because of increased use of antenatal steroids and postnatal surfactant, and a widespread acceptance of the philosophy of synchronous ventilation with paralysis where necessary. There is a strong link between air leak of any kind and CLD. Severe PIE such as that shown in Fig 13.11 is now fortunately rare but remains a predictor of severe chronic lung disease.

Aetiology

Air leaks are primarily found in babies on IPPV plus PEEP, but pneumothorax and pneumomediastinum may also occur:

- following overvigorous resuscitation at birth, with either a bag and mask or an ETT, especially if a small ETT was inserted and slipped down into a lobar bronchus (pp. 358–359);
- in association with any severe lung disease pre-IPPV, especially MAS and RDS;
- spontaneously: healthy neonates may generate inspiratory pressures exceeding 70 cmH$_2$O, which is well above the pressure at which normal lungs rupture.

When gas leaks out of an alveolus (or an acinar unit) in a neonate it rarely ruptures subpleurally but tracks along the bronchovascular bundle. If it is trapped within a bronchovascular bundle because there is more interstitial connective tissue in very premature lungs or because of damage caused by IPPV, PIE will develop (Fig. 13.11). PIE can take two forms. The diffuse form shown in Fig. 13.11 is characteristically seen in extremely low birth weight neonates. Another form with more patchy distribution and larger cystic space is virtually limited to babies who have required pressures of >30/5 cmH$_2$O for severe RDS or pulmonary hypoplasia. In both forms, the disease may be unilateral or even affect just one lobe.

If parenchymal gas gets as far as the mediastinum, it will cause a pneumomediastinum. From there it commonly ruptures into the plural cavity, giving a pneumothorax. Occasionally air in the mediastinum ruptures into the pericardium, or tracks down the mediastinal tissues, through the diaphragm and into the retroperitoneal tissues, where it may lodge or rupture out to give a pneumoperitoneum; air may also escape into the subcutaneous tissues. Terminally air may rupture into the vascular tree, causing a fatal air embolus. If babies with air leaks suddenly collapse, this diagnosis should be sought by early postmortem X-ray and at autopsy.

Clinical signs

Pneumothorax

A small non-tension pneumothorax may have little effect apart from mild respiratory difficulty or slight deterioration in the condition of a baby requiring IPPV. Radiological surveys of whole neonatal populations have shown an incidence of pneumothorax of 1.0–1.5%, most of them asymptomatic.

Tension pneumothorax is the most common cause of sudden deterioration in ventilated babies. It presents dramatically because ventilation is eventually severely compromised, with the lung collapsed on the side of the lesion and mediastinal shift compressing the contralateral lung. However, babies on HFOV may develop a tension pneumothorax slowly, with gradual deterioration over a matter of a few hours. The baby becomes increasingly dyspnoeic or apnoeic and is often pale and/or cyanosed. The mediastinal shift, by distorting the great vessels as they come through the diaphragm, may impair arterial perfusion to the lower half of the body, or dam back the venous return. This may reduce the cardiac output and may result in the baby being differentially perfused, with striking colour differences above and below the diaphragm. The affected side will be hyper-resonant on percussion, but on auscultation air entry may sound surprisingly good. The affected side transilluminates brilliantly with an appropriate bright light source. The abdomen may be distended and appear rigid, owing to the tension pneumothorax pushing the diaphragm down, compressing the abdominal contents.

Pulmonary interstitial emphysema

This is often asymptomatic, though when marked (Fig. 13.11) it causes a steady deterioration in the baby's blood gases with hypoxaemia and hypercapnia: it is one of the causes of neonates being impossible to oxygenate. The lungs may be very tympanitic and on auscultation there are often widespread fine crackles. If there are large amounts of trapped intrapulmonary gas, the lungs will transilluminate.

Pneumomediastinum

This is commonly asymptomatic, but there may be anterior bowing of the sternum and the heart sounds may be muffled. Diagnosis can be confirmed with CXR.

Pneumopericardium

This is often asymptomatic but should be considered in any seriously ill neonate known to be having problems with air leaks who becomes hypotensive (due to tamponade) or in whom the heart sounds become muffled.

Pneumoperitoneum

This also can be an incidental finding on X-ray. If large, the abdomen will become distended and tympanitic. It must be differentiated from perforation of a viscus, especially in NEC (see below).

Radiology

Diagnosis is made by appropriate X-rays, including a lateral horizontal beam film of the chest and abdomen. This is the only satisfactory way of demonstrating a pneumomediastinum and pneumoperitoneum where, with the baby lying supine, air collects under the sternum or the anterior abdominal wall. A similar view is also valuable for assessing the size of the pneumothorax in RDS where there is always a major degree of lung collapse, even without tension developing.

Differential diagnosis

There is rarely any difficulty with the differential diagnosis once the X-ray is taken. The problem is remembering to exclude air leaks such as pneumothorax and PIE by X-ray in any baby with worsening dyspnoea or hypoxaemia.

Treatment

Pneumothorax

Most babies with pneumothoraces already have severe lung disease such as RDS or meconium aspiration, and already have indwelling catheters and monitors attached when the pneumothorax develops. In the occasional baby in whom the pneumothorax is an isolated lesion, the basic routines of respiratory intensive care should be instituted. However, never leave a baby severely distressed with a tension pneumothorax while other procedures are carried out, with the exception of ventilation – if a baby with a tension pneumothorax is not already ventilated, secure the airway and establish artificial ventilation first.

All tension pneumothoraces, and all pneumothoraces in babies with primary lung disease, should be drained. In an emergency, a 17- or 19-gauge needle can be inserted anteriorly through the second intercostal space in the mid-clavicular line, but must always be followed by an FG10 or FG12 thoracentesis tube (pp. 359–361). Use local anaesthetic and give morphine unless the baby is moribund.

Since air gathers anteriorly, the tip of the drain should also be anterior and not lying in the paravertebral gutter. The tube should be firmly anchored to the chest wall and connected to an underwater seal and attached to suction of 10–20 cmH$_2$O. Without suction, removal of all the air in babies with severe lung disease is rarely possible. In sick babies the pneumothorax must be virtually completely drained. Therefore, always check the CXR after inserting the tube, and, if the pneumothorax persists, adjust the position of the tube. If this does not work, insert a second chest drain aiming towards the largest residual loculus of air.

After a baby develops a pneumothorax he is often much more difficult to oxygenate for the next 24–48 hours. Higher pressures, and the manoeuvres outlined on p. 145, are often required. Most babies after pneumothorax are much easier to manage if they are paralysed or sedated and they must be given adequate analgesia. Leave the drain in situ with applied suction until the lung has been expanded for at least 24 hours, and longer in babies on IPPV. When removing the drain the suction should be stopped, the tube clamped and then removed, checking with an X-ray to ensure that the pneumothorax has not reaccumulated. In the spontaneously breathing baby with a small non-tension pneumothorax, no underlying lung disease, minimal respiratory distress and satisfactory blood gases, the pneumothorax can be allowed to resolve spontaneously.

Pneumomediastinum

This commonly co-exists with pneumothorax. It cannot be drained, since it consists of multiple small locules of air within the connective tissue matrix of the mediastinum. If it causes symptoms, routine management of respiratory illness should be carried out.

Pulmonary interstitial emphysema

In the diffuse generalized form of this disease seen early in the course of RDS, the best initial approach is to paralyse the baby and ventilate him at 80–100 breaths/min using as low a MAP as possible, allowing the $PaCO_2$ to run at 8–9 kPa (60–65 mmHg) if necessary. It is in this situation that HFOV may be valuable if available.

If PIE is unilateral, the affected lung can be bypassed by selectively intubating the contralateral bronchus. The interstitial bubbles of gas are absorbed within 2–3 days and do not usually reappear when the lung reflates. Disappearance of the PIE has also been reported after lying the neonate for several days on the side of the affected lung. Large discrete cysts can be drained using a thoracentesis tube or differential bronchial intubation can be used. Occasionally a lobectomy is necessary.

Pneumopericardium

This is usually an incidental finding on CXR in a baby with other major air leaks (e.g. tension pneumothorax). If large it may cause cardiac tamponade. The pericardium can be drained via the sub-xiphoid route, using a FG17–19 Medicut, which can be left in situ if necessary until radiological proof of clearing is obtained.

Pneumoperitoneum

If this is under tension and is causing diaphragmatic splintage, it should be drained by paracentesis.

Subcutaneous emphysema

This should not, and in fact cannot, be treated.

■ Massive pulmonary haemorrhage

Aetiology

The following factors have been implicated: severe birth asphyxia, hypothermia, rhesus haemolytic disease, left heart failure especially with PDA or CHD, fluid overload, oxygen toxicity and coagulopathy. The unifying concept for all these factors is that they combine left-sided heart failure with pulmonary capillary damage. Initially this will cause pulmonary oedema, but eventually red cells will leak out of the capillaries. The haematocrit of pulmonary haemorrhage fluid is usually less than 10%, i.e. it is a haemorrhagic pulmonary oedema.

Clinical signs

The baby, usually seriously ill with one of the above conditions, suddenly deteriorates and becomes pale, cyanosed and limp, often over a 2–5-minute period. If he is being ventilated, bloody fluid will be found welling up his ETT. If not, he will usually become apnoeic and at laryngoscopy bloody fluid is seen welling up the trachea.

Radiology

In the acute phase the X-ray usually shows homogeneously opaque lungs, with some cardiac enlargement.

Treatment

All such babies should be intubated and ventilated, irrespective of whether or not they show any inclination to breathe spontaneously after resuscitation. If they are already on IPPV, the inflating pressure may need to be raised by 5–10 cmH$_2$O. The ventilator settings and the general management are those required for RDS.

Treat the underlying condition and in addition:

- Treat the baby for heart failure with diuretics in the first place.
- Arrange an echocardiogram to assess the size of the ductus arteriosus.
- Muscle relaxants such as pancuronium are virtually always necessary.
- Blood transfusion is usually required to correct the blood loss from the haemorrhage and the ensuing hypotension.
- Check blood coagulation studies. The baby often has disseminated intravascular coagulation following resuscitation. If this is present, treat accordingly (pp. 318–319).
- Control fluid intake very carefully. Fluid overload is often an iatrogenic component in the aetiology of the disease.
- If there is significant flow through the ductus (see above), give indomethocin once the coagulopathy is controlled and the platelet count is above 100×10^9/L.
- Surfactant – one or two doses depending on response – can be tried.

Persistent pulmonary hypertension of the newborn

Key points

- Pulmonary hypertension is a common complication in babies with severe lung disease (respiratory distress syndrome, meconium aspiration syndrome). In general, treatment in this group should be aimed at the respiratory problem.
- Persistent pulmonary hypertension of the newborn (PPHN) as a diagnosis should be restricted to those babies in whom pulmonary hypertension is the main (if not the sole) cause of their hypoxaemia, and in these babies treatment should be aimed at lowering the pulmonary artery pressure.
- The initial management of PPHN is conservative, keeping all physiological variables within the normal range in a paralysed baby. In particular, keep the PaCO$_2$ no higher than 5 kPa (37 mmHg) and use strict minimal handling (no physiotherapy).
- Babies with PPHN who remain persistently hypoxaemic may respond to inhaled nitric oxide.
- Weaning nitric oxide and intermittent positive pressure ventilation needs to be done slowly and carefully.

This condition is sometimes called persistent fetal circulation. We prefer the term PPHN because the placenta is no longer in the circulation. PPHN has an incidence of one in 1400 live births, and refers to the clinical situation that results when a newborn baby fails to complete the normal cardiorespiratory adaptation necessary for extra-uterine life (pp. 287–289). The basic problem in PPHN is a failure of the normal rapid decrease in pulmonary vascular resistance with the accompanying increase in pulmonary blood flow. Pulmonary vasodilation is mediated by prostacyclin, nitric oxide, endothelin 1 and PaO_2. Nitric oxide has recently been shown to be an effective treatment for PPHN (see below). Oxygen is an extremely potent pulmonary vasodilator, and PPHN can occur as a primary entity or accompany many conditions in which hypoxaemia is present (Table 13.9).

Pathophysiology

Histological examination of the pulmonary arterioles in babies who die from PPHN reveals an excessively muscular media, which extends further than usual down the small arteriolar branches. In animal models, chronic intra-uterine hypoxia produces similar medial hypertrophy of the peripheral pulmonary arteries.

Clinical signs

PPHN presents with cyanosis in the first 12 hours of life; the babies are blue but the respiratory distress is minimal. P2 may be loud, and a soft systolic murmur of tricuspid incompetence is occasionally heard. Cardiomegaly and heart failure are not features. The CXR usually shows a normal-sized heart with pulmonary vascularity normal to decreased. Characteristically there is a marked variability in the PaO_2 early in the course of the disease. Once PPHN is established there is persistent severe hypoxaemia.

Investigations

There may be a mild decrease in lung markings on the CXR, but unless the PPHN is secondary to hypoxaemia accompanying lung disease (Table 13.9) the CXR is unremarkable. Cross-sectional echocardiography will demonstrate a structurally normal heart. Ventricular function may be reduced and there may be a PDA. Indirect assessment of the pulmonary artery pressure is possible with Doppler ultrasound. Colour Doppler may show tricuspid incompetence, in which case the Bernoulli equation (pressure = $4V^2$ where V = peak velocity of the regurgitant jet) can be used to estimate the pulmonary artery pressure. Colour Doppler can also demonstrate right-to-left shunting across the foramen ovale and at ductal level.

Table 13.9 Conditions in which persistent pulmonary hypertension of the newborn can develop

Chronic intra-uterine hypoxia resulting in primary PPHN	
Alveolar capillary dysplasia	
Diaphragmatic hernia	p. 276
Congenital heart disease	pp. 287–306
Meconium aspiration syndrome	pp. 155–157
GBS septicaemia	pp. 197–198
Pulmonary hypoplasia	p. 165
Hypoxic ischaemic encephalopathy	pp. 220–224
Respiratory distress syndrome	pp. 130–135
Maternal prostaglandin synthetase inhibitor treatment	
Maternal lithium treatment	

GBS, group B beta-haemolytic *Streptococcus*.

Treatment

1. Maintain as many physiological variables within the normal range as possible, paying particular attention to:
   - blood gases;
   - blood pressure (mean arterial pressure should be initially maintained around 50 mmHg but higher levels may be necessary in severe cases); dopamine is the first-line inotrope of choice, with noradrenaline as second line (dobutamine should be avoided);
   - electrolytes and calcium;
   - blood glucose;
   - PCV.
2. Give antibiotics after taking cultures (risk of GBS).
3. Minimal handling is crucial because slight interference from suction, physiotherapy or a CXR can cause a dramatic increase in pulmonary artery pressure and clinical deterioration.
4. Monitor all variables as outlined on pp. 51–62. Continuous PaO_2 and SpO_2 monitoring is essential, ideally recording from both pre- and post-ductal sites.
5. Use paralysis, sedation and analgesia liberally.

If the pulmonary artery pressure (and oxygen requirement) does not fall with this conservative management, physiological pulmonary artery vasodilatation should be attempted using nitric oxide.

Formerly many other drugs, including tolazoline and prostacyclin, were used, but all have the disadvantage of reducing systemic BP as much as (or more than) they reduce the pulmonary arterial pressure. They may still need to be used in emergency when nitric oxide is not available while awaiting transfer to a specialist centre. Magnesium sulphate has been used and it is certainly of value to measure magnesium levels and consider giving intravenous magnesium sulphate to bring plasma levels to the upper end of the normal range.

Using nitric oxide in persistent pulmonary hypertension of the newborn

- In significant PPHN nitric oxide should be started at 20 ppm.
- Measure the methaemoglobin concentration after 1 hour of nitric oxide administration (reduce the concentration if the levels are above 5%).
- If no response there it is often worth trying to increase to 30 ppm, but if no significant improvement discussions should be had with an ECMO centre (see p. 157).
- Once the inspired oxygen concentration is down to 40%, begin weaning nitric oxide.
- Wean by 1 ppm every hour while the blood gases remain stable (use transcutaneous/continuous monitoring if possible to reduce the number of samples) until 3 ppm is reached.
- Wean the last 5 ppm more slowly, say 1 ppm every 2–3 hours. This is because in some babies endogenous manufacture appears to be inhibited during nitric oxide therapy.
- Watch for rebound. Some babies need nitric oxide restarting.

Extracorporeal membrane oxygenation

ECMO is a modification of heart–lung bypass technology which has been developed for use in babies with severe pulmonary or cardiopulmonary failure. The main indications for use are MAS and PPHN, and these babies do best. ECMO candidates must be >2 kg in weight and >34 weeks' gestation because of the risk of intracerebral haemorrhage associated with heparin anticoagulation. Infants who are ventilated with an oxygenation index greater than 30–40 (Appendix 2) should be considered for ECMO and discussed with an ECMO centre because their predicted mortality is very high.

Survival after ECMO in babies with PPHN and MAS is over 90%; mortality in this group was reduced by a half in the UK randomized controlled trial (UK Collaborative ECMO Study Group 1996). Outcome remains poor for babies with congenital diaphragmatic hernia who require ECMO; these babies usually have irreversible pulmonary hypoplasia. The most feared and common complication of ECMO is bleeding; platelet consumption is inevitable. Neurological sequelae (including hearing loss) are quite common, with 16% of this severely ill group having CNS abnormality detectable at a year.

Pulmonary hypoplasia

Pulmonary hypoplasia can be due to an underlying syndrome such as Potter's or one of the short-limbed dwarfism syndromes which are associated with a small chest. In this situation pulmonary hypoplasia is one part of a lethal malformation, should be recognized as such, and intensive care is inappropriate. Pulmonary hypoplasia may also occur as an insolated and lethal abnormality which will be recognized only if, at autopsy, lung weights are carefully measured. Two groups of babies with pulmonary hypoplasia are important and should be treated:

- preterm babies delivered after prolonged preterm rupture of the membranes; in general this type of pulmonary hypoplasia develops only if the membranes rupture before 26 weeks' gestation;
- congenital diaphragmatic hernia.

Pulmonary hypoplasia secondary to prolonged preterm rupture of the membranes

These babies can be identified from the history and by the presence of small-volume lungs on the initial CXR, which may or may not show parenchymal changes, the respiratory failure in some babies being due simply to the small alveolar volume. The management of the (usually) preterm baby in respiratory failure from this variant of pulmonary hypoplasia is the same as that for RDS. The following points should be noted:

- There is a high risk of co-existing infection. Always give antibiotics.
- Surfactant is beneficial in some cases and should be tried.
- High peak pressures (>30 cmH_2O) and longer inspiratory times (up to 1.0 second) may be required for 24–48 hours to 'open up' the lungs.
- When pressures >25 cmH_2O are being used, give pancuronium.
- If, despite high pressures, long T_i, an FiO_2 of 0.95 and surfactant, the baby remains hypoxic and hypercarbic, a trial of HFOV and nitric oxide is worth attempting. If these measures fail to improve the blood gases and the lungs remain small on a CXR, the prognosis is hopeless and intensive care should be withdrawn.

Pulmonary hypoplasia associated with congenital diaphragmatic hernia

There is usually severe pulmonary hypoplasia on the ipsilateral side and some hypoplasia on the contralateral side, which is squashed *in utero* by the mediastinal shift. The lung hypoplasia causes severe respiratory failure, which usually presents within minutes of delivery as a cyanosed dyspnoeic baby who may need active resuscitation in the labour ward with IPPV and high concentrations of oxygen.

Up to 50% of babies with congenital diaphragmatic hernia, no matter what is tried, never become adequately oxygenated and die within 12–24 hours. Among the remainder are some who respond to full intensive care with nitric oxide, paralysis and ventilation and a further subset who are easy to ventilate. Babies should be stabilized for some days before carrying out corrective surgery and should generally be off inotropes and on conventional ventilation before considering surgical intervention. The surgical management is outlined on pp. 276–277.

Pleural effusions (chylothorax)

These may be part of generalized hydrops. Isolated neonatal pleural effusions usually become chylous once the baby is feeding. Treatment is recurrent pleural taps, often combined with feeds containing medium chain triglycerides to reduce chyle formation. In refractory cases, and in discussion with respiratory specialists, octreotide may be of value. The prognosis is good.

■ Congenital malformations affecting the respiratory tract

Congenital lobar emphysema

This condition can present at any age in infancy with respiratory distress, cyanosis and a characteristic CXR showing severe emphysema, usually of an upper lobe, with a mediastinal shift. Differential diagnosis from localized PIE is usually easy on the basis of the history. Treat cases presenting as an emergency by resection of the affected lobe.

Congenital cystic adenomatoid malformation

Congenital cystic adenomatoid malformations (CCAMs) are now usually recognized during antenatal ultrasound examinations, although the diagnosis is not completely reliable. Antenatally the diagnosis relies on imaging a solid/cystic area within the thorax. An antenatally diagnosed CCAM can disappear during pregnancy. A few enlarge and cause fetal death, hydrops or pulmonary hypoplasia, which is fatal after birth. The majority cause minimal neonatal respiratory illness or are asymptomatic. Those causing symptoms should certainly be resected. A CXR is normally performed as a postnatal investigation but often appears normal. Asymptomatic babies should remain with their mother on the postnatal ward and be discharged as normal. A post-discharge CT should be performed in all cases and a referral made to the surgeons. Whether all these cases should be operated to prevent infection or the potential for malignant change remains controversial.

Upper airway obstruction

Choanal atresia

In this rare condition the baby can breathe only through his mouth. Since most neonates are obligate nose breathers, babies with choanal atresia are fine when they are crying, but go blue and breathless when their mouths are closed. This characteristic clinical picture usually presents immediately after birth and should be recognized instantly despite its rarity (1:60,000 live births), otherwise the baby may die of respiratory obstruction rather than keep his mouth open. The baby should be forced to breathe through his mouth by inserting a Magill airway, or even an ETT, until appropriate surgery can be carried out on his posterior choanae.

Babies with unilateral atresia, or those who are able to breathe through their mouths, may present much later in infancy with a purulent discharge from the obstructed nostril.

Pierre Robin syndrome (micrognathia, midline cleft palate and glossoptosis)

This syndrome may cause acute neonatal upper respiratory tract obstruction owing to the tongue falling back and obstructing the oropharynx. An airway can usually be sustained in the short term by inserting a Magill airway and lying the baby prone, often with his head extended, allowing the tongue and small mandible to fall forward. If problems persist, a long nasopharyngeal tube connected to a CPAP circuit is often successful. Small laryngeal airways are available and have been used successfully in emergencies in this situation. The laryngeal airway is like a small mask on the end of an ETT and is designed to sit over the larynx when inserted. There is a soft air-filled 'hovercraft' skirt which is blown up when the mask is in situ. If all these do not work and intubation cannot be achieved (intubation of such babies can be exceptionally difficult owing to the small mandible), emergency tracheostomy should be considered.

In the first week or two of life, with various combinations of palatal obturators, lying the baby prone, nasopharyngeal airways and spoon or tube feeding, it is usually possible to achieve normal growth and often to get the baby home. However, in severe forms of the malformation, tracheostomy and long-term hospital stay may be necessary to allow the baby to breathe, feed and grow before surgical repair is possible. There is a risk of sudden death in Pierre Robin syndrome.

In the long term the mandible grows and the cleft palate can be repaired. The modern tendency is to close the palate as soon as possible, once the baby is thriving.

Congenital laryngeal stridor/laryngomalacia

Severe forms of this disorder may present in the neonatal period. So long as the baby feeds well and thrives, does not have severe choking episodes, has a normal $PaCO_2$ and does not develop signs of cor pulmonale, a watching brief can be held in the expectation that as his larynx grows the stridor will lessen. In the very small percentage of babies in whom this is not the case, a tracheostomy is necessary in the neonatal period and is likely to be in situ for 6–12 months.

■ References

Ceruti, E (1966) Chemoreceptor reflexes in the newborn. *Pediatrics*, **37**: 556–64.

Crowley, PA (1997) Corticosteroids prior to preterm delivery. In Neilson JP, Crowther CA, Hodrett ED, *et al.* (eds) *Pregnancy and Childbirth Module of the Cochrane Database of Systematic Reviews.* The Cochrane Collaboration. Issue 3. Oxford: Update Software.

Dawes, GS (1966) Pulmonary circulation in the fetus and newborn. *British Medical Bulletin*, **22**: 61–5.

Dawson JA, Kamlin COF, Vento M, *et al.* (2010) Defining the reference range for oxygen saturation for infants after birth. *Pediatrics*, **125**: e1340–7.

Godfrey, S (1981) Growth and development of the respiratory system: functional developments. In Davis, JA, Dobbing, J (eds) *Scientific Foundations of Paediatrics,*

2nd edition. London: William Heinemann Medical Books, pp. 432–9.

Gribetz, I, Frank, NR, Avery, ME (1959) Static volume pressure relations of excised lungs of infants with hyaline membrane disease; newborns and stillborn infants. *Journal of Clinical Investigation*, **38**: 2168–75.

Morley CJ (1997) Systematic review of prophylactic versus rescue surfactant. *Archives of Disease in Childhood*, **77**: F70–4.

Soll, RF (2009) Synthetic surfactant for respiratory distress syndrome in preterm infants. *Cochrane Database of Systematic Reviews*, **1**: CD001149.

Stevens, TP, Sinkin, RA (2007) Surfactant replacement therapy. *Chest*, **131**(5): 1577–82.

UK Collaborative ECMO Study Group (1996) UK collaborative trial of neonatal ECMO. *Lancet*, **348**: 75–82.

Vain, NE, Prudent, LM, Stevens, DP, *et al.* (1989) Regulation of oxygen concentration delivered to infants via nasal cannulas. *American Journal of Diseases of Children*, **143**: 1458–60.

Ziegler, JW, Ivy, DD, Kinsella, JP, Abman, SH (1995) The role of nitric oxide, endothelin and prostaglandins in the transition of the pulmonary circulation. *Clinics in Perinatology*, **22**: 387–403.

◼ Further reading

Ahluwalia, J, White, DK, Morley, CJ (1998) Infant flow driver or single nasal prong continuous positive airway pressure: short-term physiological effects. *Acta Paediatrica*, **87**: 325–7.

Baumer, JH (2000) International randomised controlled clinical trial of patient triggered ventilation in neonatal RDS. *Archives of Disease in Childhood*, **82**: F5–10.

Blayney, MP, Logan, DR (1994) First thoracic vertebral body as a reference point for endotracheal tube placement. *Archives of Disease in Childhood*, **71**: F32–5.

Bourchier, D, Weston, PJ (1997) Randomised trial of dopamine compared with hydrocortisone for the treatment of hypotensive very low birthweight infants. *Archives of Disease in Childhood*, **76**: 174–8.

Cools, F, Offringa, M (1999) Meta-analysis of elective high frequency ventilation in preterm infants with respiratory distress syndrome. *Archives of Disease in Childhood*, **80**: F15–20.

Crowther, CA (1997) Antenatal thyrotropin-releasing hormone (TRH) prior to preterm delivery. In Neilson JP, Crowther CA, Hodnett ED, *et al.* (eds) *Pregnancy and Childbirth Module of the Cochrane Database of Systematic Reviews*. Oxford: Update Software.

Davis, PG, Henderson-Smart, DJ (1998) Extubation of premature infants from low-rate IPPV vs extubation after a trial of endotracheal CPAP. In Neilson JP, Crowther CA, Hodnett ED, *et al.* (eds) *Pregnancy and Childbirth Module of the Cochrane Database of Systematic Reviews*. Oxford: Update Software.

Dunn, PM (1965) The respiratory distress syndrome of the newborn. Immaturity versus prematurity. *Archives of Disease in Childhood*, **40**: 62–5.

Greenough, A, Milner, AD (2006) *Neonatal Lung Disease*, 2nd edition. London: Edward Arnold.

Greenough A, Dimitriou G, Prendergast M, Milner AD (2008) Synchronized mechanical ventilation for respiratory support in newborn infants. *Cochrane Database of Systematic Reviews*, **1**: CD000456.

Greenough, A, Milner AD (2012) Acute respiratory disease. In Rennie, JM (ed.) *Rennie & Roberton's Textbook of Neonatology*, 5th edition. Edinburgh: Elsevier pp. 468–551.

Henderson-Smart, DJ, Davis, PG (1998) Prophylactic methylxanthine for extubation in preterm infants. In Neilson JP, Crowther CA, Hodnett ED, *et al.* (eds) *Pregnancy and Childbirth Module of the Cochrane Database of Systematic Reviews*. Oxford: Update Software.

Jobe, AH, Mitchell, BR, Gankel, JH (1993) Beneficial effects of the combined administration of prenatal corticosteroids and postnatal surfactant on preterm infants. *American Journal of Obstetrics and Gynecology*, **168**: 508–13.

Keszler, M, Donn, SM, Bucciarelli, RL (1991) Multicenter controlled trial comparing high frequency jet ventilation and conventional mechanical ventilation in newborn infants with pulmonary interstitial emphysema. *Journal of Pediatrics*, **119**: 85–93.

Klaus, MH, Fanaroff, AA (1979) *Care of the High Risk Neonate*. London: WB Saunders, p. 214.

Neonatal Inhaled Nitric Oxide Study (NINOS) Group (1997) Inhaled nitric oxide in full-term and nearly full-term infants with hypoxic respiratory failure. *New England Journal of Medicine*, **336**: 597–604.

Nio, M, Haase, G, Kennaugh, J, *et al.* (1994) A prospective randomised trial of delayed versus immediate repair of congenital diaphragmatic hernia. *Journal of Pediatric Surgery*, **29**: 618–21.

Robertson, PA, Sniderman, SH, Laros, RK, *et al.* (1992) Neonatal morbidity according to gestational age and birthweight from five tertiary care centres in the United States 1983–1986. *American Journal of Obstetrics and Gynecology*, **166**: 1629–45.

Schmidt, B, Roberts RS, Davis P, *et al.* Caffeine for Apnea of Prematurity Trial Group (2007) Long-term effects of caffeine therapy for apnea of prematurity.

New England Journal of Medicine, **357**(19): 1893–902.

Seid, AB, Canty, TG (1985) The anterior cricoid split procedure for the management of subglottic stenosis in infants and children. *Journal of Pediatric Surgery*, **20**: 388–96.

Sinha, SK, Donn, SM (1996) Advances in neonatal conventional ventilation. *Archives of Disease in Childhood*, **75**: F135–40.

Subhedar, NV, Ryan, SW, Shaw, NJ (1997) Open randomised controlled trial of inhaled nitric oxide and early dexamethasone in high risk infants. *Archives of Disease in Childhood*, **77**: F185–90.

van den Berg E, Lemmers PM, Toet MC, *et al.* (2010) Effect of the 'InSurE' procedure on cerebral oxygenation and electrical brain activity of the preterm infant. *Archives of Disease in Childhood. Fetal and Neonatal Edition*, **95**(1): F53–8.

Wheeler K, Klingenberg C, McCallion N, *et al.* Volume-targeted versus pressure-limited ventilation in the neonate. *Cochrane Database of Systematic Reviews*, **11**: CD003666.

Whyte, S, Birrell, G, Wyllie, J (2000) Premedication before intubation in UK neonatal units. *Archives of Disease in Childhood*, **82**: F38–41.

14

Chronic lung disease

Key points

- Chronic lung disease (CLD) develops in up to 30% of very low birth weight and 50% of extremely low birth weight babies.
- Prevention is difficult; steroids, surfactant and a low-fluid regimen do not prevent CLD, but 'gentle' ventilation and avoidance of infection probably do.
- Rescue treatment after 14 days with systemic steroids is currently the most effective therapy.
- Long-term treatment with diuretics, inhaled steroids or bronchodilators or other agents is not of proven benefit.
- Babies who are still ventilator dependent at 50 days have a poor prognosis, with a high chance of death or disability.

The terms chronic lung disease (CLD) and bronchopulmonary dysplasia (BPD) are often used interchangeably. A National Institute of Health (NIH)-sponsored workshop recommended using the term BPD to clearly distinguish this condition from the multiple chronic lung diseases of later life (Jobe and Bancalari 2001), yet CLD is still in common parlance in many neonatal intensive care units (NICUs). CLD remains one of the major problems of neonatal medicine. Every neonatologist is all too familiar with the very preterm infant who initially does well, but who then spends many months in the neonatal unit (NNU) oxygen dependent.

The definition of CLD consists of a combination of oxygen requirement and changes seen on chest X-ray (CXR). The original description referred to babies who remain oxygen dependent for more than 28 days after earlier requiring mechanical ventilation in the first week, with persistent X-ray changes. With the increasing survival of extreme preterm infants these criteria have been applied to babies at 36 weeks post-conceptional age. The NIH-sponsored workshop suggested a combined definition of 'new BPD' based on the gestation at birth. This classification further defines the condition into mild, moderate and severe (Table 14.1).

CLD is rare in babies born at more than 30 weeks of gestation or over 1000 g, although the occasional case is seen in term infants who require ventilation. Among the UK EPICure cohort of babies born at less than 26 weeks' gestation in 1995, 50% were still in oxygen at their expected date of delivery, and of these children 16% remained in oxygen at a year.

Aetiology

The typical infant who develops CLD is the extremely premature baby who initially required only gentle ventilation with air at low pressures, more for poor respiratory effort than severe respiratory distress syndrome (RDS). Babies who are born when

Table 14.1 Definitions and diagnostic criteria for bronchopulmonary dysplasia (BPD) (from Jobe and Bancalari 2001)

Gestational age at birth	<32 weeks	≥32 weeks
Time of assessment	36-week corrected gestational age or discharge to home, whichever comes first	>28 days but <56 days postnatal age or discharge to home, whichever comes first
	Treatment with oxygen >21% for at least 28 days plus	
Mild BPD	Breathing room air at 36-week PMA or discharge, whichever comes first	Breathing room air by 56 days postnatal age or discharge, whichever comes first
Moderate BPD	Need for <30% oxygen at 36-week PMA or discharge, whichever comes first	Need for <30% oxygen at 56 days postnatal age or discharge, whichever comes first
Severe BPD	Need for ≥30% oxygen and/or positive pressure (PPV or NCPAP) at 36-week PMA or discharge, whichever comes first	Need for ≥30% oxygen and/or positive pressure (PPV or NCPAP) at 56 days postnatal age or discharge, whichever comes first

NCPAP, nasal continuous positive airway pressure; PMA, postmenstrual age; PPV, positive pressure ventilation.

their lungs are at the canalicular or saccular stages of development – that is, at 23–30 weeks of gestation – are at the greatest risk (Baraldi and Filippone 2007, Fig. 14.1). As the weeks go by the baby cannot be weaned off intermittent positive pressure ventilation.

To the classic description of the aetiology of CLD 'oxygen plus pressure plus time' can now be added genetic predisposition, immature lung structure, infection, poor nutrition and fluid overload often associated with patent ductus arteriosus (PDA). Mechanical ventilation is clearly important, either because of pressure (barotrauma) or volume

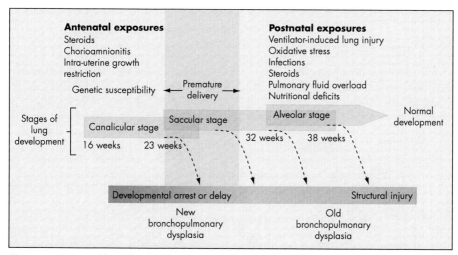

Fig. 14.1 Stages of lung development, potentially damaging factors and types of lung injury. From Baraldi and Filippone (2007), reproduced with permission from Massachusetts Medical Society

Table 14.2 Aetiological factors in chronic lung disease

1.	High-pressure, long inspiratory time ventilation with or without air leak
2.	Ventilation with variable volume delivery, perhaps because of insufficient positive end expiratory pressure
3.	Pulmonary oxygen toxicity
4.	Persisting immaturity of the surfactant system
5.	Very immature lungs (easily damaged by 1 and 2 and 3)
6.	Patent ductus arteriosus and fluid overload
7.	Infection, including chorioamnionitis, via inflammatory cytokine release
8.	Disturbance of the elastase/protease system in the lung destroying the parenchyma
9.	Gastro-oesophageal reflux and inhalation of gastric contents
10.	Genetic factors including male sex and genetic polymorphisms

(volutrauma) damage to the lungs. The effects of oxygen, positive pressure ventilation and inflammation combine to cause a cascade of destruction and abnormal repair in the lung during a critical period of active growth. Exposure to an antenatal fetal inflammatory response results in local production of potentially damaging pro-inflammatory mediators. How these factors interact and the pathway or pathways of injury have yet to be defined. The factors implicated are summarized in Fig. 14.1 and Table 14.2.

Natural history

The fact that a ventilated neonate is developing CLD is usually apparent by 7–14 days of age. He either stops improving or actually deteriorates both clinically and radiologically. The CXR shows increasing haziness with or without cysts. At this stage marked bronchorrhoea may occur, the aspirate consisting of dysplastic and metaplastic epithelial cells, macrophages and polymorphs. Infection probably contributes to increased bronchoconstriction via inflammatory mediators, and increased neutrophil counts, elevated levels of leukotrienes and platelet activating factor have all been found in the tracheal aspirate of babies developing CLD.

Clinical features

If still ventilated, the baby has a falling PaO_2 and rising $PaCO_2$. If not ventilated he is permanently dyspnoeic, often with an overinflated chest. Crackles and wheezes are frequently heard throughout both lung fields even in the absence of heart failure. If heart failure does develop there will be tachycardia, a triple rhythm, hepatosplenomegaly and peripheral oedema. Cor pulmonale should be suspected when there is a pronounced right ventricular heave, a loud and sometimes the murmur of tricuspid regurgitation. Feeding is hard work for these babies and is often accompanied by episodes of desaturation, vomiting and increased breathing difficulties.

Investigations

The electrocardiogram may show right ventricle overload and echocardiography can be used to measure the size of the right ventricle and to estimate the degree of pulmonary hypertension. Pulmonary function tests show increased airways resistance, increased airway reactivity and reduced compliance.

Differential diagnosis

The definition of CLD is given above. On this basis there is effectively no differential diagnosis. The radiological changes of Wilson–Mikity syndrome (p. 178) are not dissimilar from the cystic changes of milder CLD, but the antecedent history clearly differentiates the two conditions.

Histology

In established disease there is widespread destruction of the pulmonary tissue, which is replaced by areas of collapse and emphysema, surrounded by organizing fibrous tissue. There is peribronchial fibrosis, and the bronchial walls are thickened with muscular hypertrophy. There is often necrosis proceeding to musocal hyperplasia and squamous metaplasia of the bronchial lining. Smaller bronchi may be obliterated. There are changes of pulmonary hypertension in the arteries.

Radiology

Northway *et al.* (1967) described four distinct radiographic appearances:

- Stage 1: radiographically indistinguishable from severe RDS (1–3 days).
- Stage 2: marked radio-opacity of the lungs (4–10 days).
- Stage 3: clearing of the radio-opacity into a cystic, bubbly pattern (10–20 days).
- Stage 4: hyperexpansion, streaks of abnormal density and areas of emphysema with variable cardiomegaly (from 1 month). By 4–5 months the changes may still be severe, with a characteristic broad chest and high diaphragm.

Interventions for chronic lung disease

Prevention

- Much effort has gone into trying to prevent or minimize CLD. There has been little success. Antenatal steroids, antenatal thyrotrophin releasing hormone and

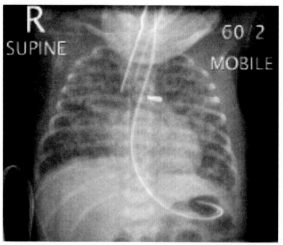

Fig. 14.2 Chest X-ray of severe chronic lung disease

surfactant therapies have had little effect. Minimizing barotrauma/volutrauma using modern invasive and non-invasive ventilation techniques is important.

■ Meticulous control of fluid balance and early treatment of a PDA may also reduce the incidence of CLD. Furthermore, nutrition plays a key role in supporting normal lung growth and development.

■ Prophylactic measures such as vitamins A and E, and superoxide dismutase have not proved successful.

■ There is a considerable difference in the incidence of CLD in different units and there is a widely held belief that this is related to careful fluid balance and/or 'gentler' ventilation techniques in extremely low birth weight babies.

Monitoring

Babies with CLD should have electrolytes and a blood count measured once or twice a week. Regular monitoring of C-reactive protein (CRP) may provide early warning of infection, and blood and endotracheal tube secretion cultures should be obtained if there are concerns regarding infection. Acid–base status in these babies can be monitored effectively by capillary samples, and pulse oximetry comes into its own as the ideal way of monitoring oxygenation in this group. X-rays should be taken if there are any signs of increasing respiratory distress or concerns about deterioration.

Infection

In the fluctuating clinical course characteristic of CLD it can be formidably difficult to decide whether an episode of deterioration is due to infection. Changes in the temperature, white blood cell (WBC) count, CRP, CXR and the nature of any aspirate from the airway can be very helpful.

Because one cannot afford to ignore the possibility of infection in babies with CLD who deteriorate, these babies inevitably get many courses of broad-spectrum antibiotics (after taking appropriate cultures, of course). Fungal infection can emerge and needs prompt treatment. Antibiotics should be stopped after 2–3 days if there is no laboratory confirmation of infection.

Intercurrent viral infections, especially respiratory syncytial virus (RSV) bronchiolitis, are a major threat. Care should be taken to protect babies with CLD from contact with staff or relatives with respiratory infections. Influenza vaccine should be given to babies with CLD in the winter months in addition to the usual vaccines, including pertussis.

The use of palivizumab is recommended for preterm infants with CLD (defined as oxygen dependency for at least 28 days from birth) at the chronological ages at the start of the RSV season and gestational ages at birth covered within the shaded area in Table 14.3.

Management

There is no specific treatment other than to keep the baby alive without further damage to his lungs, in the hope that the restrictive changes in his airways will resolve or can be controlled pharmacologically, pulmonary hypertension and cor pulmonale (and other complications, see Table 14.4) can be prevented, and the normal growth of alveoli from 30×10^6 at 28/52 to 250×10^6 at 8 years will steadily progress. The chief aspects of management are discussed below and are:

■ management of oxygen therapy and respiratory support, preventing pulmonary hypertension;

Table 14.3 Cost-effective use of palivizumab (shaded area) for preterm infants with chronic lung disease (CLD) by chronological age (months) at the start of the respiratory syncytial virus season (beginning of October) and gestational age at birth (weeks) (from the UK Joint Committee on Vaccination and Immunisation)

Gestational age at birth (whole weeks)							
Chronological age (months)	≤24	>24 to ≤26	>26 to ≤28	>28 to ≤30	>30 to ≤32	>32 to ≤34	≥35
1.0 to <1.5	█	█	█	█	█	█	
1.5–3	█	█	█	█	█		
3–6	█	█	█				
6–9	█						
>9							

The definition of CLD is oxygen dependency for at least 28 days from birth. All gestational ages are based on whole weeks.

- management of nutrition and fluid balance;
- prevention and treatment of infection;
- steroid therapy;
- other measures, e.g. bronchodilators.

Respiratory support

The most important single factor in getting the baby with CLD off the ventilator is being prepared to accept $PaCO_2$ values in the 8–9.5 kPa (60–70 mmHg) range or even higher so long as PO_2, pH and vital signs are stable ('permissive hypercarbia'). The process of weaning should progress exactly as outlined on pp. 152–153, albeit slowly. Use the lowest possible peak inspiratory pressure; high levels of positive and expiratory pressure may help to maintain alveoli at a constant volume. Caffeine and other drugs (see below) are helpful.

Oxygen

Oxygen is the mainstay of treatment for CLD. See Table 7.2 for our recommendations regarding target saturation readings in babies receiving oxygen. Basically, for babies

Table 14.4 Complications associated with chronic lung disease

Poor growth
Airway hyper-reactivity
Airway problems – tracheomalacia, subglottic stenosis from prolonged intubation
Neurodevelopmental delay
Respiratory tract infection
Pulmonary hypertension
Systemic hypertension
Metabolic bone disease
Gastrointestinal reflux, vomiting
Steroid side effects (see Table 14.5)
Nephrocalcinosis from diuretic therapy

of ≤32 weeks post-conceptional age, aim for saturations of 91–95%. The pooled results of several large trials (BOOST, SUPPORT) have shown survival to 36 weeks to be higher when SpO_2 targets of 91–95% were chosen rather than 85–89% (Stenson *et al.* 2011). Once the baby is ≥33 weeks there is less risk of retinopathy of prematurity (ROP), and for babies with CLD the aim is to avoid pulmonary hypertension, so we aim for a saturation of >94%. Cor pulmonale secondary to pulmonary hypertension is much less common than previously but is still a potential risk in CLD. To minimize the degree of hypoxic pulmonary vasoconstriction, although CO_2 can be allowed to rise to 9.5 kPa (70 mmHg) PaO_2 should be kept in the 8–12 kPa range (SpO_2 90–95%). The oxygen-carrying capacity of the blood should be maintained by transfusion, and we aim to keep the packed cell volume above 35% when the baby requires >35% oxygen.

Fluids/nutrition

These need to be carefully supervised, balancing the risks of overhydration and heart failure against the increased caloric requirements of these babies. Most CLD babies tolerate enteral feeds, which should be given at 150–180 mL/kg/24 h and of sufficient caloric density to ensure a weight gain of approximately 15 g/kg/day.

Every effort should be made to encourage oral (breast) feeding once it is possible to nurse a baby with CLD in nasal cannula oxygen. Experience has taught us that unless this is done early they can become phobic of any stimuli round their mouths and become extremely difficult to feed orally in the weeks and months ahead. In some babies, vomiting and gastro-oesophageal reflux is a problem. If this cannot be controlled easily by inclining the head of the cot and possibly anti-reflux medications, fundoplication will have to be considered.

Diuretics

These improve lung compliance and airways resistance in the short term in CLD. A single dose of furosemide is useful as an interim measure when babies are breathless, with increased oxygen requirements and excessive weight gain. Those babies with signs of incipient right heart failure who respond to furosemide should be considered for a short course of chlorthiazide and spironolactone. Using diuretics long term can have serious consequences and there is no evidence that they shorten the course of CLD. Furosemide may cause hypercalciuria, nephrocalcinosis and haematuria, although these usually resolve when the drug is stopped.

Hyponatraemia, hypocalaemia and hypochloraemia are also common with any diuretic regimen. Hypochloraemia with the resultant metabolic alkalaemia can be a particular problem and is an adverse prognostic finding.

Steroids

Since first introduced 20 years ago the use of steroids in CLD has generated controversy. The initial wave of enthusiasm for dexamethasone as a treatment for CLD was followed by concerns about the long-term neurodevelopmental effects of this treatment. More recently the use of hydrocortisone as an alternative to dexamethasone has become more prevalent.

The neurodevelopmental concerns have resulted in a dramatic reduction in steroid use in the last 10 years associated with an increase in BPD (Yoder *et al.* 2009). The risk may be related to the age at which the treatment is given; a meta-analysis of 20 randomized trials demonstrated that only early and not late treatment was associated with a significant excess of cerebral palsy (Doyle *et al.* 2010).

Steroids are clearly of some value in CLD (Watterberg 2010), and we currently use hydrocortisone in babies who are at least 14 days old, with severe lung disease and who are ventilator dependent with high oxygen requirements. If there is no response within 72 hours then steroids are stopped; if the baby responds with a significant reduction in oxygen/ventilatory requirements then steroids are continued for up to 7–10 days (or until successfully extubated) before slowly weaning over approximately 3 weeks.

Whenever starting parenteral steroids there is always anxiety about sepsis. Baseline cultures should be taken and a WBC count and CRP measured. We do not use antibiotics routinely when starting steroids, but would choose to be cautious in a baby who was already on an antibiotic cocktail and in these we would continue antibiotic treatment. Steroid treatment of CLD has accumulated a formidable list of side effects (Table 14.5). Most of these are reversible by drug withdrawal.

Bronchodilators

Giving β-mimetics and occasionally ipratropium by inhalation may improve these babies. On the NICU, bronchodilators are rarely necessary and should be administered only to those infants with symptomatic wheeze and in whom respiratory support requirements are reduced as a consequence of bronchodilator administration.

Airway intervention

Some babies with CLD have tracheomegaly and/or peripheral airway collapse: tracheobronchomalacia. This can be diagnosed only by bronchoscopy or tracheobronchography. Nevertheless, the possibility should be borne in mind because treatment can be offered in the form of balloon dilatation of the stenosed airway, or aortopexy.

Baby stimulation and parental support

Babies with CLD spend many months in the nursery and thought needs to be given to the provision of an appropriate environment for them and their parents.

Table 14.5 Side effects of steroids in chronic lung disease

| Reduced growth, including lung growth |
| Increased protein catabolism (raised urea) |
| Hypertension |
| Hyperglycaemia[a] |
| Cardiomyopathy |
| Sepsis (especially fungal) |
| Possible later neuromotor effects, including cerebral palsy |
| Osteomalacia |
| Cataract |
| Gastrointestinal haemorrhage[b] |
| Adrenal suppression[c] |
| Reduced immunological response to immunizations |

[a]Treatment, p. 244.

[b]Treatment, p. 284.

[c]Treatment, pp. 255–257.

Discharge

Some babies make a full recovery within 3–4 months. Others by this stage are still oxygen dependent. If they are requiring less than 30% inspired oxygen, are stable, off steroids and diuretics, and feeding orally they can be discharged home, receiving nasal cannula oxygen. This is obviously a major exercise involving the family, the NNU, the GP and the community services, and the management is beyond the remit of this book.

Prognosis

The longer the baby stays on the ventilator, the less likely he is to survive. Babies still ventilator dependent at 3 months or in more than 50% oxygen at 6 months have a very poor prognosis. Pre-discharge mortality is usually caused by infection, cardiac or respiratory failure. Infants with BPD require a prolonged hospital stay and require a median of two (range 0–20) re-hospitalizations in the first 2 years (Greenough *et al.* 2001). However, the hospitalization rate declines after the second year, such that hospitalization is infrequent in prematurely born children at 14 years of age, regardless of BPD status (Doyle *et al.* 2001).

The average weight and height at term of babies with severe BPD are frequently at or below the third centile, growth failure being partially the result of increased metabolic demands from increased work of breathing. Delays in development have been reported to be common with poor developmental outcome correlating positively with prolonged hospitalization and requirement for oxygen in babies with severe BPD.

■ Wilson–Mikity syndrome

This is a disease of very low birth weight (VLBW) (<1.20 kg) babies who, characteristically, have not had any serious respiratory disease in the first week of life.

Aetiology

This is not known, but it has been suggested that it is due to air trapping behind the highly compliant and collapsible airways in VLBW babies. Trapped air causes alveolar distension, rupture and fibrosis. Pulmonary function studies confirm an increased thoracic gas volume and airways resistance. Implicated factors include intra-uterine infection/chorioamnionitis.

Clinical signs

A previously healthy low birth weight baby becomes progressively dyspnoeic during the second and third weeks of life and requires supplementary oxygen. There may be a few fine crepitations in his lungs. His blood gases initially show hypoxaemia and mild CO_2 retention. In most babies the disease spontaneously begins to recover by the sixth to eighth week of life, and the babies are asymptomatic by the age of 3 months. A small percentage have progressive disease, culminating in death from respiratory failure and cor pulmonale at 3–4 months.

Radiology

The CXR shows a honeycomb appearance, with coarse interstitial fibrosis outlining areas of hyperaeration. These changes are most prominent in the upper lobes and may take more than 12 months to clear.

Histology

This shows areas of emphysema, septal thickening and fibrosis corresponding to the honeycomb appearance of the chest X-ray. The bronchial tree is histologically normal.

Treatment

There is no specific treatment other than supplementary oxygen and treating heart failure if it develops. Most cases of the disease occur at a gestation where ROP is still a major hazard, but the baby is too old for umbilical artery catheterization. SpO_2 measurements are valuable in monitoring these babies, and if the baby is in more than 40% O_2, peripheral arterial samples from an indwelling peripheral arterial line should be taken regularly for blood gas analysis.

■ References

Baraldi E, Filippone, M (2007) Chronic lung disease after premature birth. *New England Journal of Medicine*, **357**: 1946–55.

Doyle, LW, Cheun, MM, Ford, GW, *et al.* (2001) Birth weight <1501 g and respiratory health at age 14. *Archives of Disease in Childhood*, **84**: 40–4.

Doyle, LW, Ehrenkranz, RA, Halliday, HL (2010) Postnatal hydrocortisone for preventing or treating bronchopulmonary dysplasia in preterm infants: a systematic review. *Neonatology*, **98**: 111–17.

Greenough, A, Boorman, J, Alexander, J, *et al.* (2001) Health care utilisation of CLD infants related to hospitalisation for RSV infection. *Archives of Disease in Childhood*, **85**: 463–8.

Jobe, AH, Bancalari, E (2001) Bronchopulmonary dysplasia. *American Journal of Respiratory and Critical Case Medicine*, **163**(7): 1723–9.

Northway, WHJ, Rosan, RC, Porter, DY (1967) Pulmonary disease following respiratory therapy of hyaline membrane disease: bronchopulmonary dysplasia. *New England Journal of Medicine*, **276**: 357–68.

Stenson, B, Brocklehurst, P, Tarnow-Mordi, W (2011) Increased 36 week survival with high oxygen saturation target in extremely preterm infants. *New England Journal of Medicine*, **364**: 1681.

Watterberg, KL; Committee on Fetus and Newborn (2010) Postnatal corticosteroids to prevent or treat bronchopulmonary dysplasia. *Pediatrics*, **126**(4): 800–8.

Yoder, BA, Harrison, M, Clark, RH (2009) Time-related changes in steroid use and bronchopulmonary dysplasia in preterm infants. *Pediatrics*, **124**: 673–9.

■ Further reading

Greenough, A, Milner, AD (2012) Chronic lung disease . In Rennie, JM (ed.) *Rennie & Roberton's Textbook of Neonatology*, 5th edition. Edinburgh: Elsevier pp. 552–570.

■ Web link

UK Joint Committee on Vaccination and Immunisation. Palivizumab recommendation:

www.dh.gov.uk/prod_consum_dh/groups/dh_digitalassets/@dh/@ab/documents/digitalasset/dh_122751.pdf

15

Apnoeic attacks

Key points

- The definition of a clinically significant apnoea is a pause in breathing for more than 20 seconds, or any apnoea associated with a bradycardia or colour change.
- Apnoea must be distinguished from periodic breathing, which is very common in newborn babies.
- Primary apnoea is a diagnosis of exclusion; any baby who develops clinically significant apnoeic attacks must be carefully assessed to exclude the causes of secondary apnoea, including sepsis.
- Primary apnoea of prematurity may be obstructive, central or mixed and usually stops by 34 weeks' gestational age.
- Babies with apnoeic attacks have normal lungs and retinopathy of prematurity is a significant risk if oxygen is administered indiscriminately.
- Most premature babies with apnoeic attacks respond to oral methylxanthines.

■ Definition of apnoea and periodic breathing

Most entirely normal babies, both term and preterm, have periodic breathing in which periods of regular breathing are separated by short episodes of apnoea (3–15 seconds). The American Academy of Pediatrics defines apnoea as a pause in breathing of greater than 20 seconds or one of less than 20 seconds and associated with bradycardia and/or cyanosis. Clinically significant apnoea is associated with swallowing movements (never seen in periodic breathing), and with bradycardia and desaturation. In some babies desaturation occurs after very short apnoeas, leading to one proposed definition of apnoea as 'that non-breathing interval which a given infant cannot tolerate without bradycardia and cyanosis'. The bradycardia usually starts after a time lag and is probably caused by the reduced oxygenation, although there may be a common brainstem pathway which gives rise to the apnoea and bradycardia together. Apnoea is more common in active sleep and may be associated with episodes of gastro-oesophageal reflux. Feeding hypoxia is also a common problem in preterm babies who are learning to swallow, and can cause apnoea. Monitoring for apnoea is described in pp. 55–56, and in clinical practice most apnoea monitors are set to alarm after 20 seconds of apnoea.

■ Clinically significant apnoea

Apnoeic attacks in a baby who is already unwell are a sign of deterioration. In a previously asymptomatic baby the onset of apnoea may be the first indication of serious disease. Whenever a baby develops apnoeic attacks the following causes should be considered, and if necessary excluded by investigation:

1. Infection (Chapter 16).
2. Metabolic disorders, e.g. hypoglycaemia (pp. 236–243), hypocalcaemia (pp. 89, 251); inborn errors of metabolism (pp. 244–249).
3. Upper airways obstruction; obstruction of the neck by flexion.
4. Central nervous system disorders; germinal matrix–intraventricular haemorrhage (GMH-IVH) (pp. 226–230); seizures (pp. 217–220); Arnold–Chiari malformation; very occasionally congenital central hypoventilation syndrome (Ondine's curse).
5. Respiratory depression from drugs.
6. Gastro-oesophageal reflux (p. 284); aspiration of feed; feeding hypoxia.
7. Wrong environmental temperature setting (p. 52).
8. Anaemia of prematurity (pp. 306–308).
9. Respiratory distress syndrome can present with apnoea but should have been diagnosed much earlier by the usual criteria (p. 130).
10. Other lung disease; remember, apnoea can recur with viral infections, especially respiratory syncytial virus.
11. Post-operative; all preterm babies must be monitored for apnoea post-operatively.
12. Heart failure, especially pulmonary oedema with a patent ductus arteriosus.

◼ Recurrent apnoea of prematurity

When all the problems outlined above have been excluded, one is left with a group of otherwise entirely healthy preterm babies who develop apnoeic attacks. Characteristically the attacks develop on the fifth or sixth day of life, and irrespective of the gestation at birth usually disappear by 34–36 weeks' gestational age (Fig. 15.1).

◼ Pathophysiology

In babies who are otherwise well and have recurrent apnoea of prematurity there are three types of apnoeic attack: obstructive, central and mixed (Fig. 15.2). In obstructive apnoea the upper airway becomes occluded by laryngeal adduction while the baby

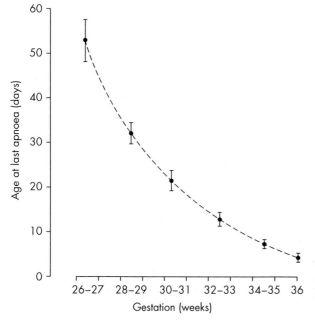

Fig. 15.1 Mean postnatal age (±SE) when last apnoea was detected versus gestational age at birth. From Henderson-Smart (1981)

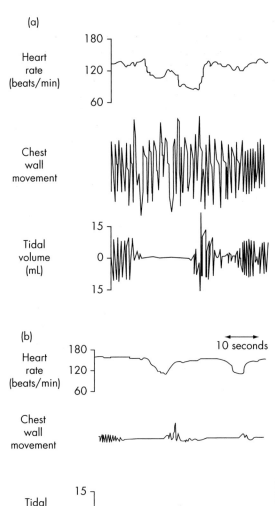

(a)

Heart rate (beats/min)

180
120
60

Chest wall movement

Tidal volume (mL)

15
0
15

(b)

Heart rate (beats/min)

180
120
60

10 seconds

Chest wall movement

Tidal volume (mL)

15
0
15

Fig. 15.2 (a) Obstructive apnoea: breathing movement is maintained while tidal flow ceases. (b) Central apnoea: breathing movements and tidal flow cease simultaneously

continues to make (ineffective) respiratory movements. About 10% of neonatal apnoeic attacks are of this type, which are more common in babies with a neurological problem, either congenital (e.g. Down syndrome, neural tube defect) or acquired (post GMH-IVH). In the common central apnoea the baby just stops breathing at end expiration with his larynx open, but in a proportion of these the larynx adducts during the attack, converting it into a mixed attack (Upton *et al.* 1992). About 10% of short attacks are mixed, but the proportion is greater in the more prolonged attacks.

The exact aetiology of apnoea of prematurity is unknown and is probably multifactorial. The potential factors are as follows:

■ *Neurological immaturity:* this is undoubtedly important, and the incidence of apnoeic attacks can be shown to decline in association with maturation of various brainstem functions. Brainstem compression, as in the Arnold–Chiari malformation, can cause apnoeas.

Apnoeic attacks

- *Hypoxia*: this depresses respiration in neonates (p. 38).
- *Abnormal CO$_2$ response:* preterm babies have a flattened CO$_2$ response curve (p. 120).
- *Anaemia*: once the packed cell volume is below 40%, the frequency of attacks increases.
- *Reflexes from the upper airway:* it can be shown that liquids other than liquor amnii, saline or species-specific milk applied to the upper airway induce reflex apnoea. This may be the mechanism of gastro-oesophageal reflux-induced apnoea.
- *Airway obstruction*: curiously this may actually perpetuate the apnoea – the baby just gives up when his airway is occluded. Examination of the upper airway with an ultrathin fibreoptic scope has shown that the aryepiglottic folds are large and obstructing the airway in some babies.
- *Sleep state*: respiration is much more irregular and apnoeic attacks much more common in active sleep. In part this is a manifestation of the inherent tendency for respiratory rate to cycle in active sleep, but an additional factor is that, with the marked hypotonicity of active sleep, the rib cage may be distorted sufficiently during inspiration that the chest wall mechanoreceptors inhibit the inspiratory drive (p. 120).
- *Temperature change*: it is an old observation that, if the incubator gets too hot, the frequency of apnoeic attacks increases.
- *Feeding*: a common observation is that the number of apnoeic attacks increases in the 20–30 minutes after a bolus nasogastric feed.
- *Handling*: one of the reasons for the minimal handling rule is the recognition that disturbing the baby for anything – changing his nappy, taking blood – may precipitate a run of apnoeic attacks.
- *Post-operative*: any surgical procedure/anaesthetic, no matter how trivial, may be followed by an increase in the number of apnoeic attacks.
- *Immunizations/viral infections:* surviving ex-preterm babies who are given their routine immunizations while still on the neonatal unit (particularly those with chronic lung disease) can have frequent apnoeic attacks in the 24–48 hours after immunization.

Radiology

The chest X-ray in babies with recurrent apnoea is usually normal, but should always be done to exclude other diseases.

Treatment

As many as possible of the triggering factors for apnoea which are present should be corrected, including changing to continuous pump feeding, but not resorting to intravenous feeding in the first place.

Anaemia should be corrected and the incubator temperature controlled. The baby should lie with his head well supported and his neck comfortably extended by putting a small folded nappy under his neck and shoulders. Check the blood gases and if these show a mild hypoxaemia – say PaO_2 of 6.6–8 kPa (50–60 mmHg) – the inspired oxygen concentration can be very cautiously increased, 2% at a time.

Great care must be taken with oxygen therapy. These very premature babies usually have normal lungs, and once they are breathing normally in an oxygen-enriched atmosphere may achieve PaO_2 values well in the retinopathy of prematurity (ROP)-inducing range.

Recurrent apnoea should be treated with a methylxanthine intravenously or orally (theophylline and caffeine).

For the few babies in whom recurrent apnoea persists despite theophylline, low-pressure (3–4 cmH$_2$O) nasal continuous positive airways pressure (CPAP) will usually control the attacks. CPAP works by slightly increasing the functional residual capacity and reducing the distortion of the rib cage during inspiration, and partly by keeping the upper airways open. It is rare to need to ventilate a baby with apnoea. However, if this is necessary, since the lungs are normal and very compliant, the initial ventilator settings should be 25% O_2, rate 25 breaths/min, inspiratory time 0.3 second, pressures 13/2 cmH$_2$O. Once the baby is intubated and attached to the ventilator at these settings, the blood gases can be checked, and it is then usually possible to drop back to a rate of 5–10 breaths/min in most cases. It is often very difficult to wean a baby with recurrent apnoea off ventilation, and it may take 10–14 days in some cases. The methylxanthines should always be used to help the process. Anti-reflux medication is often given to babies with apnoea. Many preterm babies suffer from gastro-oesophageal reflux as well as apnoea, and at the present time there is no good evidence to support the view that apnoea and reflux are temporally or causally related or that anti-reflux medications decrease the frequency of apnoea (Finer *et al.* 2006).

Treatment of an apnoeic attack

As soon as an apnoeic attack is detected, the baby's head should be gently extended, and if he has aspirated a feed his upper airways should be carefully sucked out. All this may provide enough stimulus to restart breathing, but, if not, the soles of the feet should be flicked while checking his heart rate. Most babies will respond to these simple remedies. If they do not, and their heart rate is falling, they should be ventilated, using a bag and mask, with the gas mixture they are normally breathing. *At no time should they be given 100% oxygen by face mask since this carries a risk of ROP.* Oxygen should be given only if there is a progressive bradycardia despite adequate lung inflation with the bag and mask, and then only under medical supervision, with careful monitoring of SpO$_2$ during the resuscitation and rapid reduction of the F_iO_2 after resuscitation. It is rare for such a baby to need intubation, provided that the attack is detected early and bag and mask ventilation is properly administered.

■ References

Finer, NN, Higgins, R, Kattwinkel, J, Martin, RJ (2006) Summary proceedings from the Apnea-of-Prematurity group. *Pediatrics*, **117**: S47–51.

Henderson-Smart, DJ (1981) The effect of gestational age on the incidence of recurrent apnoea. *Australian Pediatric Journal*, **17**: 273–6.

Upton, CJ, Milner, AD, Stokes, GM (1992) Upper airway patency during apnoea of prematurity. *Archives of Disease in Childhood*, **67**: 419–24.

■ Further reading

Hannam, S (2012) Apnoea and bradycardia. In Rennie, JM (ed.) *Rennie & Roberton's Textbook of Neonatology*, 5th edition. Edinburgh: Elsevier, pp. 571–580.

Miller, MJ (1986) Diagnostic methods and clinical disorders in children. In Edelman, N, Santiago, T (eds) *Breathing Disorders of Sleep*. New York: Churchill Livingstone.

16

Infection

Key points

■ Meticulous hand washing and the use of alcohol gel is the best way to prevent cross-infection in a neonatal unit.

■ Infection remains an important cause of morbidity and mortality at all birth weights and gestations, but is particularly important in very preterm babies.

■ Perinatal infection is an important contributor to neuronal damage and adverse outcome in preterm babies, even without meningitis ('cytokine'-mediated damage).

■ The bacterial organisms that most commonly infect babies are group B beta-haemolytic *Streptococcus* and *Escherichia coli*, with coagulase-negative staphylococci a frequent cause of late-onset sepsis in very low birth weight babies.

■ Any baby suspected of sepsis must have investigations, including a blood culture, carried out immediately, and antibiotics (usually penicillin and an aminoglycoside) started straight away.

■ Although herpes infection is rare, it is important to think of the diagnosis and start intravenous aciclovir; one clue is the absence of bacterial organisms on a gram stain of cerebrospinal fluid (CSF) when the CSF also contains a high number of white cells in a baby who has not been previously treated with antibiotics.

■ Neonatal bacterial meningitis has a high risk of adverse outcome. All cases should be managed in large centres with appropriate expertise.

■ Infection control in neonatal units

Babies usually emerge from a sterile intra-uterine environment, and it follows from this that most infections in babies admitted to neonatal units (NNUs) are hospital-acquired, or nosocomial, infections. The risk of nosocomial infection is directly proportional to the number and crowding of babies in the unit, the number of infections in those babies, and the number of people (visitors and staff) going in and out of the unit. Staff who are overworked have less time for hand washing. NNUs should be spacious and designed so that only those who need to enter them pass through, and with plenty of sinks. Babies should be admitted to the NNU only if absolutely necessary, and staffing levels should be maintained.

Scrupulous attention to hand washing is the single most important factor in the prevention of cross-infection. Hands and forearms should always be washed with a suitable preparation, dried and alcohol gel applied before and after handling a baby. Gel should be applied after touching notes, keyboards or door handles. Watches and jewellery must be removed so that staff are 'bare below the elbows'. There is no evidence that the use of gowns, masks and overshoes by staff or parents makes any difference to the level of cross-infection in an NNU. Gowns and masks should be used only when it is necessary to protect the staff during outbreaks of serious infection.

Staff with a current infectious disease such as a respiratory illness, boils, gastroenteritis or weeping dermatitis should be excluded from the unit. Staff with cold sores or herpetic whitlows should cover them, treat with aciclovir and cannot work in a clinical area until the lesions have crusted over. Mothers with wound infections, cold sores, vaginal discharge or known pathogens on their high vaginal swab (HVS) should be allowed in, but any exposed lesions should be covered and their hand washing should be supervised and particularly fastidious. Topical aciclovir should be applied to any cold sores. Mothers of babies with *Listeria* are inevitably faecal carriers and should be isolated themselves, as should their affected baby.

Communal equipment such as stethoscopes and thermometers is a major source of cross-infection. Individual pieces of equipment must be provided. Disposable equipment should be used where possible, for example blood pressure cuffs.

Neonates with infections which could be a hazard to other babies should be nursed in separate rooms if possible. An incubator provides a moderately secure microenvironment for most infected neonates if the hand-washing technique is rigorous, and is adequate for asymptomatic carriers of pathogenic organisms.

When confronted by epidemic infectious disease (e.g. recurrent *Serratia* septicaemia or enterovirus infections), there is no alternative but to close the unit to new admissions. Occasionally outbreaks of particular organisms require investigation to locate them, or a change in practice to eradicate them – e.g. *Pseudomonas* can contaminate taps, and gentamicin resistance can spread rapidly between different gram-negative organisms requiring a change of first-line antibiotic policy.

With the current trend to early discharge, babies can be readmitted to the NNU from the community, but we would always 'isolate' such infants in incubators pending surface swabs and cultures. Babies who require readmission and who have symptoms of viral infections such as respiratory syncytial virus (RSV) must not be readmitted to NNUs unless they can be isolated, as epidemics can follow. Viral infections can be life-threatening to babies with chronic lung disease (CLD).

■ Host defences in the newborn and the inflammatory response

The newborn baby has a 'good enough' immune system for his needs, which are usually limited. He depends on his mother for 'immune protection' via transplacental antibody transmission and the protection provided by breast milk. The newborn immune system, like that of the adult, can be described as 'innate' and 'adaptive' (Table 16.1). The system is 'downregulated' in the newborn, but the baby is still capable of mounting a robust, even an exaggerated, pro-inflammatory response to infection in some circumstances. It is this inflammatory response, involving interleukins and other cytokines, which is thought to be potentially damaging to neuronal development, particularly the pre-oligodendrocytes. These are the cells which will make myelin when fully mature. Both the fetal and neonatal inflammatory response have been linked to brain injury in preterm babies, and babies who have mounted an inflammatory response at term may be 'preconditioned' and more susceptible to hypoxic ischaemic injury than entirely healthy babies (Malaeb and Damman 2009).

Physical defences

The neonatal skin is very thin, easily damaged and infected. The umbilical stump becomes necrotic after birth and acts as a locus for infections which can then disseminate. The passage of an endotracheal tube, a nasogastric tube or an intravascular catheter provides a route for pathogenic organisms to enter the body.

Table 16.1 Comparison of innate and adaptive immune systems

	Innate	Adaptive
Characteristics	Non-specific response	Highly specific response
	Response is fast (minutes)	Response is slow (days)
	Has no memory	Has memory
Components	Natural barriers, e.g. skin Complement Neutrophils and macrophages Pattern-recognition molecules, e.g. Toll-like receptors and Nod proteins on dendritic cells	T and B lymphocytes Major histocompatibility complex restricted antigen- recognition molecules

The newborn baby is virtually germ-free at birth, apart from organisms that become smeared over him as he passes through the vagina. He therefore lacks the protection afforded by having a resident flora of non-pathogenic organisms. A normal neonate is colonized by generally non-pathogenic organisms acquired from his mother, including those in her vagina and rectum, to which he was exposed during delivery. However, particularly if he is in an NNU, he may also be colonized by, and subsequently infected with, potentially pathogenic organisms acquired from the hospital environment. The gut is a particularly important organ in this respect due to gut-associated lymphoid tissue, and early feeding with fresh 'mother's own' breast milk is a very important way of establishing a colony of 'friendly' bacteria. Approximately 80% of the body's entire immune system is in the intestine, and nutrition and immune function are closely linked in the newborn period (and remain so throughout life). Much current research is directed at evaluating the role of probiotics in preventing gut-associated lymphoid tissue (necrotizing enterocolitis (NEC)). Probiotics are strains of 'friendly' bacteria such as *Lactobacillus* CG or *Bifidobacterium* given by mouth, which multiply in the gut and colonize it. However, concerns remain about the emergence of resistant strains, cross-colonization in the nursery and the possibility of septicaemia due to the strain used (Millar *et al.* 2012).

Cellular immunity

Cells involved in the immune system are macrophages, neutrophils, eosinophils and mast cells. Lymphocyte function is well developed even in the 28-week fetus. The absolute number of T-cells present is similar to adult values. T-cells are able to mount a response from the third trimester, and antigen-specific T-cells are found in cord blood.

A full complement of B-lymphocyte types is present by the end of the second trimester, and these cells can respond by synthesizing antibodies, although their function is still suboptimal (De Vries *et al.* 1999). A swift antibody synthetic response by the neonatal lymphocyte is dependent on the presence of some immunoglobulin G (IgG) in the plasma to help process the antigen. The response of the neonate will be improved if he has an adequate level of transplacental maternal IgG.

Phagocyte function

Polymorphonuclear leucocytes from healthy preterm and full-term babies when suspended in normal adult serum show normal phagocytosis and bactericidal activity, but some reduction in chemotaxis and adherence. There is some evidence that phagocytic ability against *Escherichia coli* is less in cells from cord blood than at 3 days of life, when it reaches adult levels.

Humoral immunity

The normal neonate, irrespective of gestation, has virtually no circulating IgA, IgD, IgE or IgM. If any of these are present in cord blood or the early neonatal period, they have been manufactured by the fetus and imply fetal infection. In general, IgA responses protect against inflammation, while IgG is more pro-inflammatory and serves to 'opsonize' bacteria (make them more 'tasty' to phagocytes). IgE responses may also promote inflammation by disrupting epithelial barrier and neural function. IgG, meanwhile, is both actively and passively transported across the placenta from about the twentieth week of gestation, and by full term the baby's IgG level is higher than that of his mother. Following delivery, the level of IgG in the baby's plasma falls with a half-life of about 3 weeks, and until he produces adequate amounts of IgG, IgM and IgA there is a transient postnatal hypogammaglobulinaemia. This is rarely clinically important in a term baby, but a premature baby is born before much IgG has crossed the placenta and is therefore at increased risk of infection from the time of birth for several weeks until after the postnatal hypogammaglobulinaemia has been corrected. At the trough, about 3–4 weeks after delivery, the preterm baby may have IgG levels less than 0.2 g/L.

Since the neonate acquires his IgG from his mother, he is immune to the infections to which she is immune, except for those conditions in which immunity is IgM mediated or cell mediated (*E. coli*, tuberculosis (TB)). The levels of the components of the complement cascade and the alternative complement pathway in the neonate are 50–80% of adult values, and even lower in premature babies. The neonate is technically immunodeficient because he lacks these defence mechanisms. However, it is important to recognize that he is immunocompetent since he can, and does, respond to the antigenic challenges he receives postnatally, particularly if he has adequate levels of IgG.

■ Bacterial infection in the newborn

The major bacterial pathogens now encountered are *E. coli*, the group B β-haemolytic *Streptococcus* (GBS; *Streptococcus agalactiae*) and *Staphylococcus epidermidis* (coagulase-negative staphylococci (CONS)), which are responsible for 80–85% of severe neonatal infections. Many NNUs contribute data to national or international infection-surveillance networks, which are able to monitor changes in infecting pathogens and antibiotic resistance over time. The UK NeonIN data demonstrate that, with the inclusion of CONS, the incidence of all neonatal infection is 0.8% of live births. Other bacteria which are commonly responsible for serious infection are:

1. *Pseudomonas aeruginosa*;
2. other gram-negative bacilli (*Klebsiella, Proteus, Enterobacter, Haemophilus*);
3. *Staphylococcus aureus*;
4. *Pneumococcus* and other streptococci (groups A, D, G and viridans);
5. *Listeria monocytogenes*;

Superficial infections

Bacterial infection of the umbilicus and skin

Effective umbilical cord care is important. Maternity units no longer treat the umbilical cord stump with antibiotic powder or spray, but the umbilicus should be kept clean and dry. A slightly sticky cord can usually be treated with alcohol wipes.

If infection does occur, with periumbilical redness and local discharge, it is usually due to staphylococci or *E. coli*. Systemic antibiotics are indicated if the discharge is copious or oedema and inflammation are spreading onto the abdominal wall.

Staphylococcal skin infection is now rarely seen. It is important to recognize the condition of neonatal pustular melanosis for the benign condition that it is, and not to treat these babies with antibiotics. Neonatal pustular melanosis is quite common in babies with deeply pigmented skin, and the rash is present at birth. In addition to the pustules, look for older lesions with a freckle-like appearance and a flaky collar to them; characteristically, there are lesions at different stages of development. All paediatricians should also be familiar with the appearance of erythema toxicum. Occasionally toxic epidermal necrolysis (Ritter's disease) develops. This responds to adequate parenteral fluid replacement and intravenous flucloxacillin. Group A *Streptococcus* can cause extensive tissue loss owing to 'nectrotizing fasciitis' and toxic shock, resulting in very serious illness, albeit rare.

Thrush (usually *Candida* infection)

This is usually a trivial oral or perianal infection in otherwise healthy term babies. It presents as white plaques on the buccal mucosa and tongue which cannot be wiped off, or as the typical bright erythematous perianal rash with discrete lesions looking like the base of thin-roofed blisters, lying peripheral to the confluent rash. This usually responds promptly to treatment with topical miconazole gel or nystatin suspension.

Thrush is more common in very low birth weight (VLBW) babies who are on broad-spectrum antibiotics for a prolonged period of time, especially if they are also receiving steroids for CLD (see Chapter 14). In such babies systemic candidiasis may occur. We use prophylactic fluconazole intravenously in babies of birth weight less than 1 kg with long lines or umbilical catheters in place, and there is some evidence to support this practice.

Conjunctivitis

The diagnosis and management of this condition is outlined in Table 16.2.

Superficial abscesses

These develop at the site of intravenous infusions, heel sticks or any other place where the skin is damaged. The local lesion is obvious, but care should be taken to ensure that

Table 16.2 Management of neonatal conjunctivitis

Organism	Age at presentation	Diagnosis	Treatment
Gonococcus	1 day (some recognized in 1st week)	Maternal history Profuse conjunctival discharge Urgent gram stain on pus shows gram-negative intracellular diplococci. Culture of swab sent in transport medium	Single dose of ceftriaxone, 25–50 mg/kg IV or IM to a maximum dose of 125 mg is effective and topical treatment is not then necessary. Older regimens of IV and topical penicillin are also effective. Notifiable disease. Remember to isolate baby with mother, organize treatment and contact tracing for mother

(continued)

Table 16.2 (Continued)

Organism	Age at presentation	Diagnosis	Treatment
Chlamydia trachomatis	5 days or more	No distinguishing clinical features. May be maternal history Conventional cultures can be sterile. Antigen detected in eye swab by immunofluorescence	Systemic erythromycin (45 mg/kg/24 h in three divided doses) for at least 2 weeks to prevent pneumonia. Well absorbed orally. Also use 1% chlortetracycline eye ointment or drops
Others; most common are Staphylococcus aureus, Escherichia coli, Haemophilus, Streptococcus pneumoniae	3–5 days peak, but may be at any time including day 1	Culture of swab	If mild, sterile saline cleaning. If discharge persists for more than 48 hours and there is lid oedema, use chloramphenicol eye drops

IM, intramuscular; IV, intravenous.

the underlying bone is not affected. If fluctuant, the abscess should be aspirated and the pus sent for gram stain and culture. The other routine investigations for infection should also be carried out (pp. 192–193). Treatment with intravenous flucloxacillin and gentamicin should be given initially for 7 days or until the lesion is healed.

Systemic bacterial infection

The comparative immunodeficiency of neonates not only predisposes them to infection but also means that when infection occurs it may disseminate rapidly, with septicaemic shock and death occurring within 12 hours of the first signs of illness. This dissemination, which is particularly rapid in the most immature, has two major implications:

1. Early diagnosis is essential. Even very trivial clinical findings that suggest infection demand full laboratory evaluation.
2. Initial therapy must be started on the basis of clinical suspicion. There is not time to wait for the laboratory results to come back 24–48 hours later.

Shrewd and vigilant observation by the nurses and parents who are with the babies all the time is the cornerstone of early diagnosis. Woe betide the neonatal resident who ignores such observations made by an experienced nurse.

History

Apart from verifying the presenting history, the following points should always be checked:

1. Is the baby compromised in any way that would predispose him to infection (e.g. very premature, indwelling catheter, endotracheal tube)?
2. Was there anything in the perinatal history suggesting an infectious risk (e.g. maternal illness or pyrexia, prolonged rupture of membranes, pathogens known in the mother's HVS)?
3. Is there a risk of nosocomial infection from relatives, staff or other sick babies on the unit?

Early symptoms and signs

- *Temperature change.* Hypothermia and hyperthermia are often due to deficiencies in the control of the environmental temperature (Chapter 7). A body temperature below 36°C or above 37.5°C sustained for more than an hour or two in an appropriate environmental temperature is due to infection until proved otherwise. The higher or lower the temperature, the more significant it is.
- *Reluctant to feed.* When a term baby is reluctant to feed from breast or bottle, infection should be suspected, particularly in a baby who was previously feeding well.
- *Listlessness, lethargy, hypotonia, pallor, mottled skin.* These are often the first, mild, non-specific signs that a baby is unwell. The baby just does not seem 'right'. Very preterm babies are often described as 'not handling well' or 'going off' – non-specific terms that neonatal nurses use when the baby has an increase of apnoeas and bradycardias, particularly when moved or touched.
- *Irritability.* A baby who is irritable and will not stop crying or whimpering, even for a feed, may be developing septicaemia or meningitis. A high-pitched monotonous cry is a neonatal danger sign.
- *Jaundice.* If this develops rapidly in a baby without haemolytic disease, sepsis is present until proved otherwise, although the yield of infection screens when jaundice is the *only* presenting sign in a well baby is very low.
- *Vomiting.* If persistent, this is suggestive of infection (as well as intestinal obstruction). Diarrhoea and vomiting are not necessarily signs of gastroenteritis in neonates, and are much more commonly non-specific features of early infection.
- *Ileus/intestinal obstruction.* Sepsis may present as vomiting, abdominal distension and constipation due to an ileus, particularly when there is intra-abdominal infection (e.g. NEC, pp. 278–283).
- *Pseudoparalysis.* The lack of movement owing to limb pain may alert the clinician to the presence of arthritis or osteomyelitis before local or generalized signs develop.
- *Apnoea.* Commonly the first sign of infection in premature babies.
- *Tachypnoea.* Tachypnoea accompanying any of the above signs is often the first sign of pneumonia or septicaemia.
- *Cardiovascular signs.* Tachycardia is common in any infection and marked in cardiac infections. Delayed capillary filling is a useful early sign. Skin blanched by pressure should return to normal colour within 1–2 seconds.

Late signs and symptoms

These are usually specific to one organ system. If infection presents in this way it suggests that the diagnosis could have been made earlier if the baby had been more carefully and expertly observed.

- *Respiratory:* cyanosis, grunting, respiratory distress, cough.
- *Abdominal:* bilious or faeculent vomiting, gross abdominal distension, livid flanks, indurated abdominal skin and periumbilical staining, absent bowel sounds.
- *central nervous system (CNS):* high-pitched cry, retracted head, bulging fontanelle, convulsion.
- *Haemorrhagic diathesis:* petechiae, bleeding from puncture sites.
- *Sclerema:* this is a late feature of any serious illness, especially in preterm neonates. It has no specific significance or specific therapy.

Clinical examination

The baby should be completely undressed and carefully examined, paying particular attention to the following points:

1. Confirm the presenting signs (e.g. fever, jaundice, pallor, grunting).
2. Are there any lesions on the skin, subcutaneous tissues or scalp?
3. Is there periodic breathing or tachypnoea at rest?
4. Is there tachycardia or murmurs suggesting cardiac disease?
5. Are there added sounds on auscultation of the chest?
6. Is there hepatosplenomegaly which accompanies generalized infection as well as hepatitis?
7. Is there kidney enlargement? Cortical swelling of the kidneys may be present in early septicaemia as well as urinary tract infection (UTI).
8. Is the umbilicus red and tender with a thickened cord of inflamed umbilical vein extending up the falciform ligament?
9. Can osteomyelitis and arthritis be excluded by the presence of full and painless limb movements?
10. Are bowel sounds present? Does the baby cry during palpation of his abdomen, suggesting peritonitis?
11. Meningism is rare in neonatal meningitis, but check the back and skull for pits or other skin defects that might be the entry site for spinal infection.
12. Assess the baby's overall neurological state.
13. Babies do not have dysuria or frequency, but with pyelonephritis they may have loin tenderness which can be detected by gentle pressure on the renal angle.
14. Is the baby dehydrated? Has he lost more than 10% of his birth weight, suggesting major gut fluid loss?

Investigations

Whenever there is any suspicion of infection on the above features, the following tests should *always* be carried out:

1. Take swabs. There is little benefit from taking swabs from any site other than the ear and throat when assessing babies in the first 6–12 hours. Gastric aspirate reflects the liquor and the contents of the birth canal, is not helpful after the first feed, and has largely been abandoned. Swab any skin wound or spot. Remember viral cultures.
2. In the presence of early-onset sepsis, a maternal HVS should always be cultured.
3. In late-onset sepsis or NEC, stool culture or rectal swabs can be helpful.
4. Endotracheal tube aspirate (if applicable).
5. Bag urine in investigation after 24 hours of age. The vulva or penis should be cleaned as carefully as possible and any infection noted, to assist interpretation of the result. The urine should be decanted from the bag into a sterile container as soon as possible after voiding. Results from bag specimens of urine collected from neonates should always be viewed with grave suspicion unless pus cells or bacteria were seen immediately on examination of the sample. If any doubt exists, urine must be obtained by suprapubic bladder puncture.
6. Blood culture. The 'gold standard' test. Use a strict aseptic technique with a closed system and aim for at least 0.5 mL of blood. Great care should be taken in interpreting positive results when more than one organism is grown or the organisms grown are also skin commensals. Unless these grow in pure culture within 24–48 hours, they are probably contaminants.

7. White blood cell (WBC) count and differential. Polymorph counts above $7.5–8.0 \times 10^9$/L (7500–8000/mm³) or below 2×10^9/L (2000/mm³), more than 0.8×10^9 myelocytes/L (800/mm³) an I:T ratio of >0.2 (the ratio of immature to total neutrophils) and a left shift or toxic granulation of the white cells are all suggestive of neonatal bacterial infection after the third day of life, but the range is wide. On the first day of life a polymorphonuclear leucocytosis is not usually due to infection, but neutropenia, an I:T ratio of >0.2 and the presence of immature cells, and toxic granulation are. Thrombocytopenia ($<100 \times 10^9$/L) is common in infected babies.

8. C-reactive protein (CRP). A CRP above 10 mg/L suggests infection, but the levels often take 12 hours to rise. The CRP doubling time is 8 hours, and the half-life is about 19 hours. CRP is more helpful for monitoring progress than for establishing the diagnosis.

The following investigations should also be carried out in most situations:

1. *Lumbar puncture*: this should be carried out in all babies with suspected sepsis with the exception of babies with respiratory distress syndrome in whom antibiotics are started at birth (p. 149) or those with CLD on intermittent positive pressure ventilation (IPPV) who develop lung infection (p. 174).
2. *Chest X-ray (CXR)*: this often gets forgotten – unwisely! CXR should be done unless there is an obvious extrapulmonary focus of infection.
3. *Abdominal X-ray*: if the symptoms suggest intra-abdominal pathology, if there is any abdominal distension, or if there is blood in the stool. The main diagnosis of importance is NEC.
4. *Blood gases*: a metabolic acidaemia is often present in severe infections, and if the base deficit is above 8 mmol/L not only does it suggest sepsis but it may need correction. Hypoxia, hypercapnia or apnoeic attacks are indications for ventilation in sepsis.
5. The plasma electrolytes, urea, glucose, calcium and albumin should also be checked – not only may they be abnormal when sepsis presents, but also a baseline measurement is important when planning fluid and electrolyte balance in the next few days.

Interpretation of results

When the baby first presents, a quick decision has to be made about whether or not to treat with antibiotics. Of the tests initially carried out, those which give the definitive answer – the cultures – take 24–48 hours to come back, so neonatologists have to rely on tests with a turn-around time of an hour or two to help them make that decision. Basically, if there has been a good reason to perform the infection screen in the first place then antibiotics should be started.

If in doubt, treat

Treatment of systemic bacterial infection

Antibiotics

Any baby in whom it is remotely possible that an infection is responsible for the abnormal clinical and laboratory findings should be given antibiotics. These can be stopped in 2 days if the baby's condition rapidly improves and cultures are negative. CRP is particularly helpful in this regard; there is a lag in the rise, but if the level remains below 10 mg/L, bacterial infection is unlikely. Taken together with negative culture results (or culture results suggesting contamination) in a well baby, a low level of CRP supports a decision to stop antibiotics after 48 hours of treatment.

Proven infections should be treated for at least 7 days, rising to 14 days in babies with *S. aureus* septicaemia, because of its propensity to seed to other tissues, and at least 21 days in meningitis (see below). In virtually all cases the antibiotic should be given intravenously; intramuscular antibiotics in a neonate may cause nerve and muscle damage. Oral antibiotics have no place other than in the treatment of UTI, chlamydial conjunctivitis (Table 16.1) or trivial superficial skin infections in babies who are systemically well.

The choice of antibiotics in the neonatal period is becoming increasingly difficult, with the rising incidence of CONS sepsis and the emergence of multiple antibiotic-resistant organisms such as meticillin-resistant *S. aureus*, ampicillin-resistant *E. coli* and gentamicin-resistant gram-negative organisms. However, penicillin plus an aminoglycoside (usually gentamicin) remain the most suitable antibiotics for routine use in the neonatal period. Cephalosporins are useful second-line antibiotics, but drug resistance can rapidly emerge when they are used as first line. The suggestions in Table 16.3 may be helpful.

Our current practice is to give penicillin and amikacin to babies less than 48 hours old in whom streptococci (particularly GBS) and pneumococci are a problem. Most units use gentamicin; we changed to amikacin because of a problem with gentamicin resistance. This combination provides good cover for most early-onset infections apart from *S. aureus*, which is not currently a major clinical problem. Beyond 48 hours we use flucloxacillin plus an aminoglycoside to cover staphylococcal disease unless the baby has a long line in situ, in which case we use teicoplanin and ceftazidime. In babies with intra-abdominal sepsis and NEC, we add metronidazole to deal with any potential anaerobic infections.

Third-generation cephalosporins are very effective against most gram-negative bacilli, and they penetrate the cerebrospinal fluid (CSF) well. However, they are not effective against *Streptococcus faecalis*, *Listeria*, *Enterobacter* species and (with the exception of ceftazidime) *Pseudomonas*, and there is anxiety about their efficacy against gram-positive cocci (Goldberg 1987). Furthermore, their routine use often results in alterations in the resident flora in the unit, selecting for multiple antibiotic-resistant gram-negative organisms and anaerobes, such as *Bacteroides*.

The disadvantage of using an aminoglycoside is the need to monitor plasma levels. Standard practice is to monitor the levels around the third dose, although levels should

Table 16.3 Summary of suggested antibiotic regimens

Early or late infection	Choice of antibiotic
Early <48 hours–1 week	**First line** Benzyl penicillin with gentamicin or amikacin Consider amoxicillin if *Listeria* suspected Consider flucloxacillin if *Staphylococcus aureus* suspected
Late >48 hours–1 week	**First line** Flucloxacillin with gentamicin **Second line** Ceftazidime and teichoplanin **Third line** Meropenem, ciprofloxacin
Meningitis	**First line** Cefotaxime with amoxicillin or benzylpenicillin +/– gentamicin **Second line** Meropenem

Table 16.4 Drug levels of some commonly used antibiotics

Drug	Sampling time	Target range
Amikacin	1 hour post dose	15–20 µg/mL
	Pre dose	<4 µg/mL
Gentamicin	1 hour post dose	6–10 µg/mL
	Pre dose	<2 µg/mL
Netilmicin	1 hour post dose	10–12 µg/mL
	Pre dose	<2 µg/mL
Tobramycin	1 hour post dose	4–8 µg/mL
	Pre dose	<2 µg/mL

be checked earlier in babies with poor renal function. The trough level should be taken just before a dose is due and a peak level 1 hour later. Acceptable levels are given in Table 16.4. With once-daily dosing, a pre-dose level is considered clinically adequate. If the trough level is too high, the dose frequency needs to be decreased. The genetic link between gentamicin and sensorineural hearing loss is also of concern, following the finding that approximately 1:500 of the population carry the mitochondrial DNA mutation m.1555A→G. Carriers of this mutation have permanent and profound hearing loss after receiving aminoglycosides even when drug levels are within the therapeutic range (Bitner-Glindzicz *et al.* 2009; Vandebona *et al.* 2009).

Plasma levels do not need to be measured when giving cephalosporins or penicillins.

Whichever antibiotic policy is decided upon, a close watch must be kept on which organisms are actually responsible for the serious infections in the unit and whether their antibiotic resistance pattern is changing. The routine antibiotic cocktail can then be continuously adapted and updated. As discussed, we have been using amikacin for over a year now as first-line treatment because of an emergence of gentamicin-resistant gram-negative organisms.

Adjuvant treatments

Antibiotics alone do not always treat infection in the newborn, and various immunomodulating treatments have been tried. These include immunoglobulins, exchange transfusion, haemopoietic growth factors (recombinant human granulocyte colony-stimulating factor (rhG-CSF) and recombinant human granulocyte–macrophage colony-stimulating factor (rhGM-CSF)), pre- and probiotics (see above) and pentoxyfilline.

Immunoglobulin

Since the last edition of this book, much further work has been done using intravenous immunoglobulin (IVIG) as prophylaxis or as an adjunct to treatment in babies with infection. So far, no study has shown that pooled IVIG is of any benefit in the prophylaxis or treatment of neonatal sepsis (Ohlsson and Lacy 2006). One factor behind the disappointing response is probably the fact that there is considerable batch-to-batch variation in the antibody profile of IVIG, and the CONS-specific activity is often low. In a study of an intravenous immune globulin derived from donors with high titres of antibody to surface adhesins of *Staphylococcus epidermidis* and *S. aureus* (INH-A21), immunoglobulin infusion was well tolerated but there was no reduction in the incidence of these infections (De Jonge *et al.* 2007).

Recombinant DNA technology has been used to make an anti-staphylococcal antibody directed against a component of the bacterial cell wall (pagibaximab). Early results show that babies can tolerate the drug and future trials are awaited.

Exchange transfusion

This is a complex way of infusing immunoglobulins and white blood cells, and its use in severe sepsis is limited. However, exchange transfusion gives many other opsonins, as well as coagulation factors, and 'washes out' assorted toxic metabolites, so a single-volume exchange using blood which is as fresh as possible still has a place in the management of the occasional baby with fulminating sepsis.

Recombinant human G-CSF and GM-CSF (rhG-CSF and rhGM-CSF)

Severely septic neonates of all gestations may have a marked neutropenia. Granulocyte transfusions were used in the past with varying degrees of success, but their use has now been superseded by G-CSF and GM-CSF. Both these agents raise the neutrophil leucocyte count in septicaemic neutropenic babies and these agents may have a role in septic neutropenic neonates. However, the authors of the Cochrane review of rhG-CSF and rhGM-CSF for treating or preventing neonatal infections concluded that there is no evidence to support the introduction of either rhG-CSF or rhGM-CSF for the treatment or prophylaxis of infection (Carr *et al.* 2006). The PROGRAMS trial demonstrated that, while early postnatal rhGM-CSF corrects neutropenia, short-term outcomes, survival and sepsis rates are not improved (Carr *et al.* 2009).

■ Maintenance of homeostasis

Fluid and electrolyte balance

All babies being treated with antibiotics will have an intravenous line in situ for administration of drugs. In babies in whom the infection is mild, or in whom the antibiotics are being given on suspicion of infection only, it is usually possible to continue breast feeding, or feed by nasogastric tube. However, in the seriously ill baby with septicaemia or meningitis, an ileus lasting several days usually develops so that feeding should be stopped and fluid balance will need to be maintained intravenously, taking great care to avoid fluid overload. Plasma biochemistry should be checked at least daily during the acute illness.

Acidaemia/blood gases

Septicaemic babies are often acidaemic and hypoxic, and should be ventilated. Umbilical arterial catheters should probably be removed from babies with blood-stream infection, but peripheral arterial cannulae are very useful in this situation in order to monitor blood pressure and acid–base balance.

Cardiovascular support

Hypotension is common in septicaemic babies, and the mean blood pressure should be kept above a suitable level based on the baby's gestation and postnatal age (Appendix 3). This is usually at least 40–50 mmHg in term babies and around 30 mmHg in preterm babies. Hypotension should be treated initially with plasma expanders or blood giving 15 mL/kg, but intravenous dopamine 5–10 µg/kg/min or dobutamine are often required. In severe sepsis, persistent pulmonary hypertension of the newborn (PPHN) may develop (pp. 162–163).

Haematology

The full blood count should be checked daily and the baby transfused if the haemoglobin is less than 12 g/dL. Haemolysis after blood transfusion due to the agglutination of neonatal red cells by normal adult serum (T-activation) can occur in neonatal sepsis and NEC. Disseminated intravascular coagulation (DIC) may also occur in severe septicaemia, and clotting studies and a platelet count should always be done. If DIC is confirmed, it should be treated with infusions of fresh frozen plasma, platelets or blood.

Rapid-onset neonatal septicaemia

The most dramatic form of neonatal septicaemia is the fulminating pneumonic/septicaemic illness which can develop in babies of all gestations. Characteristically this is caused by GBS, but many organisms may be responsible.

Group B streptococcal septicaemia

It is convenient to divide neonatal GBS infections into the following three categories:

1. Acute postpartum disease presenting at birth or within 2–4 hours of delivery; septicaemic and pneumonic; all GBS serotypes.
2. Early-onset disease: average age of onset 20 hours; all serotypes of GBS; equal numbers of cases with meningitis, pneumonia and septicaemia; all serotypes.
3. Late-onset disease: usually greater than 7 days old, predominantly GBS serotype III; 85% of cases are meningitis.

The group 1 babies who have been infected *in utero* are often in poor condition at birth and difficult to resuscitate. More typically, with intrapartum infection the baby presents at age 1–2 hours with mild grunting and recession, but then rapidly deteriorates if not promptly and vigorously treated, soon becoming apnoeic, hypotensive and oliguric, and dying during the first 24–48 hours. The pathogenesis of neonatal GBS infection is illustrated in Fig. 16.1. The treatment for groups 1 and 2 is identical and is outlined in Fig. 16.1.

Prevention of early-onset group B beta-haemolytic *Streptococcus*

Screening is not currently recommended in the UK, but all units should have a policy in place to offer intrapartum antibiotic prophylaxis (IAP) to mothers based on the Royal College of Obstetricians and Gynaecologists (RCOG) Green Top guideline (no. 36) of 2012 and the National Institute for Health and Clinical Excellence intrapartum care guideline of 2007. Treatment is not required if a woman is undergoing an elective caesarean section in the absence of ruptured membranes.

The RCOG guideline recommends offering IAP treatment to the following high-risk groups:

■ women whose previous baby had early-onset GBS disease;
■ women found to carry GBS in the current pregnancy;
■ raised maternal temperature in labour (RCOG defines maternal pyrexia as >38°C);
■ GBS bacteriuria in pregnancy.

The RCOG no longer recommends IAP for prolonged membrane rupture at term in women with no other risk factors.

Neonatal treatment

1. Babies of ≥37 weeks' gestation whose mothers received prophylaxis more than 4 hours (some say 2 hours) before delivery do not need to be investigated

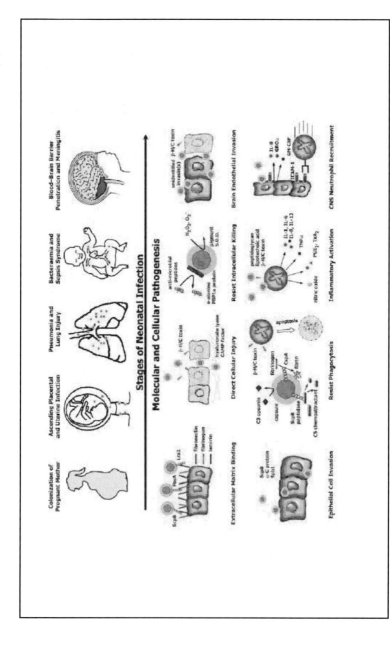

Fig. 16.1 Stages in the molecular and cellular pathogenesis of neonatal group B *Streptococcus* (GBS) infection. β–H/C, beta-haemolysin/cytolysin; S.O.D., superoxide dismutase; IL, interleukin; TNFα, tumour necrosis factor-alpha; PGE₂, prostaglandin E₂; TXA2, thromboxane A₂; GRDα, growth-related oncogene-alpha; ICAM-1, intercellular adhesion molecule 1; GM-CSF, granulocyte–macrophage colony-stimulating factor. From Doran and Nizet (2004) with permission

or treated because IAP is largely effective. Opinions differ on whether these babies can be offered early discharge from the hospital; our own practice is to observe them for 24 hours.

2. All babies with respiratory illness should have cultures taken at presentation and receive penicillin and gentamicin until the cultures are known to be sterile.
3. Babies <37 weeks' gestation born to carrier mothers who received any prophylaxis should have a full blood count, including a differential white count, and a blood culture performed. They should be treated with intravenous penicillin and gentamicin until the cultures are known to be negative, and a lumbar puncture (LP) should be done if they are in any way unwell.
4. Babies of mothers with evidence of infection – temperature >38°C or persisting temperature over 37.8°C (chorioamnionitis/systemic sepsis) – should be screened.
5. Term babies with one risk factor who remain well can be observed without investigation or treatment for 24 hours and discharged if they remain well. Exceptions would be those with a sibling suffering from invasive GBS or twins of affected babies who have started treatment.
6. Term babies with two or more risk factors who were not exposed to IAP for more than 4 hours should be screened and treated.

Supportive treatment

Babies with severe early-onset GBS are often critically ill. They need full neonatal intensive care support. Artificial ventilation is virtually always necessary, as is correction of metabolic acidaemia and support for the blood pressure with transfusion plus dopamine and/or dobutamine.

These babies often develop PPHN, probably as a result of the release of vasoactive agents such as thromboxane A from the pulmonary vascular epithelium in response to the infection, and are hence sometimes helped by nitric oxide.

Other causes of rapid-onset septicaemia

Many other organisms acquired from the maternal birth canal have been isolated from babies with an identical clinical picture to that seen with the group B *Streptococcus*. Organisms responsible for this type of illness include the following:

1. pneumococci;
2. groups A, D and G streptococci;
3. *Enterococcus faecalis;*
4. *Haemophilus* species (*H. influenzae, H. parainfluenzae, H. aphrophilus*);
5. anaerobes;
6. coliforms, including *E. coli.*

These are all usually treated by penicillin and gentamicin initially; to optimize treatment these antibiotics need to be tailored to sensitivities once the microbiology results become available.

In particular, ampicillin should be given for *S. faecalis* and ampicillin or a cephalosporin for *Haemophilus* species.

Coagulase-negative staphylococcal septicaemia

In most NNUs this is the single most important cause of late-onset neonatal septicaemia. The reasons for this include the necessary vascular lines, and the fact that the bowel acts a reservoir for CONS in the newborn. CONS are the main organisms colonizing the skin of newborn babies in neonatal intensive care units. There are more than 20 species of CONS, although in clinical practice 80% of infections are caused by *S. epidermidis* or *Staphylococcus haemolyticus*. Slime-producing strains cause particular problems with line and shunt infections because the slime enables the organism to migrate along the catheter. The risk of line infection is a function of time and the number of times the catheter is used for injections.

Clinical features

These organisms do not usually cause fulminating illness, although CONS may be grown from blood cultures in babies with NEC. Rarely, CONS may cause meningitis, especially in babies with shunts. Characteristically the infection presents after the first week in extremely low birth weight neonates with indwelling lines for total parenteral nutrition or arterial access. The signs are the more subtle ones listed on p. 191, with just a gradual decline in the baby's condition, pallor, worsening blood gases and decreasing tolerance of feeds. Often there are no signs initially, and the infection is detected because of changes in routinely collected blood tests.

Investigation

As well as growing the organism from the blood culture, there will often be a rise in the WBC count and CRP, and a fall in the platelet count. Acid–base, electrolyte or radiological changes are rare.

Treatment

Vancomycin or teicoplanin are the antibiotics of choice for CONS infection. Unfortunately their excessive use has been associated with the development of vancomycin-resistant enterococcal infections and of gram-negative infections. Central lines should preferably be removed, but if vascular access is a problem the line can be left in situ and teicoplanin 'locks' used in an attempt to sterilize it.

Outcome

CONS is usually a mild infection and few babies should die as a result of it.

Pneumonia

The organisms responsible for pneumonia are those responsible for neonatal septicaemia (p. 188). Viral pneumonia also occurs in the neonate. Neonatal pneumonia presenting within 2–4 hours of delivery, and caused by one of the many organisms that are resident in the maternal birth canal, is discussed in the preceding section. Pneumonia that develops in babies on IPPV is discussed on pp. 151–152. Pneumonia, often viral, is a major problem for the long-term baby with severe CLD.

Respiratory distress developing after 4 hours of age in any neonate who does not have some other diagnosis readily made on clinical examination or CXR – such as pneumothorax, some lung malformation or heart failure – is due to pneumonia until proved otherwise. Cultures should be taken and the baby started on the antibiotic cocktail appropriate for his age and the known bacterial flora in the NNU. These should be continued for 7–10 days. Irrespective of the organisms responsible, the other aspects of management are those for any severe respiratory illness described in Chapter 13.

Endocarditis

This can occur in critically ill VLBW neonates with central lines. Vegetations form on the valves or the endocardium. The organisms responsible are usually staphylococci

(*S. aureus* and CONS) and *Candida*. In addition to the standard features of infection (p. 191) these babies characteristically have murmurs, haematuria and thrombocytopenia. The vegetations can be demonstrated echocardiographically, and the other investigations are those listed on p. 192. Treatment is with a 6-week course of an appropriate antibiotic. Occasionally valve damage requires surgery.

Osteomyelitis/arthritis

These conditions frequently co-exist. Multiple bone involvement may occur in babies with central lines, the usual organism being *S. aureus*. If a single site is involved, GBS is more common. The condition presents with the usual signs of infection together with pseudo-paralysis. Sometimes the diagnosis is made serendipitously when the affected bone is X-rayed. Ultrasound examination can be helpful in establishing the diagnosis, and MRI can be valuable.

The usual workup for infection is indicated and the appropriate antibiotics should be given for 4–6 weeks. Survival is the rule, but early advice from a paediatric orthopaedic surgeon must be sought if the diagnosis is confirmed. The infection often ruptures into a joint (e.g. the hip) or into soft tissue, in which case drainage is important. Permanent damage to the growth plate of the bone or the joint is common, and the effects of these serious complications can be reduced by correct early orthopaedic management.

Neonatal meningitis

Clinical signs

The traditional signs of this disease, namely a bulging fontanelle, head retraction and a high-pitched cry, are the signs of established meningitis. Ideally, the disease should be treated before these signs appear. The mortality and long-term neurological morbidity of such babies is high, and every effort should be made to detect neonatal meningitis on the basis of the early and non-specific signs of infection listed on p. 191. For this reason it is important always to have a low threshold for carrying out a LP in sick babies. Basically, there has to be a very good reason *not* to perform a LP when sepsis is suspected.

Organisms

About 40% of neonatal meningitis is due to *E. coli* and a further 40% to GBS. *Listeria* causes about 10%, but the remaining 10% can be caused by any organism including (rarely) *Haemophilus, Pneumococcus* and *Meningococcus*. Gram-negative bacillary meningitis is usually complicated by ventriculitis, and *Proteus* has a particular propensity to abscess formation.

Diagnosis

The normal neonatal CSF may contain up to 21 white cells/mm^3 at term, and up to 30 white cells/mm^3 in preterm babies (Appendix 5). A WBC count greater than this is highly suspicious of meningitis, particularly in clinical context and if the protein is elevated and the glucose level is lowered. However, following an intracranial haemorrhage, especially a GMH-IVH, the polymorph count may exceed 100/mm^3, and the picture is further confused by the CSF glucose level, which in these babies is often less than 1.0 mmol/L (18 mg%). It has been suggested by various authors that it is possible to apply a formula to compare observed and predicted WBC counts in CSF samples with high red cell counts thought to be due to a 'traumatic tap'.

However, none of the formulas can be used with confidence, and most recent reports doubt their value (Greenberg *et al.* 2008). A baseline brain ultrasound examination should be performed looking for cerebral oedema, ventricular size and ventriculitis.

Antibiotic treatment

It cannot be emphasized too strongly that neonatal meningitis is a major emergency, with a high complication rate, and such babies should be transferred to a centre with all the microbiological, neurosurgical and neuroradiological facilities required to carry out the therapy described below.

The baby often has a concomitant septicaemia, and his basic treatment should follow the routine described for severe infection. Certain additions to the treatment are required if meningitis is present. The third-generation cephalosporins have revolutionized the treatment of neonatal meningitis and improved the outlook. Before the organism is identified, initial treatment should be with cefotaxime, amoxicillin or penicillin, and gentamicin. Give aciclovir if there is a high WBC count on the CSF and no organisms are identified on the gram stain in a baby who was not previously exposed to antibiotics, and ask for a herpes polymerase chain reaction (PCR) test (see below).

GBS meningitis
For this, give benzyl penicillin 100 mg/kg/24 h combined with a standard dose of intravenous gentamicin, as the two drugs have a synergistic effect on the organism. Most babies respond clinically to antibiotic therapy within 48 hours, but consider repeating the LP if there is no clinical improvement.

Listeria *meningitis*
This will respond to large doses of intravenous ampicillin 200–300 mg/kg/24 h given in two or three divided doses. As with GBS meningitis, it is probably worth adding intravenous gentamicin in conventional doses.

E. coli *and other gram-negative enteric organisms*
An appropriate initial therapy is cefotaxime 150 mg/kg/24 h in three divided doses, plus gentamicin in conventional doses. A repeat LP at 24–48 hours should be done in gram-negative meningitis because there is a significant failure rate after systemic treatment. If the CSF fails to sterilize and the WBC count remains high, alternative antibiotics such as meropenem should be discussed.

Intraventricular therapy
There is no point in putting antibiotics into the lumbar theca, since they rarely penetrate beyond the basal cisterns. Intraventricular therapy is the most contentious area in the treatment of neonatal meningitis. However, if meningitis is not responding to systemic therapy after 24–48 hours, as assessed by changes in the CSF, ventricular puncture should be considered, particularly if the ventricles are enlarged. The ventricular puncture should be performed under ultrasound guidance. If the ventricular CSF is clear then all is well and the baby's poor condition is presumably due to overwhelming sepsis. If ventriculitis is present, then a suitable antibiotic to which the organism is sensitive should be instilled, and consideration given to repeating the test and discussing insertion of a ventricular reservoir for repeated instillation of antibiotic if the CSF is not sterilized.

Assessment of progress

Every sample of CSF must be subjected to microscopy, biochemistry and culture. A LP following cessation of treatment in a clinically well baby is unnecessary (Heath *et al.* 2003). If aminoglycosides are being used they must be monitored by measuring serum levels. It is particularly important to check ventricular aminoglycoside levels if these drugs are being given directly into the CSF.

A careful neurological examination of the baby should be carried out daily – including head circumference measurements – so that hydrocephalus in particular can be rapidly detected and dealt with. Regular cranial ultrasound imaging will also help to detect complications, and MRI should be done in babies who are not responding to treatment in case of abscess formation.

Duration of treatment

Intravenous antibiotics should always be given for 21 days in neonatal meningitis. The only exceptions to this rule are GBS and *Listeria* meningitis with a rapid clinical, laboratory and microbiological response and a normal cranial ultrasound scan, in which 2 weeks of treatment may be adequate. If there is any suggestion of ventriculitis in GBS meningitis, with strands seen within the ventricular cavity on cranial ultrasound images, we treat for 3 weeks.

Supportive treatment

Many babies with meningitis have seizures and cerebral oedema. Seizures should be treated with the usual anticonvulsants, beginning with phenobarbitone (p. 220). If raised intracranial pressure (ICP) is clinically apparent, then the blood pressure should be supported in order to maintain cerebral perfusion rather than attempting to reduce ICP. Consideration should be given to an intraventricular tap or insertion of an intraventricular reservoir to measure the pressure and drain CSF. At present there is insufficient evidence to justify steroid treatment in neonatal meningitis.

Fluid and electrolyte balance should be monitored carefully, since these babies are particularly susceptible to inappropriate antidiuretic hormone secretion (see chapter 10). Fluid intake should be reduced to 40–60 mL/kg/24 h for the first few days of the illness.

Problems in the treatment of neonatal meningitis

- *Treatment failure*: with modern antibiotic therapy given as outlined above, this is rare, although it may be necessary to continue treatment for 4 or occasionally 6 weeks with unusual gram-negative organisms. If the lumbar CSF is slow to clear and the baby is not responding as expected, careful assessment of the baby initially by ultrasound but then by MRI is indicated. Consider intraventricular antibiotics, via a Rickham reservoir.
- *Abscess*: intracerebral abscesses are particularly common with *Citrobacter* and *Proteus* meningitis. If these organisms are grown, serial ultrasound assessments and MRI should be performed. Most abscesses respond to prolonged (6–8 weeks) intravenous antibiotics but often require operative drainage.
- *Hydrocephalus*: this will be detected using occipitofrontal circumference measurements and ultrasound. If infection is present in the ventricles, an intraventricular device is usually required in order to give antibiotics and control the ventriculomegaly. If hydrocephalus persists after bacteriological cure, a shunt will need to be inserted.

Outcome

Despite the improvements in care and imaging, around 25% of survivors still have a significant disability, including deafness, cerebral palsy or learning difficulties. Seizures worsen the prognosis, and the results are worse in preterm babies, and for gram-negative infections.

Urinary tract infection

This commonly presents with mild symptoms such as vomiting, poor weight gain, persisting anaemia or mild jaundice, although sometimes all the signs of severe sepsis are present. The danger of diagnosing UTI purely on the basis of results of bag urine has already been emphasized. If culture of a bag urine is sterile then the baby does not have a UTI. Bag urine samples with no more than 50 cells/mm^3 without bacterial growth, or significant bacterial growth ($>10^5$ organisms/mL) without sufficient pus cells, should not be treated as a UTI without confirmation from urine obtained by suprapubic bladder puncture. However, a bag urine with a pure growth of more than 10^5 organisms/mL, with a WBC count of more than 100–200/mm^3, is adequate proof of UTI, provided that there was no local infection of the perineum or foreskin when the bag sample was collected. In urine obtained by a suprapubic stab, anything grown in pure culture, irrespective of the numbers of organisms present, indicates a UTI.

Whenever a UTI is diagnosed, the baby should be carefully examined to exclude renal, bladder or genital abnormalities, and in particular posterior urethral valves should be considered in male babies (p. 328). In babies with few or no symptoms, treat with oral antibiotics such as trimethoprim; but if the baby is more seriously ill a parenteral aminoglycoside should be used. The antibiotic can be altered appropriately once sensitivities are available, and should be given for 7–10 days.

Once a UTI has been diagnosed, all neonates should have their blood pressure measured and their urea and electrolytes checked, and these tests should be repeated following completion of therapy. The renal tract must be investigated because 30–50% of these babies will have abnormalities, mainly reflux. All cases of neonatal UTI should be investigated with a renal ultrasound scan within 6 weeks. Abnormal ultrasound scan, atypical or recurrent UTI are indications for a dimercaptosuccinic acid scan 4–6 months after acute infection and a micturating cysto-urogram.

Gastroenteritis

Severe nursery epidemics of gastroenteritis due to *Salmonella*, *Shigella*, enteropathogenic *E. coli* and viruses still occasionally occur, although most of the cases of gastroenteritis that are now seen in the neonatal period are sporadic. Infection with rotavirus is endemic in some NNUs without the babies becoming symptomatic. Norovirus remains a threat in winter months.

Diagnosis

Stool cultures should be sent from all babies with diarrhoea, although the yield of positive cultures is low.

Treatment

Whenever any neonate develops mild gastroenteritis he should be isolated. In most cases milk feeds can continue and oral rehydration fluids can be used. If the diarrhoea and vomiting do not settle, or if dehydration develops, intravenous therapy will be required for 24–48 hours before restarting oral fluids. Gastroenteritis in preterm babies usually requires a 24–48-hour period of intravenous therapy before symptoms subside.

If a term baby develops gastroenteritis on the postnatal ward, he should not be admitted to the NNU. If he can be managed with oral treatment, transfer him with his mother to the isolation unit in the maternity hospital; but if the baby requires intravenous therapy he should be transferred to the unit that manages infectious gastroenteritis in older babies. If the baby is already on the NNU he should be kept there, but full barrier nursing routines must be used.

Babies who have recovered, but who are still shedding pathogens in their stools, can go home if they are feeding and gaining weight well. If, however, they have to stay in the NNU they should be isolated. Two other points to note about gastroenteritis in the newborn:

1. Severe diarrhoea without vomiting which responds to clear fluids but relapses when milk is reintroduced suggests lactose (or other sugar) intolerance.
2. Many completely asymptomatic babies carry enteropathogenic *E. coli* (usually derived from their mothers) in their stools. No action is required.

Prolonged rupture of membranes

In the absence of maternal GBS carriage, if a term baby is asymptomatic, no matter how long the period for which the membranes were ruptured, no cultures need to be done or therapy given. If a baby who is born after prolonged (>18 hours) rupture of the membranes develops any symptoms in the first 24 hours of life, these should be attributed to infection until proved otherwise. Cultures should be taken from the mother and the baby, and antibiotic treatment started.

Preterm babies (<37 weeks) born after preterm premature rupture of the membranes should be investigated for infection and treated until culture results are available.

Listeriosis

Neonatal listeriosis is rare in the UK since advice about not eating unpasteurized cheese in pregnancy became widespread and the food industry developed better techniques for sterilizing cook–chill foods and paté. The Health Protection Agency has recorded only about 20 cases of pregnancy-associated *Listeria* infection per year since 1990, the year after government advice regarding these foods was released. Maternal listeriosis can result in fetal infection and premature labour (with meconium-stained liquor), severe early-onset sepsis or neonatal meningitis. Women with HIV are more susceptible to *Listeria* infection. Mothers of babies with *Listeria* should be isolated because they carry the organism in their bowel, and nosocomial spread of *Listeria* is well documented.

The infection can be transmitted across the placenta, leading to a presentation at birth, and maternal infection can trigger preterm labour. These babies are often very ill at birth, with features of generalized sepsis and pneumonia together with, in some cases, characteristic 2–3 mm pinkish-grey granulomata in the skin. These granulomata are widespread throughout all tissues, hence the name 'granulomatosis infantisepticum' for this form of the disease.

Later-onset sepsis with meningitis is initially indistinguishable from similar illness caused by other organisms.

The investigations are those conventionally carried out, and there are no findings specific to *Listeria*. The diagnosis is made by culturing the gram-positive coccobacillus from blood or CSF. Treatment is with ampicillin and gentamicin for at least 2 weeks. *Listeria* is resistant to all third-generation cephalosporins.

Tuberculosis

The prognosis is best when infected mothers have been detected by antenatal screening and anti-tuberculous treatment instituted during pregnancy (Mnyani and

McIntyre 2011). The management of an infant of a mother with active TB infection poses special problems. Isolation of the baby from the infected mother is usually not feasible and is in any case undesirable, because it would mean that breast feeding was no longer possible. The following policy is advocated for asymptomatic infants of mothers with sputum-positive TB:

- Test mother for HIV (with her permission).
- Treat the mother for TB.
- Maintain breast feeding (except where this is precluded by the gravity of the maternal illness).
- Exclude congenital tuberculosis with chest X-ray and LP.
- If no congenital TB, give the infant prophylactic isoniazid 10 mg/kg once daily for 3–4 months.
- Consider immunizing the infant with isoniazid-resistant bacillus Calmette–Guérin (BCG), if available, or BCG vaccine if not.
- At 3–4 months of age, perform a tuberculin skin test (TST) on the infant: if the TST is negative and the infant is well, stop isoniazid.
- If the TST is positive at 3 months, re-evaluate the infant for TB.

Neonatal TB infection is rare and treatment is empiric. One recommended regimen is isoniazid (10 mg/kg/day) plus rifampicin (15 mg/kg/day) and pyrazinamide (25 mg/kg/day) for 2 months, followed by 4 months of isoniazid and rifampicin. If isoniazid resistance is suspected, usually on the basis of the likely geographical source of the infection, at least one additional drug should be used until sensitivities are known. Ethambutol (20 mg/kg/day) is one possibility. Steroids have no place in treatment because of the lack of a host reaction. Isoniazid prophylaxis is recommended for skin test-negative neonatal contacts.

Virus infections

Viruses are the cause of many severe neonatal infections. The signs and symptoms are identical to those seen in bacterial infections. Antibiotics are given to such babies, since the clinical signs are identical to those seen in bacterial sepsis. They can be stopped once a viral aetiology is established.

Any baby who shows the signs and symptoms of serious infection but in whom no bacteria are found after 48 hours of culture should be suspected of a viral infection. Samples of stool, CSF and nasopharyngeal aspirate should be sent to the laboratory for appropriate PCR tests. Give aciclovir early while awaiting the PCR results if there is any suspicion of viral infection, and particularly (as above) if no organisms are seen on a gram stain in babies with high CSF white cell counts.

Coxsackie group B myocarditis

This condition presents in full-term babies towards the end of the first week with fever, listlessness, tachycardia, tachypnoea, cyanosis, mottling and poor peripheral circulation. The baby is in heart failure with a triple rhythm, hepatosplenomegaly and a soft systolic murmur. He is usually hypotensive and oedematous. CXR shows cardiomegaly and the electrocardiogram (ECG) shows changes of cardiomyopathy. There may be co-existing aseptic meningitis. In such a baby samples of stool and CSF should be sent for viral cultures.

Differential diagnosis from other forms of septicaemia is usually easy, because of the primarily myocardial impact of the disease and the co-existence of an aseptic meningitis. Differentiation from other cardiac diseases, including congenital heart disease, can usually be made on the basis of the associated clinical signs of infection, the ECG changes and echocardiography.

Treatment

The baby should receive all possible intensive care support, taking particular care to avoid fluid overload. Specialized advice is essential in these cases and may involve the use of digoxin (with great care), diuretics, dopamine or captopril. Some babies will recover and their long-term prognosis is good, although digoxin and captopril may be needed for several months or years. The majority, despite all forms of therapy, die in low-output heart failure.

Neonatal herpes

Herpes simplex is the virus which causes cold sores and genital herpes; it should not be confused with herpes zoster, which causes shingles. About 75% of cases are due to the type II (genital) strain, with 25% caused by the type I (oropharyngeal) strain. The risk is greatest in the babies of women who are suffering their first herpetic infection, because these women will not have protected their infants with transplacental immunoglobulin. The RCOG has produced a helpful guideline on the management of herpes in pregnancy (RCOG 2007). Women who do present with primary herpes lesions within 6 weeks of the due date should be offered caesarean section. Women with recurrent lesions late in pregnancy can be treated with daily aciclovir, but if active lesions are present when labour starts they should be managed according to the RCOG guideline (avoid scalp clips, long periods of membrane rupture, etc.). Team work should allow the neonatologist to be alert to these babies and there must be a low threshold for initiating investigation and starting intravenous aciclovir if the baby has any clinical signs, however subtle.

The majority of cases of neonatal herpes occur in babies born to women who were asymptomatic in pregnancy, never knowingly having suffered from herpes. A small number of cases are acquired nosocomially from oral or cutaneous herpes. Health care workers with herpetic whitlows or active cold sores should not work in the clinical area.

Clinical features

Neonatal herpes is fortunately rare in the UK, with an incidence of about 1 in 60,000 live births. The disease can present in three forms. Infection confined to the skin, eye and mouth has the best prognosis; disseminated disease or disease confined to the CNS is worse. Disseminated disease still has about a 30% mortality rate, with 17% suffering long-term sequelae, and babies with herpes meningitis have a high risk (70%) of permanent disability, particularly if they present with seizures.

Investigation

The diagnosis rests on demonstration of viral DNA with PCR; few laboratories now attempt viral culture. Blood, CSF, urine and fluid from any skin lesions should be sent to the laboratory. An ophthalmology consult should be obtained to assess any retinal or corneal lesions.

Treatment

In any baby in whom herpes is a possibility, including the asymptomatic baby born through an overtly infected birth canal, intravenous aciclovir should be given (60 mg/kg/24 h in three divided doses) for at least 14 days, or until the possibility of herpes has been excluded. Skin or mucous membrane lesions can progress to involve the CNS or other organs, so all herpetic lesions should be aggressively treated.

In addition, all the usual intensive therapy for the hypotensive seriously ill neonate with a coagulopathy may be required.

Recurrence of the disease is quite common, and recent research supports continuing oral treatment with aciclovir after the intravenous course is over. Outcome is improved after oral treatment 100 mg/day for 6 months. These babies should be monitored for neutropenia.

Outcome

Babies with localized disease usually survive intact, but with disseminated and CNS disease the mortality is 20–30%, with a similar proportion being handicapped. The outlook is better for those with type I herpes. Even after 2 weeks of intravenous aciclovir, relapses are not uncommon, and require a further 2-week course of therapy.

Viral meningitis

In the neonate the CSF findings are identical to those for viral meningitis in older children, with a normal CSF sugar level and a CSF cell count of less than $1000/mm^3$. It is not possible to infer from the type of white cells present in CSF whether the infecting organism is viral or bacterial. Appropriate viral PCR should be sent in the presence of these findings. The disease is rarely severe, no specific treatment is required, and neurologically intact recovery is the rule.

Enterovirus infections

Echoviruses of serotypes 6, 7, 12, 14, 17 and especially 11 have been responsible for several epidemics of severe and often fatal neonatal disease over the years. The babies often present with the non-specific signs, but characteristically have some abdominal distension and tenderness. In severe cases the course is rapidly downhill, with apnoea, hypotension, jaundice and DIC unresponsive to all therapy. Milder cases have an aseptic meningitis.

Respiratory viral infections

Neonates, particularly VLBW survivors who require long-term IPPV and have CLD, may be in the NNU for 3–4 months, and during this time they may well develop a viral respiratory infection contracted from their parents or the staff. The treatment of these babies is no different from that of any other baby with a viral upper respiratory tract infection or bronchiolitis.

Respiratory syncytial virus

Infections with RSV in babies with CLD can be devastating. The severe bronchiolitis often precipitates apnoea, and the neonates once more need IPPV and high oxygen concentrations – often for a further 1–2 weeks – before they can be weaned off. In other babies it provokes terminal respiratory failure from which the baby cannot be retrieved by long-term IPPV, antibiotics and further courses of steroids or diuretics. We currently use immunoglobulin prophylaxis for babies at home in oxygen, and this is in line with national recommendations.

Cytomegalovirus

Many babies acquire asymptomatic cytomegalovirus (CMV) in the neonatal period, and a small number who are preterm and have been transfused with blood from a

CMV-positive donor may develop CMV hepatitis or pneumonitis, the latter making the prognosis in CLD very much worse. The disease is largely untreatable – although ganciclovir can be tried – and is occasionally fatal in CLD. Attempts at prevention must include transfusing neonates only with blood from CMV-negative donors, but occasionally babies with CLD acquire CMV from a nursery visitor.

Hepatitis

The various forms of hepatitis can all be transmitted to the neonate at the time of birth, but because of their long incubation period they rarely present in the neonatal period. Babies born to mothers carrying hepatitis B must be immunized. Immunization effectively prevents the babies becoming chronic carriers with the attendant risk of hepatocellular carcinoma in later life.

The current shortage of specific immunoglobulin in the UK means that only babies of mothers with high infectivity are offered this treatment. Mothers with high infectivity are defined as those who are e antigen positive, e antibody negative or both e antigen and e antibody negative. Their babies must be given 200 IU of immunoglobulin as well as vaccine, ideally within the first 12 hours of life. Vaccine is not always effective in babies, so that four doses are recommended at birth, 1, 2 and 12 months, with a blood sample at 14 months to check antibody levels. There are two vaccines available in the UK: Engerix B (GlaxoSmithKline) and H-B-VaxII (Pasteur Merieux MSD). The dose is contained in 0.5 mL of vaccine for both preparations; the dose of Enerix B is 10 µg and that of H-B-VaxII is 5 µg.

Hepatitis C

Hepatitis C virus (HCV) can be transmitted vertically, especially when the mother is co-infected with HIV. Breast feeding, however, seems relatively safe. HCV RNA should be measured at 3–6 months and serology (and HCV RNA) at 12–18 months. This follow-up is recommended for all babies of all HCV mothers. Although maternal viral load in pregnancy determines the risk of transmission, negative results are reassuring and, if the baby becomes infected with HCV, prompt referral to the children's liver unit is indicated.

Systemic fungal infection

The baby may be colonized initially by maternal vaginal candidiasis, and fungal infection of the skin and lungs is more common in babies born to mothers with an intra-uterine contraceptive device in situ which has failed to prevent pregnancy. Fungal septicaemia and/or meningitis is a particular problem in ill preterm babies who have received multiple courses of antibiotics. We use fluconazole prophylaxis in babies less than 1 kg who have long lines or umbilical catheters in situ, and have not seen a case of invasive fungal sepsis or meningitis since we began using this regimen. There is concern that use of prophylaxis will encourage the emergence of resistant strains.

The presenting features are those of any severe neonatal infection, though endophthalmitis and endocarditis are specific manifestations. Skin lesions are common – many babies have a patchy erythematous skin rash on their trunk.

The usual investigations for sepsis should be carried out. In addition, appropriate samples – endotracheal tube aspirates, urine – can be examined microscopically for budding yeasts and hyphae, and the blood should be cultured in a special medium. Microscopic examination of the buffy coat of blood can also help.

Treatment should begin with liposomal amphotericin B 1.0 mg/kg/day to a total dose of 20–30 mg/kg. Liposomal amphotericin (AmBisome) is well tolerated and effective (Friedlich *et al.* 1997). If the infection does not respond, consider adding flucytosine 100 mg/kg/day. Image the renal tract and the brain as well as performing ophthalmoscopy and an echocardiogram to look for organ infection with fungus.

■ Congenital infections

Congenital rubella, cytomegalovirus, toxoplasmosis

In their severe form these three conditions have relatively similar clinical findings:

1. Low birth weight for gestational age.
2. Jaundice.
3. Hepatosplenomegaly.
4. Thrombocytopenia and purpura.
5. Cataract.
6. Chorioretinitis.
7. Abnormalities of head growth/intracranial calcification.
8. Osteitis.
9. Congenital heart disease.

If combinations of these abnormalities are present, appropriate serological tests should be carried out. A congenitally infected neonate will have the same high titre of IgG in his plasma as his mother, but the diagnostic test is the titre of specific IgM in his plasma against the micro-organism in question. In addition, throat swabs and samples of urine or swabs from any lesions should be sent for PCR.

Congenital rubella

This disease is now extremely rare owing to the measles–mumps–rubella vaccine being offered to all children in the UK. Most reported cases are born to immigrant mothers who were not vaccinated. The babies should be treated symptomatically. In particular, a patent ductus arteriosus should be closed, cataracts extracted and hearing tests done early to identify and treat those who are deaf. There is no other treatment.

Congenital cytomegalovirus

Most cases of congenital CMV are asymptomatic in the neonatal period. Such babies are at increased risk of deafness in later life, and if congenital CMV is diagnosed, hearing testing must be offered. Ganciclovir should be considered for babies with active disease, although this cannot reverse existing damage and has to be given intravenously.

Congenital toxoplasmosis

This may present with many of the features listed above or with isolated chorioretinitis. Many countries, but not the UK, screen pregnant women for this infection. If congenital infection of any form is found, the baby should be given spiramycin 100 mg/kg/day for 4–6 weeks alternating with pyrimethamine (1 mg/kg/day) plus sulphadiazine (50 mg/kg/day) for 3 weeks for a whole year. This will reduce the likelihood of long-term sequelae, particularly chorioretinitis.

Congenital varicella

This is a rare complication of maternal varicella in the first 20 weeks of pregnancy and affects mainly female fetuses. It causes widespread damage to the CNS, eyes, limb atrophy and cutaneous scars. Most cases die in early infancy.

Congenital parvovirus B19 infection

This is the virus of erythema infectiosum (fifth disease) and it also causes aplastic crisis in patients with haemolytic anaemias such as spherocytosis and sickle cell anaemia. Most maternal infections cause no problems, but a small number will abort, and about 1% of their fetuses will develop hydrops. If such a baby is born he has a treatable condition.

Congenital human T-cell lymphotropic virus 1 infection

This virus, common in patients from Japan or the Caribbean, causes T-cell lymphoma and leukaemia in adults. It is transmitted in breast milk. Sero-positive women from these communities should therefore be advised not to breast feed their babies.

Congenital syphilis

This disease is still rare in the UK, though increasing in other parts of the world. In clinical practice the most common problem occurs with positive serology in mothers who had yaws in childhood. If the mother's serology is consistent with this, and she gives an accurate history, our practice is to monitor the baby for falling antibody titres as an outpatient but not to treat the baby.

Diagnosis in the neonatal period is difficult owing to the poor specificity and sensitivity of all the antitreponemal tests (e.g. IgM fluorescent treponemal antibody test) when used in the neonate. All babies with symptoms and positive tests, who are born to mothers not treated adequately during pregnancy, should receive benzyl penicillin intravenously for 10 days. This also treats congenital neurosyphilis. However, because of residual uncertainty, asymptomatic babies, even of fully treated mothers, should receive a single dose of benzathine penicillin 30 mg/kg (Risser and Hwang 1996). Do not forget to check the treatment status of the mother – and her consorts!

HIV/AIDS

Worldwide, HIV infection remains a pandemic problem, with an estimated 420,000 children newly infected in 2007 and 33 million people living with the infection. Fortunately congenital HIV infection is still a relatively rare disease in the UK, and there has been considerable success in reducing mother-to-child transmission. Nevertheless, the neonatal resident is often faced with immediate management of the baby born to an HIV-positive mother. Most of these women have already been extensively counselled and offered several options for reducing the chance of transmission of the virus to their fetus, including the option of an elective caesarean section delivery. A plan for treatment of the baby should have been made, taking into account any particular drug resistance of the mother's disease. UK guidelines for management of paediatric HIV infection (the Children's HIV Association guidelines) have been published (www.chiva.org.uk). The British HIV Association has recently published detailed guidelines for managing HIV infection in pregnancy and preventing mother-to-child transmission (de Ruiter *et al.* 2008). Highly active antiretroviral therapy has led to improved survival.

In perinatal HIV:

1. All babies born to HIV-infected mothers have transplacentally acquired antibody. If they do not become infected, the antibodies disappear by 18 months of age (often by 9 months). This means that other tests, including estimation of HIV RNA viral load and PCR for HIV pro-viral DNA, are required to make the diagnosis.
2. Perinatal transmission can be reduced by caesarean section delivery combined with antiviral drugs (see next point). However, in women with an undetectable viral load, vaginal delivery is now routine.
3. Perinatal transmission can be reduced by two-thirds by giving zidovudine to HIV-positive mothers antenatally and continuing this treatment to the baby for 6 weeks (Connor *et al.* 1994). The first dose needs to be given within 4 hours of delivery.
4. Additional antiviral drugs are indicated in some cases, where the mother is already on combination treatment. These include nevirapine 2 mg/kg as a single dose after birth at 48–72 hours and didanosine (DDI) 20 mg twice a day. Lamivudine (3TC) has caused neonatal death as a result of mitochondrial toxicity.
5. Cross-infection routines on the labour ward, especially in high-risk areas (London, Glasgow), must be designed to assume that all women are HIV-positive. Gloves should be worn for resuscitation procedures and for testing the suck reflex during the newborn examination.
6. For babies of women known to be HIV-positive, hospital guidelines must be followed. The baby should stay with his mother who should not breast feed him.
7. Babies of HIV-positive women are at risk from other problems, including other sexually transmitted diseases and drug-withdrawal syndromes.
8. BCG vaccination should be withheld until the results of testing are known. Infants of HIV-positive mothers should be immunized at the normal times using diphtheria–pertussis–tetanus vaccine using the Salk killed-polio vaccine.
9. Confidentiality is an important issue. The mother's HIV status may not be known by her partner or her immediate family.

Tests to be performed on the baby's blood (not cord blood, which may be contaminated) after birth include a full blood count, liver function tests, immunoglobulins and T-cells, HIV viral load, P24 antigen and PCR for proviral DNA.

■ Effect of perinatal maternal infections

In most situations a maternal infectious illness, such as UTI or respiratory infection, poses no risk to the baby. In other situations (e.g. meningitis) the mother will be too ill to keep her baby. If the mother is suffering from one of the illnesses listed in Table 16.5, appropriate precautions should be taken while allowing access to a normal baby. If, however, the baby is on an NNU, mothers with conditions marked by an asterisk in Table 16.5 should not be allowed to visit the unit because of the risk to other babies.

Table 16.5 Effect of perinatal maternal infections and their effect on breast feeding and access to the baby

Illness	Access to baby and desirability of breast feeding	Treatment to baby
Acute enteric infections (cholera, typhoid)	Nil during acute phase, mother too ill	Nil, encourage breast feeding if possible; immunize baby if appropriate
*Acute respiratory infection (respiratory syncytial virus, flu)	Access with masking and hand washing; breast feeding allowed no restrictions	Nil
Chlamydia	No restrictions	Nil if baby is asymptomatic, but see p. 190
Cytomegalovirus	No restrictions on access or breast feeding	Nil
*Gastroenteritis	Access with meticulous hand washing; no access to NNU if norovirus suspected	Nil
Hepatitis A	No restrictions but meticulous hand washing	250 mg of immunoglobulin to baby
Hepatitis B	No restriction, breast feeding not contraindicated if full immunization given	Give first dose of vaccine within 12 hours. In addition give 200 IU. (2 mL) of hepatitis B immunoglobulin stat to high-infectivity groups (p. 209)
Hepatitis C	No restriction	Nil recommended, but 250 mg standard immunoglobulin may reduce the risk of transmission
Herpes simplex (genital)	No restriction, but meticulous hand washing and gloves	Aciclovir orally to mother (see also p. 207 – treat symptomatic babies aggressively)
Herpes simplex (labial, whitlow, etc.)	No restriction, but mother to treat lesions with aciclovir	None unless symptomatic, when herpes must be excluded
HIV	Free access, no breast feeding	Start antiretroviral therapy (p. 212)
Leprosy	No restrictions	Continue maternal treatment
Malaria	No restrictions on access or breast feeding if mother's general health acceptable	Test baby's blood for parasites, especially if mother has falciparum malaria or the baby develops symptoms; treat congenital infection with chloroquine or quinine
*Measles	No restrictions, but no access to NNU	Give 250 mg normal immunoglobulin to the baby (hyperimmune if available)
*Mumps	No restrictions, but no access to NNU	Nil

(continued)

Table 16.5 (Continued)

Illness	Access to baby and desirability of breast feeding	Treatment to baby
Rubella	No restrictions, but no access to NNU	No problem to neonate, but keep mother away from other antenatal patients
Sexually transmitted diseases (gonorrhoea, syphilis)	Access with meticulous hand washing; no restrictions on breast feeding if mother being treated	Assess baby carefully to check that he is not infected, especially with maternal syphilis (p. 211) and give eye prophylaxis for gonococcus (p. 189)
Skin infections (boils, impetigo)	Access; meticulous hand washing; antibiotics to mother	Nil
Streptococcal illness or carriage	No restrictions. Meticulous hand washing and masking, especially for group A *Streptococcus* respiratory infections	Nil
Toxoplasmosis	No restrictions	Treat the baby (p. 210)
Tropical diseases (trypanosomiasis, schistosomiasis, filariasis)	Usually no restrictions	Nil, but consult local tropical diseases hospital
*Tuberculosis – open	No restriction if mother's general health satisfactory; drugs do not pass in sufficient quantity into breast milk to contraindicate breast feeding but no access to NNU	INAH to baby; BCG at 6 months if baby PPD negative or give INAH-resistant BCG at once
Tuberculosis – closed	As above	As above; normal BCG routine to baby
Ureaplasma colonization	No restrictions	Nil
*Varicella	Access restricted until lesions crusted; mother gowned, masked and gloved. NO access to NNU	Give 250 mg (one vial) ZIG to baby if maternal disease develops between 7 days before and 14 days after delivery; give aciclovir if vesicles appear
*Zoster	Access to own baby, no access to NNU	Nil; baby immune from transplacental IgG

BCG, bacille Calmette–Guérin; INAH, isoniazid; PPD, purified protein derivative; ZIG, zoster immunoglobulin.

*Conditions where mother may have access to her own term baby, but is not allowed into the neonatal unit (NNU) or to have access to other babies.

References

Bitner-Glindzicz, M, Pembrey, M, Duncan, A, et al. (2009) Prevalence of mitochondrial 1555A—>G mutation in European children. *New England Journal of Medicine*, **360**(6): 640–2.

Carr, R, Modi, M, Dore, C (2006) G-CSF and GM-CSF for treating or preventing neonatal infection. *Cochrane Database of Systematic Reviews*, Issue 3.

Carr, R, Brocklehurst, P, Doré, CJ, Modi, N (2009) Granulocyte-macrophage colony stimulating factor administered as prophylaxis for reduction of sepsis in extremely preterm, small for gestational age neonates (the PROGRAMS trial): a single-blind, multicentre, randomised controlled trial. *Lancet*, **373**: 226–33.

Connor, EM, Sperling, RS, Gilbert, R (1994) Reduction of maternal infant transmission of human immunodeficiency virus type 1 with zidovudine treatment. *New England Journal of Medicine*, **331**: 1173–80.

De Jonge, M, Burchfield, D, Bloom, B, et al. (2007) Clinical trial of safety and efficacy of INH-A21 for the prevention of nosocomial staphylococcal bloodstream infection in premature infants. *Journal of Pediatrics*, **151**(3): 260–5.

de Ruiter, A, Mercey, D, Anderson, J, et al. (2008) British HIV Association and Children's HIV Association guidelines for the management of HIV infection in pregnant women 2008. *HIV Med*, **9**(7): 452–502.

De Vries, E, de Groot, R, de Bruin-Versteeg, S, et al.(1999) Analysing the developing lymphocyte system of neonates and infants. *European Journal of Pediatrics*, **158**: 611–17.

Doran, KS, Nizet, V, (2004) Molecular pathogenesis of neonatal group B streptococcal infection: no longer in its infancy. *Molecular Microbiology*, **54**(1): 23–31.

Friedlich, PS, Steinberg, I, Fujitani, A, de Lemos, R (1997) Renal tolerance with the use of Intralipid-Amphotericin B in low birthweight neonates. *American Journal of Perinatology*, **14**: 377–83.

Goldberg, DM (1987) The cephalosporins. *Medical Clinics of North America*, **71**: 1113–33.

Greenberg, RG, Smith, PB, Cotton, CM, et al. (2008) Adjustment of cerebrospinal fluid cell counts for a traumatic lumbar puncture does not aid diagnosis of meningitis in neonates. *Pediatric Infectious Disease Journal*, **27**: 1047–51.

Heath PT, Nik Yusoff, NK, Baker, CJ (2003) Neonatal meningitis. *Archives of Disease in Childhood. Fetal and Neonatal Edition*, **88**(3): F173–8.

Malaeb, S, Damman, O, (2009) Fetal inflammatory response and brain injury in the preterm newborn. *Journal of Child Neurology*, **24**(9): 1119–26.

Millar, M, Wilks, M, Fleming, P, Costeloe, K (2012) Should the use of probiotics in the preterm be routine? *Archives of Disease in Childhood. Fetal and Neonatal Edition*, **97**: F70–4.

Mnyani, CN, McIntyre, JA (2011) Tuberculosis in pregnancy. *British Journal of Obstetrics and Gynaecology*, **118**(2): 226–31.

Ohlsson, A, Lacy, JB (2006) Intravenous immunoglobulins for treatment of suspected or subsequently proven infection in neonates. *Cochrane Database of Systematic Reviews*, Issue 3.

RCOG (2007) Green Top Guideline No. 30. *Management of Genital Herpes in Pregnancy* (www.rcog.org.uk).

RCOG (2012) Green Top Guideline No. 36. *Group B Streptococcal Disease, Early Onset* (www.rcog.org.uk/file/rcog-corp/grg36-gbs.pdf).

Risser, WL, Hwang, L-Y (1996) Problems with the current case definitions of congenital syphilis. *Journal of Pediatrics*, **129**: 499–505.

Vandebona, H, Mitchell, P, Manwaring, N, et al. (2009) Prevalence of mitochondrial 1555A-->G mutation in adults of European descent. *New England Journal of Medicine*, **360**(6): 642–4.

■ Further reading

Barnhart, HX, Caldwell, MB, Thomas, P, *et al.* (1996) Natural history of human immunodeficiency virus disease in perinatally infected children: an analysis from the Pediatric Spectrum of Disease Project. *Pediatrics*, **97**: 710–16.

Freeman, J, Goldman, DA, Smith, NE, *et al.* (1990) Association of intravenous lipid emulsion and coagulase negative staphylococal bacteremia in neonatal intensive care units. *New England Journal of Medicine*, **323**: 301–8.

Haque, KN, Zaidi, MH, Haque, SK, *et al.* (1986) Intravenous immunoglobulin for prevention of sepsis in preterm and low birthweight infants. *Pediatric Infectious Disease Journal*, **5**: 622–5.

Isaacs, D, Moxon, RE (1999) *Handbook of Neonatal Infections: A Practical Guide.* London: Saunders.

Mercey, D (1998) Antenatal HIV testing. *British Medical Journal*, **316**: 241–2. (This editorial is followed by a series of articles: *BMJ* 1998; **316**: 253–307.)

Regulation and Quality Improvement Authority (2012) Independent Review of Incidents of Pseudomonas, aeruginosa Infection in Neonatal Units in Northern Ireland (www.rqia.org.uk).

Remington, JS, Klein, JO, Wilson, CB, *et al.* (2011) *Infectious Diseases of the Fetus and Newborn*, 7th edition. Philadelphia, PA: Elsevier.

Stoll, BJ, Gordon, J, Korones, SB, *et al.* (1996a) Late onset sepsis in very low birth weight neonates: A report from the National Institute of Child Health and Human Development Neonatal Research Network. *Journal of Pediatrics*, **129**: 63–71.

Stoll, BJ, Gordon, J, Korones, SB, *et al.* (1996b) Early onset sepsis in very low birthweight neonates: A report from the National Institute of Child Health and Human Development Neonatal Research Network. *Journal of Pediatrics*, **129**: 72–80.

17

Neurological problems

Assessment of the nervous system

Healthy newborns spend about 50 minutes of each hour asleep, either quiet sleep (regular breathing, no eye movements; non-rapid eye movement (REM) sleep) or active sleep (irregular breathing, rapid eye movements; REM sleep). For some of the time the normal term baby is awake and alert, fixing his gaze on the examiner's face. Even when crying he is consolable and cuddly. The normal baby's movements have a fluid, elegant quality; his hands open occasionally and he can move his fingers individually. The movements are complex and variable.

Neurological assessment must *always* include measurement of the head circumference. Persistent high-pitched crying, unconsolability (irritability), paucity/poor repertoire of movement and marked jitteriness are abnormal and can indicate problems such as hypoxic ischaemic encephalopathy, meningitis, hypoglycaemia, drug withdrawal, pain or intracranial haemorrhage (ICH). Investigation is indicated. Alarm signals include:

- persisting irritability, marked jitteriness;
- difficulty in feeding;
- opisthotonus, or persistent asymmetry in posture, movements or tone;
- abnormal cry;
- states of only crying or sleeping; no quiet alert periods;
- tense fontanelle, rapidly rising head circumference;
- seizures;
- apathy and immobility, floppiness.

Convulsions in the newborn

Key points
- Fits in the neonatal period are often subtle.
- All fitting babies require full biochemical, electroencephalogram and ultrasound investigation as well as a workup for meningitis.
- The first-line anticonvulsants are phenobarbitone and phenytoin, with midazolam as the second line.
- Most babies who fit in the neonatal period stop fitting and can safely have their anticonvulsant treatment stopped before they go home.

Incidence

The incidence of clinically recognized convulsions in the neonatal period is 1–3 per 1000 live births at term, and 50–100 per 1000 in preterm births. Most seizures are recognized in the first 24 hours of life.

Types of convulsions

The most common type of seizure in the neonate, both term and preterm, involves a very subtle change in activity. The baby becomes still; there may be tiny movements of the eyes or jaw (forced blinking, eye deviation, chewing or lip smacking) and/or changes in the breathing pattern. The period of abnormal behaviour often lasts only 30 seconds or so; even electrographically most neonatal seizures are only 2–3 minutes in length. Clonic convulsions in the neonate may be focal or generalized, and boxing or cycling movements of the limbs are common manifestations of this seizure type. Babies can have short tonic seizures in which they adopt an opisthotonic posture with extended and internally rotated limbs, and their eyes deviate into a fixed position; they may become apnoeic with cyanosis and bradycardia. The neonate often exhibits electroclinical dissociation; that is, there is poor agreement between the stereotyped clinical manifestations of seizure and any discharge on the electroencephalogram (EEG). Only rarely are the two precisely temporally related.

Aetiology and differential diagnosis of neonatal convulsions

The major causes of neonatal convulsions are listed in Table 17.1. In some babies it is comparatively easy to establish the cause of the fit (for example, a small for gestational age baby fitting from hypoglycaemia at 36 hours of age). However, in many babies several of the factors listed in Table 17.1 may co-exist. For this reason any convulsing neonate should routinely have the following tests carried out as a minimum:

- blood glucose, electrolytes and urea;
- blood gases;
- calcium and magnesium;
- white blood count and differential;
- blood culture;
- lumbar puncture;
- EEG whenever possible;
- ultrasound brain scan.

On the basis of these tests and the history of, for example, birth depression, maternal group B beta-haemolytic *Streptococcus* colonization with prolonged membrane rupture, or maternal drug ingestion, an accurate diagnosis can be made in most babies. Any baby with seizures in whom the suggested first-line investigations do not yield a diagnosis should have an MRI. Stroke, particularly, is often ultrasound-negative. Very occasionally babies convulse because they suffer from rare inborn errors of metabolism. In general, these babies are acidotic and show other neurological abnormalities (see Chapter 18). In acutely ill babies, the routine outlined on p. 246 should be followed; in less ill neonates, urinary amino acid chromatography should always be carried out.

Table 17.1 Causes of neonatal convulsions

Diagnosis	Age at start and type of fit	Diagnostic clues
Hypoxic ischaemic encephalopathy	Usually 12–24 hours; can be subtle, tonic or clonic	Pathological cardiotocogram, need for resuscitation, early acidosis, obtunded, haematuria
GMH-IVH	Preterm baby, 0–72 hours; usually subtle	Decreased PCV; increased fontanelle tension; readily diagnosed with ultrasound
Aterial thrombosis or 'stroke' (usually middle cerebral artery)	24–72 hours, can be later. Baby remains alert between seizures, which are often focal	Well baby. Diagnose with ultrasound or MRI
Meningitis	Any time and type of fit	Ill baby with signs of sepsis; lumbar puncture
Hypoglycaemia	<72 hours, clonic	Small-for-dates or preterm baby; if term and normal weight, suggests rare cause of hypoglycaemia (see pp. 243–244)
Hypocalcaemia	Early or late (5–8 days)	Rare now; usually seriously ill baby <48 hours old
Hypomagnesaemia	5–8 days, clonic, multifocal	Associated with low calcium and phosphate
High or low serum sodium	Any age, usually clonic	Ill babies; hypernatraemia is linked to large postnatal weight loss
Kernicterus	Any time, any type	Very high unconjugated serum bilirubin
Congenital central nervous system malformation	Any time, any type	Increasingly recognized with imaging. Can be small head, etc.
Pyridoxine dependency	Seizures are resistant to treatment unless pyridoxine is given	Response to IV pyridoxine. Test urinary alpha-aminoadipic semialdehyde and pipecolic acid and antiquitin gene
Glycine encephalopathy	Hypotonia, 'hiccoughs' and intractable seizures	High cerebrospinal fluid and plasma glycine levels, burst-suppressed EEG
Fifth day fits	Around the fifth day, usually clonic	Have become very rare – normal investigation results
Benign familial neonatal seizures	Usually 3–7 days; brief clonic seizures	Family history (autosomal dominant). Normal investigations, associated with a microdeletion on chromosomes 20 and 8 – a 'channelopathy'
Benign neonatal sleep myoclonus	5 days on; only in sleep; only myoclonic jerks	Normal investigations, exclude inborn errors
Maternal drug withdrawal	Usually less than a week, clonic	Maternal history, hair or urine analysis
Rare inborn errors	Usually <72 hours; any type of fit	Can be a family history of previous sudden neonatal death

EEG, electroencephalogram; GMH-IVH, germinal matrix–intraventricular haemorrhage; IV, intravenous; PCV, packed cell volume.

Treatment of neonatal convulsions

Turn the baby on his side and secure the airway (intubate and give intermittent positive pressure ventilation if apnoea, cyanosis or bradycardia develop). Gently aspirate the pharynx if inhalation of milk or vomit has occurred. Give oxygen by mask if the baby is cyanosed but breathing – very carefully to babies at risk from retinopathy of prematurity. Take blood for a laboratory and ward estimation of glucose while anticonvulsants are being obtained, and give 3 mL/kg of 10% dextrose intravenously if the result is below 2.6 mmol/L.

Use phenobarbitone as the first-line anticonvulsant, remembering larger doses cause apnoea and may require intubation. If phenobarbitone does not work, try, in order, phenytoin (only if no myocardial ischaemia), then load with midazolam followed by a continuous infusion which can be titrated as required.

In most babies with neonatal convulsions, maintenance anticonvulsant therapy (usually with phenobarbitone 5 mg/kg/24 h) should be started and continued for several days. However, the half-life of phenobarbitone is long and it is often useful to check plasma levels prior to starting maintenance therapy. In general, babies who recover to a normal neurological state before going home do not need maintenance anticonvulsants, but anticonvulsants should be continued in babies with other persisting clinical or EEG abnormality or underlying central nervous system malformation.

■ Hypoxic ischaemic encephalopathy

Key points

- ■ Hypoxic ischaemic encephalopathy (HIE) causes permanent damage to the central nervous system in around 1:2000 babies born at term.
- ■ Prevention of HIE largely depends on good obstetric management.
- ■ Therapeutic hypothermia to 33–34°C commencing within 6 hours of birth and continuing for 72 hours followed by a gradual re-warming at 0.5°C every 2 hours is now recognized to be a safe and effective treatment for term neonates with HIE.
- ■ Supportive neonatal care in HIE involves maintenance of homeostasis and controlling seizures. There is as yet no specific neuroprotective regimen which has been shown to be of benefit (apart from cooling).
- ■ Predicting outcome accurately is aided by the results of electroencephalography, neuroimaging and careful clinical assessment of the worst grade of encephalopathy, with recognition that cooling therapy may alter the time at which these assessments should be interpreted.

The characteristic neurological syndrome seen in term babies after a period of perinatal asphyxia is called hypoxic ischaemic encephalopathy (HIE). The underlying insult is usually a combination of hypoxia and hypotension during late fetal life, resulting in acidosis. The insult can be an acute, profound hypoxia lasting 10–25 minutes (e.g. cord prolapse, uterine rupture) or a chronic partial hypoxia lasting for an hour or more (cord entanglement, uterine hyperstimulation) (p. 30). The diagnosis must be based on more than just a low Apgar score, for which there are many other causes (p. 40). However, in the delivery room the Apgar score may be the only piece of information available. After successful resuscitation, it is helpful to consider the factors in Table 17.2 when deciding whether to admit a baby to the neonatal unit (NNU) for observation (Portman *et al.* 1990). The clinical picture evolves over the first 12 hours;

Table 17.2 The Portman score for post-asphyxia morbidity (Portman *et al.* 1990)

	0 points	1 point	2 points	3 points
5 min Apgar score	6	5–6	3–4	0–2
Base deficit from arterial blood gas in first hour (mmol/L)	<10	10–14	15–19	>19
Cardiotocogram	Normal	Variable decelerations	Severe variable or late decelerations	Prolonged bradycardia

≥6 points, severe morbidity; positive predictive value 78%.

babies who go to the postnatal ward must be observed carefully because they can, and often do, develop symptoms between 12 and 72 hours after birth.

Diagnosis of hypoxic ischaemic encephalopathy

The severity of HIE has been divided into three grades (Table 17.3). A scoring system can also be useful in the clinical assessment of neonates with encephalopathy (Table 17.4). About six in 1000 babies in the UK suffer some form of HIE, with grades II and III each affecting one in 1000 babies worldwide. The incidence of HIE is known to be high in developing countries and the disorder makes a large contribution to the burden of childhood disability.

Table 17.3 Clinical grade of hypoxic ischaemic encephalopathy (from Levene *et al.* 1986)

Grade I (mild)	Grade II (moderate)	Grade III (severe)
Irritability 'hyperalert'	Lethargy	Comatose
Mild hypotonia	Marked abnormalities in tone	Severe hypotonia
Poor sucking	Requires tube feeds	Failure to maintain spontaneous respiration
No seizures	Seizures	Prolonged seizures

Table 17.4 Thompson score of neonatal encephalopathy (from Thompson *et al.* 1997)

SCORE:	0	1	2	3
Tone	Normal	Hyper	Hypo	Flaccid
Consciousness	Normal	Hyperalert, starey	Lethargic	Comatose
Seizures	Normal	<3 per day	>2 per day	
Posture	Normal	Fisting, cycling	Strong distal flexion	Decerebrate
Moro	Normal	Partial	Absent	
Grasp	Normal	Poor	Absent	
Suck	Normal	Poor	Absent ± bites	
Respiration	Normal	Hyperventilation	Brief apnoea	IPPV (apnoea)
Fontanelle	Normal	Full, not tense	Tense	

IPPV, intermittent positive pressure ventilation.

If the insult was mild, all that will usually occur will be that the baby will be wide eyed and irritable, making a rapid recovery within a few days. With more severe injury, fits are often difficult to control. Alternatively the baby may never breathe, be ventilator-dependent and have an isoelectric (flat) EEG. Grades II and III HIE are the most common cause of seizures in term babies (Table 17.1), but if the positive features of pathological cardiotocogram, birth depression, early metabolic acidosis and multiple organ system involvement are lacking, then one of the other diagnoses must be sought. The seizures of HIE are often very subtle and typically occur at a postnatal age of 12–24 hours.

Other organ systems are involved, and there may be hypoglycaemia and marked hypotension from myocardial depression. The chest X-ray may show a large heart with electrocardiogram changes of ischaemia. Renal failure with oliguria and haematuria is also usual.

Investigation of hypoxic ischaemic encephalopathy

Ultrasound and CT scanning in the early phases show a featureless brain with loss of the normal sulci and gyri with compressed ventricles. Evidence of cerebral oedema is not predictive of outcome, but does support a clinical diagnosis of HIE. In 'acute profound' damage the deep grey matter of the thalami and lentiform nuclei are typically affected, and produce abnormal signals on MR images. MR is more sensitive than ultrasound in detecting these abnormalities, although when basal ganglia changes are severe enough to be imaged with ultrasound, the prognosis is usually poor. The background EEG is of diagnostic and prognostic value. The EEG in HIE has an abnormal background, often with multifocal seizures of varying morphology. Doppler ultrasound studies of the cerebral circulation show a high cerebral blood flow velocity with a particularly high diastolic velocity, and can be useful in confirming the diagnosis and assisting in prognosis.

Treatment of hypoxic ischaemic encephalopathy

Over the past decade therapeutic hypothermia has emerged as the first safe and effective treatment for neonatal encephalopathy (Edwards *et al.* 2010). The criteria used for initiating cooling treatment within the large UK total body hypothermia (ToBY) trial are shown in Table 17.5. Infants that meet criteria A should be assessed for whether they meet the neurological abnormality entry criteria (B). Treatment should begin within 6 hours of life.

Table 17.5 Inclusion criteria used in the trials of therapeutic hypothermia

Criteria A	Criteria B
Infants ≥36 completed weeks' gestation admitted to the NICU with at least one of the following:	Seizures or moderate to severe encephalopathy, consisting of:
■ Apgar score of ≤5 at 10 minutes after birth ■ Continued need for resuscitation, including endotracheal or mask ventilation, at 10 minutes after birth ■ Acidosis within 60 minutes of birth (defined as any occurrence of umbilical cord, arterial or capillary pH <7.00) ■ Base deficit ≥16 mmol/L in umbilical cord or any blood sample (arterial, venous or capillary) within 60 minutes of birth	■ Altered state of consciousness (reduced or absent response to stimulation) *and* ■ Abnormal tone (focal or general hypotonia, or flaccid) *and* ■ Abnormal primitive reflexes (weak or absent suck or Moro response)

NICU, neonatal intensive care unit.

As soon as possible a cerebral function monitoring or EEG trace should be obtained, but if this is not available and the baby otherwise meets the criteria, the lack of EEG monitoring should not delay starting therapeutic hypothermia. If a baby is born outside a cooling centre, urgent transfer should be arranged and consideration given to starting passive cooling (allowing the baby to cool down naturally by removing external heat sources) if adequate and appropriate facilities are available for temperature monitoring. Babies undergoing therapeutic hypothermia require skilled nursing care, with appropriate analgesia and sedation. It is important to note that cooling without such supportive care is not neuroprotective in animal models.

Hypoxic ischemic injury is a multisystem condition with multiple sequelae (Table 17.6). Severely affected infants can be among the sickest infants on the NNU and should be cared for in units with the appropriate expertise and access to neurological monitoring and imaging.

Anticonvulsants should be stopped once the fits cease, as ongoing unnecessary treatment contributes to the hypotonia and feeding difficulty and makes the baby hard to assess. The following clinical features are worrying, and add prognostic information to that obtained from investigation:

- persisting fits or apnoeas;
- prolonged hypotonia and apathy;
- prolonged hypertonia;
- persisting failure to suck feeds.

Table 17.6 Organ systems affected in hypoxic ischaemic encephalopathy

Organ system	Manifestation of dysfunction	Management
Central nervous system	Seizures; apnoeas; raised intracranial pressure; intracranial bleeding; nerve palsies	See this chapter
Respiratory	Respiratory distress due to surfactant deficiency; ARDS; apnoea; PPHN; pulmonary haemorrhage; meconium aspiration	Ventilate; measure blood gases; correct acidosis; see Chapter 13
Cardiovascular	Shock; hypotension; cardiomegaly; heart failure; ECG evidence of ischaemia	Ventilate; give inotropes; fluid restriction; diuretics
Renal	Oliguria; haematuria; proteinuria; myoglobinuria; renal failure	Fluid restriction; careful monitoring; consider dialysis if central nervous system prognosis considered good
Haematological	DIC; raised white cell count; raised nucleated red cell count	Vitamin K; fresh frozen plasma; cryoprecipitate; fibrinogen concentrates, cover for infection
Metabolic	Hypoglycaemia; hypocalcaemia; hyponatraemia	Replace lost ions; careful fluid balance
Gastrointestinal	Ileus; necrotizing enterocolitis	Start enteral feeds cautiously; treat necrotizing enterocolitis as on pp. 281–283
Hepatic	Elevated transaminases/ammonia; prolonged coagulation times; jaundice	Vitamin K; support coagulation; phototherapy/exchange transfusion as indicated

ARDS, acute respiratory distress syndrome; DIC, disseminated intravascular coagulation; ECG, electrocardiogram; PPHN, persistent pulmonary hypertension of the newborn.

Prognosis in hypoxic ischaemic encephalopathy

The advent of therapeutic cooling has reignited the debate regarding our ability accurately to predict outcome in HIE. Many of the previously used tools, such as clinical examination on day 3, EEG at 12–72 hours and Doppler carotid blood flow at 24–48 hours, have been demonstrated to be less predictive in the post-cooling era. Currently much attention is being directed at establishing criteria on which to consider withdrawal of intensive care. Additional tests which may be of benefit include the use of magnetic resonance spectroscopy and other MR biomarkers if available.

The following are *not* helpful in the prognosis of HIE:

- neuroimaging evidence of cerebral oedema;
- the number or type of clinical or electrical seizures (unless very prolonged 'status epilepticus' is confirmed with continuous EEG monitoring);
- the degree of renal impairment;
- the cord pH;
- the Apgar score at less than 10 minutes of age.

■ Focal vascular lesions

Neonatal stroke

Neonatal cerebral artery infarction may occur if a vessel is blocked by an embolus or thrombus. The baby presents with fits but is usually alert between the episodes and even during them. Cranial ultrasound may be normal but can show midline shift and an abnormal area of echodensity, most commonly in the left middle cerebral artery territory. MRI including diffusion-weighted imaging may be required to make the diagnosis. Investigation should include a search for the inherited thrombotic disorders such as protein C or protein S deficiency or the factor V Leiden mutation. Treatment is conservative, and the outcome is often good. MRI evidence of three-site involvement of the hemisphere, the basal ganglia and the posterior limb of the internal capsule is strongly associated with later contralateral hemiplegia irrespective of the size of the infarct.

Cerebral venous thrombosis

Thrombosis of the cerebral veins can occur with dehydration, infection or the inherited thrombotic disorders. The diagnosis is probably more common than is clinically suspected and can be confirmed with CT or MRI scan. Treatment with thrombolytic therapy has been tried but the results are not encouraging.

■ Extracranial haemorrhage

Subgaleal (subaponeurotic) haemorrhage

The subgaleal space is a large potential space beneath the aponeurotic membrane, and a large amount of blood can collect here before the diagnosis is made (Fig. 17.1). Ventouse delivery increases the risk of this form of bleeding. Babies present with a boggy swelling which crosses the suture lines, and the head circumference can increase by several centimetres in less than 24 hours. In severe cases the baby can collapse with shock before the source of the bleeding is appreciated; mortality is 17–25%. Treatment with blood and volume replacement is effective and the outlook for babies who are successfully treated who do not have any associated hypoxic ischaemia is good.

Intracranial haemorrhage

- Serious intracranial haemorrhage is rare at term. Babies with subdural or intracerebral haemorrhage should be evaluated in consultation with neurosurgeons. Subarachnoid haemorrhage is common, causes minimal symptoms and has a good prognosis.
- Germinal matrix–intraventricular haemorrhage (GMH-IVH) occurs in up to 20% of very low birth weight babies. The incidence can be minimized by antenatal steroids and attention to maintaining homeostasis in critically ill neonates. We do not use any specific drug prophylaxis.
- Uncomplicated GMH-IVH is frequently asymptomatic and has few sequelae.
- Complicated GMH-IVH includes post-haemorrhagic ventriculomegaly, progressive hydrocephalus and periventricular venous infarction. Serious long-term neurological sequelae are frequent in such babies.
- Other than treating hydrocephalus, no treatment is available for these serious complications.

Bleeding can occur at many sites (Fig. 17.1). Presentation is usually with seizures, but fever can occur, although the first sign of the problem can be the associated coagulopathy (bruising, bleeding) or shock. Intracranial haemorrhage is detected with neuroimaging in 3–5% of apparently healthy term babies, but the significance of subclinical bleeding is not yet clear.

Subdural haemorrhage

The most common site for a subdural haematoma at term is around the tentorium cerebelli, where the great cerebral vein and the inferior sagittal sinus combine to give the straight sinus (Fig. 17.1). This area is easily damaged, and the vessel walls can be torn during distortion of the fetal head. Subdural bleeds can also result from tearing of the bridging veins over the vault where the bleeding coagulates to cause a convexity subdural haemorrhage.

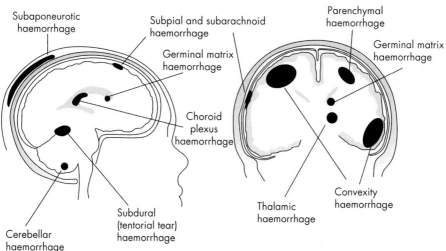

Fig. 17.1 Sites of intracranial haemorrhage. Modified from Rennie (2012) with permission

Signs

These are usually those of associated severe asphyxia (see above), raised intracranial pressure or blood loss. Although the anterior fontanelle is often bulging, this is primarily due to cerebral oedema. The diagnosis can be confirmed ultrasonically, although the subdural space is not always well seen with this technique and a CT or MRI scan is often required.

Treatment

Treat any co-existing asphyxia (see above). A convexity subdural haemorrhage under the vault can be drained by subdural tap, but draining a collection in the posterior fossa requires formal neurosurgical intervention. Small subdural collections, often little more than a film of blood over the cortex, cannot be aspirated without further traumatizing the cortex pressed up against the inside of the skull. They should be left alone. Neurosurgical input may be appropriate in symptomatic cases, particularly in the presence of an associated skull fracture, midline shift, signs of raised intracranial pressure or any focal neurological signs suggesting 'coning'.

Subarachnoid haemorrhage

This form of haemorrhage is probably much more common than is realized, with small amounts of capillary or venous subarachnoid bleeding occurring during many mildly traumatic or asphyxial deliveries. The condition is often asymptomatic, but may present with fits or irritability during the first few days. The cerebrospinal fluid (CSF) obtained is uniformly blood-stained. A cerebral ultrasound scan should be done to exclude other types of ICH, but subarachnoid bleeding cannot usually be seen with ultrasound. Symptomatic treatment of the fits or co-existing birth asphyxia is all that is required; there is no need to do repeat lumbar punctures to drain CSF. The prognosis is good.

Germinal matrix–intraventricular haemorrhage and accompanying intraparenchymal lesions

This type of intracranial bleeding is found in 20% of babies weighing less than 1.50 kg at birth; 90% of these bleeds appear for the first time within 72 hours of birth. Up to 20% will extend during the next few days.

Germinal matrix–intraventricular haemorrhage (GMH-IVH) may occur spontaneously in a comparatively asymptomatic baby weighing less than 1 kg at birth, but is most commonly seen in babies less than 1.5 kg at birth who have been hypoxic, hypotensive, hypercarbic and acidaemic in association with apnoea, severe birth asphyxia, pneumothorax or respiratory distress syndrome. The underlying problem is thought to be that of an alteration in cerebral blood flow causing bleeding into the fragile capillary bed of the germinal matrix. Fluctuations in blood pressure, or of blood flow in this area associated with the baby fighting the ventilator, are thought to be important. Vasodilatation associated with hypercarbia contributes.

Classification

In the past the term 'periventricular haemorrhage', abbreviated to PVH, was widely used to embrace germinal matrix haemorrhage, intraventricular haemorrhage and haemorrhage into the brain parenchyma. In our view, the term PVH should be abandoned; it is now realized that neither are all parenchymal lesions haemorrhagic, nor are they all periventricular. The Papile classification, which was based on CT scan appearances, is outmoded. In the Papile system, grade I described a haemorrhage confined to the subependymal region, grade II was used for bleeding into the ventricular cavity but not distending it, grade III for an intraventricular bleed with ventricular enlargement and grade IV for any parenchymal lesion. There are several disadvantages to this system, including the fact that grade IV 'lumps' all parenchymal lesions together, whereas modern neuroimaging can distinguish many different types, and the evolution of a parenchymal lesion often provides the best clue to which type of lesion it is. We prefer to term these intraparenchymal lesions (IPLs). Using ultrasound it is not possible to make a certain pathological diagnosis, so the terms 'grade IV intraventricular haemorrhage' and 'parenchymal extension of intraventricular haemorrhage' should be abandoned. As yet there is no universal agreement on how to classify GMH-IVH or intraparenchymal lesions. Table 17.7 provides a suggested classification.

Pathology

The bleeding arises in the germinal matrix, a structure which is abundant over the head of the caudate nucleus and can also be found in the periventricular zone. The germinal matrix involutes early in the third trimester, making GMH-IVH rare in babies over 32 weeks' gestation and 1.5 kg birth weight. The venous drainage of the deep white matter occurs via a fan-shaped leash of vessels, which drain into a vessel lateral to and below the germinal matrix. Obstruction to this vein is thought to be responsible for the common accompaniment of a fan-shaped white matter lesion on the same side as a GMH-IVH. These lesions are intraparenchymal venous infarctions, which often become haemorrhagic and develop into a porencephalic cyst.

IVH can occur at term. When it does, the baby has often been delivered by forceps or ventouse (Towner *et al.* 1999). Other causes are vitamin K deficiency bleeding (see Chapter 23) or a coagulopathy associated with HIE.

Signs and symptoms

In about half of the cases, mostly those with an uncomplicated GMH, the haemorrhage develops without causing any clinical signs. With bigger haemorrhages, babies are likely to have signs. They often become limp and unresponsive, and may develop fits. If babies are breathing spontaneously they may become apnoeic and are difficult to resuscitate because they have become hypotensive and acidaemic. Often the packed cell volume will drop by 5–10% after a few hours, and the baby looks pale and peripherally vasoconstricted. However, only if the GMH-IVH is very large does the neonate develop a tense anterior fontanelle or an acute increase in his head circumference.

Table 17.7 Description of neonatal intracranial lesions seen early in life with ultrasound

Description	Generic term
Germinal matrix haemorrhage	GMH-IVH
Intraventricular haemorrhage without ventricular dilatation	GMH-IVH
Intraventricular haemorrhage with acute ventricular dilatation (measure the ventricle)	GMH-IVH and ventriculomegaly
Intraparenchymal lesion – describe size, location, degree of echogenicity (Fig. 17.2b) and permanently record the image	IPL

GMH-IVH, germinal matrix–intraventricular haemorrhage; IPL, intraparenchymal lesion.

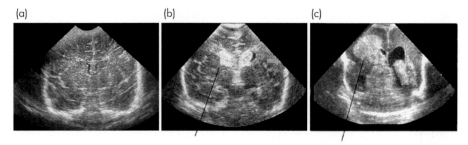

Fig. 17.2 (a) Normal ultrasound scan, (b) intraventricular haemorrhage (IVH),
(c) intraparenchymal lesion (IPL) accompanying germinal matrix–intraventricular haemorrhage

Diagnosis

GMH-IVH is readily diagnosed with cerebral ultrasonography, and many NNUs routinely screen all very low birth weight (VLBW) admissions this way. A GMH can be recognized as an echogenic area between the caudate nucleus and the ventricle, and an IVH as an echogenic clot within the normally echolucent ventricle (Fig. 17.2b). Unilateral IPL accompanying GMH-IVH (Fig. 17.2c) is usually globular and on the same side, evolving over a period of weeks into a porencephalic cyst.

Prevention

The importance of good general care, with attention to control of blood pressure and blood gases, gentle handling and gentle ventilation, has combined with the benefits of antenatal steroids and postnatal surfactant to produce a welcome decline in the incidence of GMH-IVH over the last decades. The interrelationship of clinical disturbance with GMH-IVH is one of the major justifications for the minimal handling concept (Chapter 7) and yet another reason for sucking out endotracheal tubes only if it is absolutely necessary and using ventilator techniques which reduce the incidence of pneumothorax (see Chapter 13).

The current low incidence of GMH-IVH and IPL seen in many units means that the use of specific prophylaxis has fallen. The most promising drug in this respect is indometacin, but the long-term outcome studies did not show great benefit. Our current practice does not include routine drug prophylaxis against GMH-IVH.

Treatment and management of complications

Babies with GMH-IVH are often asymptomatic and neither receive nor need treatment. In those who do deteriorate, anaemia, acidaemia and hypotension usually respond promptly to blood transfusion and dopamine. If the acidosis does not resolve, infusions of base should be given. Fits should be controlled with phenobarbitone and coagulation abnormalities corrected. There is no specific treatment for GMH-IVH.

About 30% of babies with a significant GMH-IVH develop post-haemorrhagic ventricular dilatation (PHVD) on ultrasound scan; the larger the initial GMH-IVH, the higher the risk of developing PHVD. When the initial bleed forms a cast of the whole ventricle, PHVD is a certainty. Enlargement of the ventricles can be imaged with ultrasound long before clinical symptoms or excessive head growth occur. In about half the babies with PHVD the condition is transient; the other half go on to develop hydrocephalus requiring treatment. Distinguishing between these groups is the key to management. In many babies the PHVD is mild, asymptomatic, and will

(a)

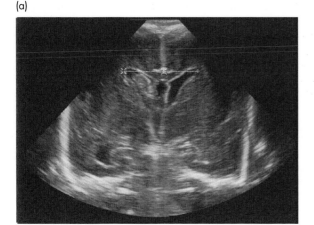

(b)

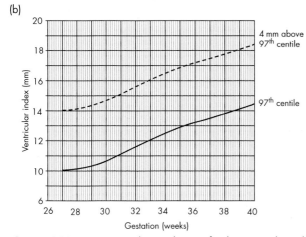

Fig. 17.3 Measurement and normal range for the ventricular index. From Levene (1981)

resolve. Progressive hydrocephalus is very likely if the CSF pressure is more than 15 cmH$_2$O; the upper limit of normal pressure in the newborn is about 7 cmH$_2$O. Once the diagnosis has been made, a lumbar puncture should be done to measure the pressure, to exclude low-grade infection as a cause of the ventricular enlargement, and to measure the CSF protein concentration in case a shunt is required.

Once PHVD has been recognized, serial measurements of ventricular size and head circumference are mandatory. There are many measurement systems available, but we recommend the Levene ventricular index (Fig. 17.3). This linear measure, of the width of the lateral ventricle on a coronal ultrasound scan in the plane of the third ventricle, has proved robust and repeatable. There is no evidence that early drainage of CSF or diuretic treatment alters the natural history of PHVD. Repeated ventricular taps are not recommended as they can result in multiple needle tracks through the brain.

Absolute indications for CSF drainage, either with a ventriculoperitoneal shunt or via a reservoir if the baby is too frail or the CSF protein too high for a definitive procedure, include:

- symptoms such as apnoea, seizures, irritability or vomiting associated with a CSF pressure of more than 10 cmH$_2$O;
- a head circumference enlarging at twice the normal rate for more than 2 weeks, or crossing two centile lines.

Prognosis

The prognosis for babies with uncomplicated GMH-IVH is good. Babies with PHVD which is non-progressive are at increased risk (about 50%) of neurodevelopmental sequelae, whereas those who require shunting do less well. Babies with an IPL which evolves into a porencephalic cyst are at high risk of a hemiplegic cerebral palsy, with or without developmental delay. The exact prognosis from an IPL depends on the exact size and location of the lesion. An MRI at corrected age of term can be very useful.

■ Preterm white matter injury/periventricular leukomalacia

Key points
- Preterm brain injury is likely to be an amalgamation of specific destructive lesions and disorders of normal brain development.
- The aetiology of periventricular leukomalacia (PVL) is still unclear; underperfusion of the periventricular white matter and the effects of excitotoxicity and cytokines (released during infective processes) on the oligodendroglia are thought to be important.
- PVL is not always diagnosed with neonatal ultrasound and later MRI detects far more cases.
- There is no treatment of proven value to prevent PVL or which can modify its prognosis once changes are seen on ultrasound or with MRI.

Preterm white matter damage was originally described from autopsy studies in the 1960s with 'white spots' seen in the periventricular white matter. This condition, described as cystic periventricular leukomalacia (PVL), probably represents the most severe end of a spectrum of injury. It can be reliably diagnosed on ultrasound with cysts seen as infants approach term-equivalent age. Bilateral occipital cystic PVL reliably predicts cerebral palsy in surviving infants. Thankfully the incidence of cystic PVL has fallen and is now present in only around 2–3% of VLBW babies. More recently a diffuse pattern of white matter injury has been recognized on MRI, which affects up to 50% of VLBW babies imaged at term-equivalent age. This pattern of injury appears as diffuse excessive high signal intensity (DEHSI) within the white matter on T$_2$-weighted MR images. Advanced MR techniques have shown that this is associated with decreased volumes within the cortex, basal ganglia, corpus callosum and the cerebral white matter. In addition there is a reduced structural organization within the brain represented by a decrease in fractional anisotropy (a measure of directional diffusion) on diffusion tensor imaging. Ultrasound is relatively insensitive at detecting diffuse white matter injury.

Pathogenesis

This is less well understood than that of GMH-IVH, and PVL is less tightly linked to gestational age. Hypoxic ischaemic or excitotoxic injury to the oligodendroglia is thought to be important. There are associations between bacterial infection, both antenatal and postnatal, necrotizing enterocolitis (NEC) and white matter injury. Hypocarbia is important and levels less than 3 kPa should be avoided. Twins are at

Neurological problems

Table 17.8 Causes of hypotonia

Condition	Differential diagnosis
Spinal cord injury	Usually breech delivery. Diagnose with MRI
Infantile spinal muscular atrophy	Often type 1 – Werdnig–Hoffman disease – when presenting in the neonatal period. Absent tendon jerks; tongue fibrillation; 'jug handle' upper limbs with bright facial expression. Genetic testing now possible and can exclude the need for muscle biopsy and electromyogram
Neonatal myasthenia	Maternal history (not always); Tensilon test
Congenital muscular dystrophy	Electromyography; muscle biopsy (see Dubowitz 1995)
Congenital myopathies	Nemaline myopathy, central core disease, etc.
Congenital myotonic dystrophy	Examine mother. Baby often oedematous with respiratory difficulty; electromyography and muscle biopsy
Malformation syndrome, e.g. Down, Prader–Willi	Characteristic facies; other abnormalities; see Chapter 5
Metabolic myopathy, e.g. glycogenoses, mitochondrial myopathy, lipid storage myopathy	
Congenital muscular dystrophy	

high risk, particularly those with twin–twin transfusion syndrome or where one twin has died. Overall a combination of specific susceptibility of developing neuronal and glial cells to injury combined with disorders of normal brain development appears to underlie the process of preterm brain injury.

Diagnosis

Clinical signs are few, although some babies exhibit abnormal neurological behaviour and/or abnormal movement patterns. Ultrasound can detect cystic change in the white matter and 'flares', but autopsy studies confirm that many areas of diffuse gliosis are missed by ultrasound imaging. MRI can detect DEHSI in addition to cystic damage. Advanced MR techniques such as diffusion tensor imaging and volumetric analysis are not currently available for routine clinical evaluation.

Prevention and treatment

In contrast to GMH-IVH, where many intervention studies have been performed both before and after delivery, hardly any data are available with regard to the prevention of PVL. Prevention of systemic hypotension is considered to be important, although evidence for hypotension as a specific risk factor is remarkably hard to find and lacks confirmation. Adjusting ventilatory settings in order to avoid severe prolonged hypocarbia is vital. There is no treatment.

Prognosis

Bilateral occipital cystic PVL is a depressingly reliable predictor of spastic diplegic cerebral palsy. Small anterior cysts, and cysts confined to the parietal region, appear to have a better outlook. Studies continue regarding the prognosis of prolonged flare which does not progress to cyst formation and regarding the importance of mild white matter hyperintensity diagnosed with MRI.

Neonatal hypotonia

The common causes for a baby being very floppy in the neonatal period are:

- perinatal or antenatal hypoxic ischaemia;
- prematurity;
- sepsis, including NEC;
- drug depression;
- hypoglycaemia;
- trisomy 21;
- any severe illness with hypoxia and acidaemia.

These diagnoses are usually obvious and the hypotonia disappears as the baby recovers.

If these common causes of hypotonia can be excluded, there are a large number of rare differential diagnoses (Table 17.8). These babies usually require sophisticated biochemical, electrophysiological or morbid anatomical investigation, and should be referred to an appropriate centre. Remember that creatine kinase levels are usually raised after birth and fall to normal levels after around 5–10 days.

Nerve palsies

Facial palsy

In the majority of cases the facial nerve has been injured by being compressed against the ramus of the mandible during the birth process, and the facial weakness rapidly resolves during the first week. Diffculty with feeding may occasionally occur, and the baby should then be tube-fed until facial power returns. Facial palsy can be due to nuclear agenesis, in which case evidence of other cranial nerve palsies is usually present (Möebius syndrome).

Congenital brachial plexus palsy

The incidence of congenital brachial plexus palsy in the UK has decreased and is currently around 1 in 2300 deliveries; there is still an association with macrosomia and shoulder dystocia. It is traditionally held that the upper cords of the brachial plexus C(4)56(7) may be torn by excessive traction when there is difficulty in delivering the anterior shoulder, or in extracting the head in a breech delivery. The most useful classification is probably that of Narakas (see Evans-Jones and Birch 2005) – groups I and II constitute classical 'Erb's palsy', with group II cases having wrist extensor involvement. The right arm is more commonly affected than the left, but the condition can be bilateral. Injury to C8 and T1 causing a claw hand (Klumpke's paralysis) is rare.

Group I   paralysis of the shoulder and biceps (C5 and C6).

Group II   paralysis of the shoulder, biceps and forearm extensors (C5, 6 and 7).

Group III   complete paralysis of the limb, flail arm (C5–T11).

Group IV   as III but with ipsilateral Horner syndrome due to sympathetic chain involvement.

Often, virtually all movement at the shoulder joint is lost and the baby cannot flex his elbow. His arm lies limply at his side in the 'waiter's tip' position. The biceps jerk is absent. The phrenic nerve may also be involved, and diaphragmatic paralysis should be considered in babies with lack of active movement of the arm who have associated respiratory difficulty. Bony injury such as fractured clavicle or humerus should be sought.

The outcome depends on the extent and severity of the lesion, with 52% of 276 cases in the British Paediatric Surveillance Unit survey having recovered fully when evaluated at a median age of 6 months (Evans-Jones and Birch 2005). Long-term effects include posterior dislocation of the shoulder, a potentially very disabling condition. Sensation can be permanently affected. If weakness persists beyond the first week, physiotherapy should be started to prevent joint contractures. Advances in microsurgical technique mean that referral for consideration of surgical repair of the plexus should be considered if there is no return of biceps function by 3 months. The prognosis for group III and IV cases is worse and the risk of a permanently flail arm justifies early referral for these infants.

▌ Central nervous system malformations

Diagnosis of malformations such as lissencephaly and schizencephaly has increased with the availability of MR scanning, and in some of these conditions the gene deletion or homeobox gene mutation is now known. Conversely, neural tube defects have become very rare in modern neonatal practice. Prenatal prophylaxis of neural tube defects with folic acid is feasible, and all women who are seeking to become pregnant are recommended to take folate supplements.

Anencephaly

This is a uniformly fatal condition, although some babies live for a few weeks or even months. No attempt should be made to resuscitate a baby with anencephaly. The disorder is rarely seen now, since antenatal diagnosis is easy and most parents opt for termination.

Encephalocele

These are usually occipital and are comparatively rare, and may be part of complex multisystem malformations which are usually fatal shortly after birth. Encephaloceles are usually skin covered, but when they are large, death may result from trauma to the lesion during an unexpectedly difficult delivery.

The prognosis for most babies is poor. With small lesions, which may just be meningoceles and contain no neural tissue, the prognosis is better and complete neuroradiological and neurosurgical appraisal should be carried out after delivery.

Holoprosencephaly

In this condition there is a single monoventricle. Sometimes there is the associated sign of a single nostril, or cyclops. The prognosis is poor.

Spina bifida with meningocele or menigomyelocele

Meningocele

Babies with these skin-covered lesions which contain no neural tissue pose few immediate problems. They usually have small defects and these can be repaired during the neonatal period or later. Orthopaedic problems are rare, and only about 10% of these babies develop hydrocephalus.

Meningomyelocele

These defects, in which the neural plate is exposed or is covered only with a thin film of easily ruptured meninges, may occur in the cervical, thoracic or lumbar regions. Undiagnosed lesions are now very rare. Immediately after delivery, an exposed lesion should be covered with a sterile, non-adhesive dressing to protect it from physical injury and to minimize the chance of infection. The baby should be admitted to the NNU for assessment by an experienced paediatrician and neurosurgeon, noting the following features:

1. Birth weight and gestation.
2. General condition (e.g. vigorous, neurologically depressed, shocked).
3. Associated malformations (e.g. heart murmur, imperforate anus).
4. Size, level and condition of the lesion.
5. Severity of the neurological deficit, aiming to identify the lowest cord segment with detectable motor and sensory function.
6. Sphincter function.
7. Associated orthopaedic malformation (e.g. developmental dysplasia of the hip, talipes).
8. Degree of kyphoscolisis – all babies should have a lateral spinal X-ray.
9. Head circumference, shape, fontanelles, degree of hydrocephalus – all babies with spina bifida should have a baseline cerebral ultrasound.
10. Eye movements and position.

Treatment

Treatment is surgical. The back is closed and a ventriculoperitoneal shunt inserted if hydrocephalus develops. The prognosis depends on the level of the lesion.

Lissencephaly/schizencephaly

The diagnosis is usually made with imaging during investigation of seizures or abnormal head size. These disorders are smooth brain (lissencephaly) or involve a cleft in the brain around the Sylvian fissure (schizencephaly).

Agenesis of the corpus callosum

This diagnosis is made antenatally or postnatally with ultrasound and confirmed on MR scanning. There is an association with trisomy 8, but often the abnormality is an isolated problem. Prognosis is then uncertain, but perhaps 50% of children are normal.

Isolated hydrocephalus

Hydrocephalus present at birth, or developing during the neonatal period, may be due to congenital infection, congenital malformations or an acquired condition such as ICH or meningitis. A baby whose head circumference is increasing abnormally quickly should be referred for neuroradiological and neurosurgical assessment. In many cases, such as those with stenosis of the aqueduct or interventricular foramina and no other cerebral abnormality, the prognosis for long-term, handicap-free survival is excellent after the insertion of a shunt.

References

Dubowitz, V (1995) *Muscle Disorders in Childhood*, 2nd edition. London: WB Saunders.

Edwards, AD, Brocklehurst, P, Gunn, AJ, *et al.* (2010) Neurological outcomes at 18 months of age after moderate hypothermia for perinatal hypoxic ischaemic encephalopathy: synthesis and meta-analysis of trial data. *British Medical Journal*, **93**: c363.

Evans-Jones L, Birch R (2005) Congenital brachial palsy. In: David, TJ (ed.) *Recent Advances in Paediatrics*, vol. 22. Edinburgh: Churchill Livingstone, pp. 55–72.

Levene, MI (1981) Measurement of the growth of the lateral ventricles in pre-term infants with real-time ultrasound. *Archives of Disease in Childhood*, **56**: 900–4.

Levene, MI (2012) Intracranial haemorrhage at term. In Rennie, JM (ed.) *Rennie & Roberton's Textbook of Neonatology*, 5th edition. Edinburgh: Elsevier, pp. 1065–1224.

Levene, MI, Sands, C, Grindulis, H, Moore, JR (1986) Comparison of two methods of predicting outcome in perinatal asphyxia. *Lancet*, **i**: 67–8.

Portman RJ, Carter BS, Gaylord MS, *et al.* (1990) Predicting neonatal morbidity after perinatal asphyxia: a scoring system. *American Journal of Obstetrics & Gynecology*, **162**: 174–82.

Thompson, CM, Puterman, AS, Linley, LL, *et al.* (1997) The value of a scoring system for hypoxic ischemic encephalopathy in predicting neurodevelopmental outcome. *Acta Paediatrica Scandinavica*, **86**: 757–61.

Towner, D, Castro, MA, Eby-Wilkens, E, Gilbert, WM (1999) Effect of mode of delivery in nulliparous women on neonatal intracranial haemorrhage. *New England Journal of Medicine*, **341**: 1709–14.

Further reading

Dyet L, Rennie, JM (2012) Preterm brain injury. In Rennie, JM (ed.) *Rennie & Roberton's Textbook of Neonatology*, 5th edition. Edinburgh: Elsevier, pp. 1156–81.

Dubowitz, V (1980) The floppy infant. *Clinics in Developmental Medicine No. 76*. Spastics International Medical Publications. London: William Heinemann.

Levene, MI, Chervenak, FA (eds) (2008) *Fetal and Neonatal Neurology and Neurosurgery*, 4th edition. Philadelphia: Elsevier.

Volpe, JJ (2008) *Neurology of the Newborn*, 5th edition. Philadelphia: Elsevier.

18

Metabolic disorders, including glucose homeostasis and inborn errors of metabolism

Key points

■ A brief period of hypoglycaemia is virtually universal in babies.
■ Term babies mount a brisk response and can use alternative fuels, and there is no evidence that a brief episode of hypoglycaemia which is not associated with neurological signs is harmful.
■ Screening for hypoglycaemia is indicated in certain high-risk groups, including premature babies, growth-retarded babies, infants of diabetic mothers and babies who have suffered from intrapartum asphyxia.
■ Symptomatic hypoglycaemia in a normally grown, term baby is unusual and full investigation, including insulin assay, is indicated.
■ Consider an inborn error of metabolism (IEM) in any baby with severe hypoglycaemia, encephalopathy or acidaemia for which there is no apparent cause after a conventional workup.
■ Early treatment of a baby with a suspected IEM includes intermittent positive pressure ventilation, stopping enteral and parenteral feeds, normalizing glucose, pH and blood pressure.
■ Investigation is initiated by screening tests including plasma ammonia, amino acids and lactate, together with urinary organic acids and ketones. Seek specialist advice early.
■ The prognosis for babies with IEMs presenting in the neonatal period is often poor, but every effort must be made to establish the diagnosis for parental counselling and in case antenatal diagnosis is possible in further pregnancies.
■ Hypocalcaemia is common in sick preterm babies, but remember maternal vitamin D deficiency as a cause in term babies.
■ Hypercalcaemia can be a serious complication of subcutaneous fat necrosis, which can occur in babies treated with therapeutic hypothermia.

■ Glucose metabolism in the newborn

The fetal blood glucose concentration is in equilibrium with, and usually about 80% of, the maternal value. Glucose is transferred to the baby by facilitated diffusion and is stored after metabolism as fat and glycogen. Human subcutaneous and body fat is deposited from 28–30 weeks' gestation onwards, and glycogen reserves are built up from 36 weeks, especially in the liver and myocardium.

The blood glucose concentration falls rapidly during the first 2 hours of life when it is the main energy source. Simultaneously, since the enzymes of glycogenolysis (release of glucose from stored glycogen) are present and active, hepatic glycogen stores fall rapidly. At the same time, gluconeogenesis from glycerol, alanine, lactate and pyruvate is switched on by the hormonal changes which follow delivery, and the neonate can use ketones and lactate for brain metabolism. After the first few hours, the baby switches to fatty acids as his principal energy source and his respiratory quotient falls to 0.7. Glucose production continues from glycogenolysis and gluconeogenesis (glucose production in the liver), producing 4–6 mg glucose/kg/min.

After birth there is a rapid rise in glucagon and catecholamine levels, but insulin levels remain low, usually less than 20 mU/mL (135 pmol/L). The result is that newborn babies, particularly if they are premature, have impaired glucose tolerance in response to both intravenous and oral glucose loads, but this may also be due to insulin resistance. Conversely, some neonates who become hypoglycaemic appear incapable of switching off insulin production and retain 'normal' but inappropriately high insulin levels.

Normal values

Blood glucose levels fall immediately after birth in all babies (Fig. 18.1) to levels <1.5 mmol/L (25 mg%). This brief period of hypoglycaemia is 'physiological' and should not be treated. Thereafter blood glucose levels rise steadily for the first few days. As with all biochemical data, values fall into three groups:

1. *Normal.* The data in Fig. 18.1 are now widely accepted. After the first 24 hours the values should lie between 2.2 and 5.5 mmol/L (40–100 mg%) for both term and preterm babies.
2. *Abnormal but harmless.* These are values outside the normal range that require treatment but which when corrected do no harm. This concept applies to hyperbilirubinaemia, hypocarbia and hyperkalaemia, for example, but for some reason people have difficulty accepting that it also applies to hypoglycaemia.
3. *Harmful.* As with hyperbilirubinaemia there is no absolute cut-off between dangerous and safe levels and there may be an 'area under the curve' phenomenon in which degree and duration of hypoglycaemia interact. A useful concept is the 'operational threshold' defining hypoglycaemia as the level of blood glucose at which treatment is required, because the body's function (particularly the brain) is compromised (Cornblath *et al.* 2000). Damaging hypoglycaemia is always associated with neuroglycopenia; in other words, it is 'symptomatic' (although newborn babies have signs, not symptoms).

In practical clinical terms this means:

1. Blood glucose must be kept above 1.5 mmol/L at all times, and above 2.0 mmol/L after the first 12 hours in both term and preterm babies.
2. If babies more than 3 days old consistently have levels below 2.5 mmol/L, a cause should be sought.
3. 'Symptomatic' hypoglycaemia is an emergency and requires intravenous treatment.
4. In 'asymptomatic' hypoglycaemia an attempt can be made to manage the problem with increased oral feeds in babies who are tolerating milk; the tempo of investigation and treatment is slower.

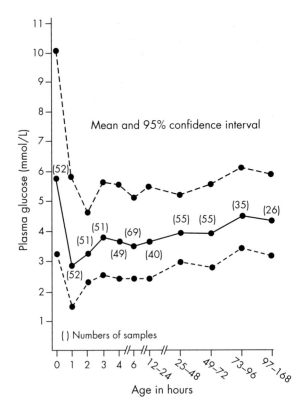

Fig. 18.1 Predicted plasma glucose values during first week of life in healthy term neonates appropriate for gestational age. Adapted from Srinivasan (1986) with permission

Symptoms of hypoglycaemia

These include the following:

1. Those due to the catecholamine response to hypoglycaemia (pallor, sweating and tachycardia). These symptoms are unusual in neonates except those with hyperinsulinaemia.
2. Signs due to the effects of hypoglycaemia on the heart, including bradycardia, hypotension and heart failure. These signs are most often seen when hypoglycaemia accompanies hypoxic ischaemic encephalopathy.
3. Signs of neuroglycopenia, including apnoea, convulsions or coma. These are signs of serious hypoglycaemia requiring urgent treatment. If in doubt the response to raising the blood glucose above 2.6 mmol/L should be tested. A prompt reduction in symptoms suggests significant symptomatic hypoglycaemia. The significance of 'softer' central nervous system (CNS) signs is more difficult to evaluate – for example, jitteriness is common in all babies whether or not they are hypoglycaemic.

Sequelae of hypoglycaemia

A striking feature of neonatal hypoglycaemia is that babies can have blood glucose values less than 1.1 mmol/L (20 mg%) without any symptoms, signs or sequelae because they are using ketones and lactate for brain metabolism (Hawdon *et al.* 1992;

de Rooy and Hawdon 2002). This fact has important clinical implications because it means that nursery routines to detect hypoglycaemia can be designed in the knowledge that asymptomatic hypoglycaemia lasting 2–3 hours will *not* cause CNS damage. However, if hypoglycaemia is prolonged, or if there are no circulating ketones or lactate, neuroglycopenia will develop with apnoea, depression of consciousness and/or convulsions. Some of these babies will have severe neurological abnormalities on follow-up, including severe intellectual retardation and spastic quadriplegia.

Screening for hypoglycaemia

Babies at risk from hypoglycaemia should be monitored as outlined in Table 18.1. A suitable method must be used. Glucose oxidase reagent sticks (Dextrostix, BM-stix) should no longer be used. These sticks are designed to use a certain volume of plasma, and the high neonatal packed cell volume and small sample size mean that the result is often inaccurate. In addition, these sticks are not accurate in the lower ranges. We currently use a Yellow Springs Laboratory standard glucometer. Glucose levels are higher in plasma than in blood by 13–18%, and they are higher in arterial blood than in capillary samples.

■ Clinical causes of hypoglycaemia

In the neonatal period there are two main groups of conditions which cause symptomatic hypoglycaemia: those in which the blood glucose falls because of depleted stores of glycogen and those that are due to hyperinsulinaemia.

Hypoglycaemia due to depleted glycogen stores

Small for gestational age

The broad definition of a small-for-gestational-age (SGA) baby is one who is below the second centile for birth weight at a given gestation. SGA babies, particularly intra-uterine growth restriction (IUGR) babies with poor body stores of both glycogen and fat, are at risk in two situations:

1. During labour the lower liver and myocardial glycogen stores give the baby little resistance to hypoxia. Much obstetric effort is put into detecting such babies

Table 18.1 Screening for hypoglycaemia

Baby diagnosis	Glucose sample timing
■ Small for gestational age (<2nd centile) ■ Maternal diabetes where glucose control has been suboptimal ■ Maternal labetalol or tolbutamide therapy ■ Preterm or sick term neonates	Pre second feed, continue until two consecutive measures >2.6 mmol/L. Then 2 hours and 6–12 hourly until levels reliably above 2.5 mmol/L, then daily when on total parenteral nutrition and at other times when clinically indicated
Hypoxic ischaemic encephalopathy	On admission; 2, 6, 12, 24 hours or regularly during intermittent positive pressure ventilation as for serious illness. Remember fluid restriction also results in glucose restriction
Haemolytic disease of the newborn	1, 2 and 4 hours after an exchange transfusion
Fitting or excessive jittering	Immediately

antenatally, and either monitoring them very carefully during labour or delivering them by elective caesarean section, although detection is not reliable.

2. Postnatally, with no glycogen stores available to be broken down to glucose, and in the absence of fat to supply ketones as an alternative brain metabolite, hypoglycaemia and neuroglycopenia may develop.

All newborn babies should be assessed using weight-for-gestation centile tables such as that shown in Table 18.2, based on the 2nd centile. Increasing the number of asymptomatic babies screened for hypoglycaemia to include those whose birth weight is between the third and the tenth centile involves screening very large numbers of healthy babies for very little gain.

Without preventative measures the peak incidence of hypoglycaemia in SGA babies occurs within the first 48 hours, often between 24 and 48 hours postnatally when the body stores of glycogen and fat have been consumed and the baby, particularly if breast fed, is still on a hypocaloric intake. Very SGA babies can develop neuroglycopenia within 6–12 hours of delivery. It follows that screening should continue for 48 hours in this population, who are not suitable for early discharge.

Prematurity

A very premature baby may develop hypoglycaemia because he was delivered before the body deposits of fat and glycogen had been laid down. Hypoglycaemia may develop at any time during the first 2 weeks if such babies are ill and the caloric intake has been inadequate.

Intrapartum asphyxia

If this is severe, even normally grown term babies may be depleted of liver and myocardial glycogen during, or immediately following, resuscitation and consequently become hypoglycaemic. In addition to neuroglycopenia, these babies may have congestive heart failure with cardiomegaly, muffled heart sounds, bradycardia and poor peripheral perfusion.

Breast milk insufficiency

There is a group of breast-fed babies in whom feeding does not become properly established. These babies present on the third or fourth day with weight loss of more than 10–12% from birth weight, a high serum sodium concentration, and are often hypoglycaemic (Moore and Perlman 1999). After the blood glucose is restored with a feed or intravenous glucose they never become hypoglycaemic again. In general the prognosis for such babies is good.

Table 18.2 Birth weight by gestational age for the diagnosis of small-for-gestational-age (SGA) babies

Gestational age[a] (weeks)	Birth weight below which the baby is SGA (g)	
	Girls	Boys
39	2400	2500
40	2600	2700
41	2750	2800
42	2900	2950

[a] Data from Usher and McLean (1969)

Hypothermia

Cold babies are often hypoglycaemic and hypoglycaemic babies will often drop their body temperature. It is therefore often impossible to know which came first. However, both conditions require treatment.

Serious illness of any type

Congenital heart disease or septicaemia may also be associated with low blood glucose levels.

Hypoglycaemia due to hyperinsulinism

Infants of diabetic mothers

These large-for-dates babies can have a characteristic chubby plethoric (cherubic) appearance and have an increased incidence of many complications (Table 18.3). Modern management of pregnant women with diabetes has improved the outlook considerably and reduced the number of babies who are overtly cherubic in appearance. However, the UK Confidential Enquiry into Maternal and Child Health reported on 3733 women who were pregnant in 2002–3 and had type 1 or type 2 diabetes. The perinatal mortality rate was increased fourfold. The caesarean section rate, the prematurity rate, the incidence of shoulder dystocia and Erb's palsy were all higher in this high-risk group. Compared with other European countries, control was suboptimal, with only 38% of diabetic mothers having a haemoglobin A1c level of <7%.

Haemolytic disease of the newborn

Newborn babies with rhesus haemolytic disease of the newborn have marked islet hypertrophy for reasons that are not clear. Babies with cord haemoglobin levels of less than 10 g/dL are particularly prone to hypoglycaemia as a rebound phenomenon after exchange transfusion, since bank blood which has a high glucose content raises the baby's glucose above 10 mmol/L (180 mg%) during the exchange and provokes further insulin release.

Maternal glucose infusion

Giving the mother glucose during labour may make both her and her fetus hyperglycaemic, which rapidly switches to hypoglycaemia after delivery when the

Table 18.3 Problems in babies of diabetic mothers

Large for dates	Delivery problems; birth trauma, shoulder dystocia; Erb's palsy
Hepatosplenomegaly	
Congenital malformations	Congenital heart disease, microcolon; sacral agenesis
Cardiac	Cardiomyopathy, cardiac septal hypertrophy
Respiratory distress syndrome	See Chapter 13
Jaundice	See Chapter 20
Hypoglycaemia	This chapter
Hypocalcaemia	This chapter
Polycythaemia	See Chapter 23

neonatal pancreas responds by releasing insulin. This hypoglycaemia is transient, self-recovering and rarely needs therapy.

Infusion of glucose into an umbilical artery catheter positioned directly opposite the coeliac axis

Glucose infusing directly into the coeliac axis can cause insulin release and hypoglycaemia.

Management of hypoglycaemia

Detection

All babies at risk from hypoglycaemia should have regular glucose estimations carried out as outlined in Table 18.1, using a reliable method. If a low value is found, blood samples should be sent to the laboratory for true glucose estimation and treatment instituted at once. In a healthy term baby of normal birth weight who presents with hypoglycaemia, samples should be collected for the estimation of insulin, cortisol, hydroxybutyrate, carnitine, amino acids, growth hormone and ammonia before treatment is started – otherwise an opportunity to make an early diagnosis of hyperinsulinism may be lost. For sick or preterm babies on intravenous fluids, calculation of the blood glucose intake in mg/kg/min is part of routine clerking:

$$\frac{(\text{glucose concentration } (\%) \ / \ 100) \times \text{infusion rate } (\text{mL/kg/day})}{1.44}$$

The normal expected glucose intake is in the range 3–8 mg/kg/min.

Prevention

Small for gestational age and very low birth weight babies
If appropriate, babies should be started on full-strength milk feeds by 2–4 hours of age, giving 60 mL/kg/24 h on day 1 and 90 mL/kg/24 h on day 2 orally or by nasogastric tube. If enteral feeding is not appropriate, 10% glucose plus appropriate electrolyte supplements should be given by an umbilical catheter or peripheral infusion.

Hypoxic ischaemic encephalopathy
The baby should be maintained on intravenous 10% dextrose until oral feeds are tolerated. We do not currently feed babies undergoing therapeutic hypothermia, although some units do maintain non-nutritive feeds during this period. Babies with hypoxic ischaemic encephalopathy are often fluid restricted to 40 mL/kg/day, here using 10% dextrose results in glucose restriction to 2.8 mg/kg/min (or less if some of the fluid volume is taken up with other infusions). Many of these babies will require stronger glucose infusions to maintain normal blood sugars.

Maternal diabetes
Feeding, by tube if necessary, should be started by 2 hours of age. Hypoglycaemia before that time can be ignored if the baby is asymptomatic. The blood glucose level usually rises by 4 hours of age if the baby feeds well, and in these babies the risk of hypoglycaemia diminishes with time (whereas the risk in an SGA baby rises in the second 24 hours).

Treatment

If a baby in the at-risk groups develops clinical signs such as apnoea, jitteriness, low temperature or lethargy, a glucose level must be measured immediately and the baby should be admitted to the neonatal unit (NNU) for urgent treatment. Any level of glucose which is associated with clinical signs is too low. In asymptomatic babies, see Table 18.4, which is a guideline only.

Table 18.4 Suggested action according to glucose level and clinical signs in babies undergoing monitoring for hypoglycaemia

If blood glucose is 2.0–2.5 mmol and baby has no clinical signs	Feed normally and continue glucose monitoring
If blood glucose <2.0 mmol/L and baby has no clinical signs	Give a further breast feed or complement and repeat blood glucose before next feed Inform the neonatal resident Record all the above, including clinical assessment and volumes of feed taken in the baby notes
If the repeat blood glucose is <2.0 mmol/L on a second occasion despite increased feeds	Refer to neonatal resident Will probably need admission to the neonatal unit for a tube feed or intravenous glucose
Blood glucose <1 mmol/L at any time, or the baby has clinical signs	Admit urgently for intravenous glucose; bolus of 3 mL/kg 10% dextrose followed by an infusion. Continue some oral feeds if at all possible

In the occasional baby, infusions of 15–20% dextrose are required to keep the glucose above 2 mmol/L (35 mg%) despite giving a total of 12–15 mg glucose/kg/min. Glucagon 30–100 µg/kg intramuscularly or intravenously may be given to such babies followed by an infusion of 5–10 µg/kg/h. A total of 100–200 µg/kg of glucagon can also be given intramuscularly in an emergency if there is difficulty or delay in starting an intravenous infusion in a symptomatic hypoglycaemic neonate. A baby who requires more than 12 mg/kg/min of glucose to maintain glucose levels is likely to be hyperinsulinaemic. The *in-utero* supply is around 6 mg/kg/min.

Glucocorticoids are rarely needed. However, if they are required, 2.5 mg of intravenous hydrocortisone/kg should be given every 12 hours; diazoxide should be used only if there is hyperinsulinaemia. Octreotide is a synthetic somatostatin analogue which suppresses insulin release in hyperinsulinism, but expert advice is required before this agent is used.

Unusual causes of neonatal hypoglycaemia

If hypoglycaemia is persistent, recurrent or difficult to treat, and in particular if one of the obvious common causes described above is not present, then the rare conditions discussed below should be considered and appropriate investigations carried out.

1. Endocrine deficiencies, which may be multiple or single (e.g. hypopituitarism, congenital adrenal hyperplasia, hypothyroidism).
2. Syndromes with hyperinsulinaemia:
   (a) Beckwith–Wiedemann syndrome;
   (b) islet cell adenoma;
   (c) idiopathic hyperinsulinism of infancy (formerly known as nesidioblastosis).
3. Inborn errors of metabolism (IEMs):
   (a) glycogen storage disease;
   (b) fructose intolerance: fructose 1,6-diphosphatase deficiency causing lactic acidaemia;
   (c) galactosaemia;
   (d) inborn errors of fatty acid oxidation (medium chain acyl-CoA dehydrogenase (MCAD) deficiency).
4. Aminoacidopathies:
   (a) maple syrup urine disease;

(b) propionic acidaemia;

(c) methylmalonic acidaemia;

(d) tyrosinosis.

The workup of such a baby is discussed by Hawdon (2012). The gene defect present in many cases of idiopathic hyperinsulinaemia has now been discovered and the problem is a defect in the potassium channels of the beta cells of the pancreas.

■ Neonatal hyperglycaemia

Neonatal diabetes mellitus

A newborn baby occasionally develops signs of juvenile diabetes with dehydration, weight loss and polyuria. The baby is usually SGA. Hyperglycaemia, acidaemia and dehydration occur, but ketosis is rare. Some insulin is present but at inappropriately low levels for the hyperglycaemia. The disease probably represents delayed maturation of the insulin-releasing mechanism of pancreatic beta cells. These babies are exquisitely sensitive to exogenous insulin; 0.5–1 units twice a day is often all that is required to control the disease. Within 1 or 2 months most babies recover completely and insulin can be discontinued. However, insulin-dependent diabetes persists in some cases.

Iatrogenic

Babies weighing <1.50 kg are often unable to metabolize glucose rapidly enough if the infusion rate exceeds 6 mg/kg/min (86 mL of 10% dextrose/kg/24 h), yet the fluid requirement of such babies often exceeds this volume and 12–14 mg/kg/min is often given with total parenteral nutrition (TPN) (see Chapter 12). Hyperglycaemia, glycosuria and dehydration may result. When high glucose infusion rates are required to maintain calorie input during TPN, babies tolerate them better if the glucose concentration is increased gradually.

If the blood glucose level exceeds 10 mmol/L (180 mg%), especially if associated with glycosuria and polyuria, the infusion should be changed to 5% dextrose. If the blood glucose does not fall rapidly on this regimen, an insulin infusion should be given, starting with 0.1 unit/kg/h. The blood glucose concentration must be monitored carefully to ensure that hypoglycaemia does not develop.

Hyperglycaemia may also be seen as a side effect of drugs used in the neonatal period, such as steroids for chronic lung disease (see Chapter 14) and theophylline. It also occurs in stressed babies after surgery.

■ Inborn errors of metabolism

As experts point out, it is worth investigating 10 babies to diagnose one, but while neonatologists are happy to adopt this approach towards infectious diseases, they have difficulty sustaining it regarding IEMs. This is a rapidly advancing area; for example Smith–Lemli–Opitz syndrome was thought to be an autosomal recessive dysmorphic syndrome for many years before it was realized that there was a defect in cholesterol metabolism with very high plasma levels of 7-dehydrocholesterol.

Acute metabolic illness

There is now an enormous list of IEMs. Each one individually is rare, but together IEMs confront the average NNU with several acutely ill babies each year. The long-term management of such cases is beyond the scope of this book, but early management in the NNU is crucial if treatable conditions are to be recognized (rare) and an accurate diagnosis made in the remainder of cases so that genetic counselling and future prenatal diagnosis can be offered to parents.

Clinical features

The range of clinical symptoms is vast, particularly for IEMs that have a major impact on a single organ such as the liver. More commonly the presentation is with an encephalopathy coupled with multi-organ involvement that develops rapidly within 48–72 hours of birth. The history often reveals previous unexplained neonatal deaths and parental consanguinity. Table 18.5 lists the clinical and biochemical features that are common at presentation, readily identified in routine neonatal intensive care, but which if they occur together and without a ready alternative should trigger investigations for an IEM.

Investigation

In the first place, the investigations listed in Table 18.6 should be carried out. They are available in most hospitals with an NNU or can be completed with a 24-hour turn-round time in regional laboratories. From the answers to these initial tests a more focused investigation can be initiated by sending samples (and often the baby) to supraregional units that specialize in IEMs. It is, of course, important not to miss intestinal obstruction as a cause of vomiting, or severe congenital heart disease (e.g. hypoplastic left heart, aortic atresia) as a cause of severe metabolic acidaemia.

Table 18.5 Common presenting features of inborn errors of metabolism (IEMs) and common differential diagnoses

Symptom/sign	Common condition to exclude
Encephalopathy – hypotonia, fits, coma	HIE (pp. 220–224), meningitis (pp. 201–203), central nervous system malformations (pp. 233–234). Exclude with history, lumbar puncture, cranial ultrasound
Persistent vomiting	Bowel obstruction, sepsis. Exclude with routine tests for sepsis and abdominal X-ray
Metabolic acidaemia	Congenital heart disease, sepsis. IEM more likely if no response to treatment with base
Hypoglycaemia	IEM more likely if no other cause, e.g. SGA, maternal diabetes, HIE
Acute liver disease – conjugated hyperbilirubinaemia	Think of alpha-1-antitrypsin deficiency; assay galactose-1-phosphate uridyl transferase (galactosaemia)
Ketonaemia, ketonuria	Both very suspicious of IEM, particularly if combined with acidaemia
Unusual smell (baby or urine)	
Neutropenia, thrombocytopenia	Sepsis, DIC. Exclude with usual tests, p. 192
Dysmorphic features	Many babies with an IEM are dysmorphic

DIC, disseminated intravascular coagulation; HIE, hypoxic ischaemic encephalopathy; SGA, small for restational age.

Table 18.6 Initial investigation in a baby suspected of an inborn error of metabolism

Blood
Glucose
Ammonia
Amino acids
Carnitine
Lactate/pyruvate
Urea and electrolytes, septic screen, liver function tests, blood gases
Urine[a]
Reducing substances
Ketones
Amino acids
Organic acids
Orotic acid
Cerebrospinal fluid
Lactate (if lactic acidaemia)
Glycine/amino acids (if glycine encephalopathy)
Electroencephalogram
Cranial ultrasound scan
Echocardiography

[a]All urine should be kept and frozen until a diagnosis is made or the baby dies; it can be used for retrospective diagnosis.

Treatment

While the diagnosis is being established, basic intensive care should be instituted as follows:

- intermittent positive pressure ventilation – controlling respiratory failure;
- intravenous bicarbonate to correct acidaemia;
- intravenous dextrose – maintain glucose above 2.6 mmol/L;
- maintain blood pressure with saline, blood or dopamine;
- control seizures with anticonvulsants.

Because many IEMs are provoked by the protein load of feeding, enteral feeds should be stopped and hydration maintained with intravenous dextrose for 24–48 hours. In selected cases, peritoneal dialysis or haemofiltration can be used to remove toxic metabolites (e.g. ammonia, amino acids). Exchange transfusions and 'blind' megavitamin therapy are no longer recommended.

Dying babies

If it appears that the baby is going to die before a diagnosis can be established, it is important to collect:

- all urine passed (and freeze it);
- at least 20 mL blood (freeze plasma);
- blood (?skin) for chromosomes.

Consider an urgent postmortem or immediate postmortem sampling, e.g. blood, skin biopsy, liver biopsy, in consultation with a specialist in IEMs and the pathologist.

■ Causes of severe early metabolic disease

Organic acidaemias

The more common ones are listed in Table 18.7. These conditions present with encephalopathy, apnoea, acidaemia, hypoglycaemia and thrombocytopenia. The relevant amino acid is elevated in blood and urine. Hyperammonaemia is also found (>500 μg/dL), but less than in the true hyperammonaemias. The treatment is that outlined above.

Glycine encephalopathy

This used to be known as non-ketotic hyperglycinaemia. The incidence is around one in 250,000; the condition is autosomal recessive and antenatal detection is possible. It is a primary defect of neuronal glycine metabolism and the symptoms are due to the very high brain levels of glycine, which acts as an inhibitory neurotransmitter.

Table 18.7 Organic acidaemias: all have acidosis and ketosis

Condition	Incidence	Enzyme deficiency	Treatment	Likely outcome	Prenatal detection
Maple syrup urine disease	1:200,000	Branched chain keto-acid dehydrogenase	May need IV glucose; dialysis if severe	Good chance of neurologically intact survival if diet started early	Yes
Isovaleric acidaemia (sweaty feet syndrome)	60+ cases	Isovaleric acid dehydrogenase	IV glucose, low leucine diet	Good outcome possible on low-protein diet; recurrent illnesses	Yes
Propionic acidaemia	Rare	Propionyl CoA carboxylase	IV glucose/bicarbonate? dialysis	Unlikely to be successful in acute neonatal form; severe handicap in survivors	Yes
Multiple carboxylase deficiency	40 cases	Deficiency of various carboxylases involved in biotin metabolism	IV glucose/bicarbonate; neonate often biotin responsive (10 mg daily)	Rarely presents neonatally	Yes
Methylmalonic acidaemia	1:40,000	Methylmalonyl CoA mutase (complex heterogeneous defect)	IV glucose/bicarbonate? dialysis. May be B_{12} responsive (1 mg daily); low-protein diet	Unlikely to result in neurologically intact survival unless B_{12} sensitive	Yes

CoA, coenzyme A; IV, intravenous.

Glycine encephalopathy presents in the neonatal period with profound hypotonia, coma, apnoea, myoclonic seizures and hiccoughing. Glycine levels are raised in blood and urine, but the increase in cerebrospinal fluid (CSF) levels is particularly striking. A markedly raised CSF–plasma glycine ratio establishes the diagnosis. The enzyme defect can be identified on lymphocytes or liver biopsy. The condition is untreatable, although some authors have claimed improvement with dextromethorphan (an N–methy–D-aspartic acid receptor antagonist).

Primary lactic acidosis

This can be due to a variety of enzyme defects, and some cases remain unexplained. The two most commonly recognized defects are fructose 1,6-diphosphatase deficiency reported (approx. 1:200,000) and deficiencies of pyruvate dehydrogenase complex (approx. 1:200,000). They are autosomal recessive disorders but only the pyruvate dehydrogenase disorders are diagnosable antenatally.

Most cases present with lactic acidaemia and pallor, with hyperventilation in some. In others there is primarily a neurological picture with hypotonia, seizures and delayed (or absent) neurological maturation. The plasma lactate level is >2 mmol/L, often being 10 times this value. Ideally, the sample should be arterial in order to avoid problems with stasis when collecting venous blood. Urinary lactate levels are also raised. Precise diagnosis requires enzyme studies of fibroblasts or a liver biopsy. A small proportion of those with pyruvate dehydrogenase complex defects do not have a lactic acidaemia and the underlying cause of the neurological syndrome may be difficult to establish.

While establishing the diagnosis in any group, treat as described above. Nutrition should be given as a high-fat, high-protein, low-carbohydrate diet, in particular avoiding fructose. Most cases that present neonatally are unresponsive to long-term therapy.

Fatty acid oxidation defects

MCAD is the most frequently recognized of these disorders in the neonatal period. The incidence is 1 in 40,000 and the disorder is autosomal recessive. The genetic mutation has been localized to chromosome 1. Babies are hypoglycaemic and hypoketonaemic, with elevated liver enzymes. Antenatal diagnosis is possible.

Peroxisomal disorders

Peroxisomes are subcellular organelles, and more than 15 different disorders of their function have been described. Several of these diseases present in the neonatal period, usually with severe neurological abnormality often combined with abnormal facies, hepatic failure and cataracts. Diagnosis is supported by high levels of very long chain fatty acids and/or deficiency of dihydroacetone phosphate acyl transferase in the plasma.

Urea cycle disorders (hyperammonaemias)

These present as shown in Table 18.8. However, acidaemia and ketosis are absent and there is gross hyperammonaemia (>1000 µg/dL, equivalent to 1400 µmol/L). Other biochemical abnormalities are absent but the urea concentration is usually very low.

Table 18.8 Urea cycle disorders

Condition and enzyme deficiency	Incidence	Genetics	Outcome	Prenatal diagnosis
Ornithine transcarbamylase deficiency	1:60,000	Sex-linked dominant	Death in males with acute neonatal form; females do well with protein restriction	Yes
Argininosuccinic aciduria	Rare <1:250,000	Recessive	Long-term survival possible on diet; amino acid supplements	Yes
Citrullinaemia	Rare <1:250,000	Recessive	Long-term survival possible	Yes
Carbamyl phosphate synthetase deficiency	Rare <1:250,000	Recessive	Neonatal forms fatal	Yes
Hyperargininaemia (arginase deficiency)	20 cases	Recessive	Long-term survival possible on diet with amino acid supplements	Yes

Emergency treatment involves reducing or stopping the protein intake, lowering the blood ammonia levels by peritoneal dialysis, and preventing ammonia release by the gut bacteria with neomycin and laxatives. Sodium benzoate (loading dose 250 mg/kg) along with sodium phenylacetate (250 mg/kg) and arginine hydrochloride (600 mg/kg) should be given to all patients. In babies with the acute neonatal form of these diseases, long-term management is problematic and rarely successful.

Transient neonatal hyperammonaemia

This has been described occasionally in seriously ill, often comatose very low birth weight (VLBW) babies who have ammonia levels above 1000 μg/dL. The cause is unknown and the babies improve steadily with vigorous treatment of the hyperammonaemia.

Phenylketonuria

The incidence is about 1 in 10,000. It is due to a deficiency of phenylalanine hydroxylase (or, rarely, dihydropteridine reductase). It is an autosomal recessive disorder. Antenatal detection is possible; neonatal screening is routine.

Babies with phenylketonuria will not be ill during the neonatal period but will present if the screening test (Guthrie test) is positive in a baby still in the neonatal unit. The test should be carried out only on babies who are receiving milk which gives a protein load and elevates the plasma phenylalanine. If the screening test is positive, before starting the diet it must be established that the hyperphenylalaninaemia detected at screening is due to genuine phenylketonuria rather than to some other cause of an elevated serum phenylalanine.

Galactosaemia

The incidence is one in 60,000–70,000. The classical disease is caused by deficiency of galactose-1-phosphate uridyl transferase; rarer variants are due to absent galactokinase or galactose-4-epimerase. All types are autosomal recessive. Antenatal detection and neonatal screening are both possible. Babies present with the following:

1. vomiting, and occasionally diarrhoea;
2. lethargy and hypotonia;
3. poor weight gain;
4. persistent jaundice;
5. hepatosplenomegaly;
6. cataracts (occasionally).

Many affected neonates become seriously ill and they may die from septicaemia before galactosaemia is diagnosed.

A baby with suggestive symptoms *must* be receiving milk for the diagnosis of galactosaemia to be considered. Galactose will be found in the urine, but this does not react with glucose reagent strips. Start all such babies without delay on a lactose-free milk such as Galactomin 17 or Pregestimil, while confirming the diagnosis by assay of galactose-1-phosphate uridyl transferase in red cells.

Neonatal hypocalcaemia

Calcium is actively transported across the placenta, so that the fetus has a higher level than the mother (levels are around 2.5–2.75 mmol/L in cord blood). Levels fall rapidly after birth, to around 2–2.25 mmol/L, and remain low for 2–4 days before rising to adult levels at around 2 weeks of age. This fall is exaggerated in sick babies (both term and preterm), whose calcium levels are often low in the first days of life. Approximately 40% of serum calcium is bound to albumin, so that the level falls by about 0.2 mmol/L for every 10 g/L fall in albumin. The definition of hypocalcaemia is usually less than 2 mmol/L or less than 1.1 mmol/L of ionized calcium.

Table 18.9 Causes of hypocalcaemia

Early hypocalcaemia – preterm, asphyxiated, infants of diabetic mothers
Associated with hypomagnesaemia
Hypoparathyroidism
Microdeletions of chromosome 22q11
X-linked
Autosomal dominant
Autosomal recessive
Mitochondrial DNA mutations
Maternal hypercalcaemia
Calcium-sensing receptor defects
Vitamin D deficiency
Vitamin D-dependent rickets
Pseudohypoparathyroidism (rare in the newborn)
Alkalosis, bicarbonate therapy
Renal failure
Malabsorption
Hypoalbuminaemia

Hypocalcaemia is associated with irritability and jitteriness and can cause seizures. The QT interval of the electrocardiogram can become prolonged (Appendix 7). Causes of hypocalcaemia are listed in Table 18.9.

Treatment

Emergency treatment is with 10% calcium gluconate 2 mL/kg by slow intravenous injection over 5–10 minutes. Extravasation of an infusion containing calcium causes extensive tissue necrosis, so the intravenous cannula must be reliable. Alternatively, add calcium gluconate to the maintenance fluid – 2.5 mL/kg/24 h of 10% is a suitable amount. If there is associated hypomagnesaemia this should also be corrected. If longer-term calcium therapy is required, switch to oral calcium and vitamin D supplements.

Neonatal hypercalcaemia

Hypercalcaemia is usually defined as a serum calcium above 2.75 mmol/L and is a relatively uncommon problem in the neonate, particularly with modern formula composition. The causes are listed in Table 18.10. The most common cause on a neonatal intensive care unit is phosphate depletion in VLBW babies, although subcutaneous fat necrosis has definitely re-emerged as a cause since the advent of therapeutic hypothermia. Williams syndrome is an important diagnosis to make; babies have a characteristic 'elfin' face and supravalvular aortic stenosis. They are usually intellectually impaired.

Hypercalcaemia is associated with irritability, poor feeding and vomiting. The main risk is of nephrocalcinosis.

Treatment

Adjust the intake and consider increased fluids and/or diuretics. Pamidronate has been tried in severe life-threatening hypercalcaemia.

Table 18.10 Causes of hypercalcaemia

Excess vitamin D
Williams syndrome
Phosphate depletion in low birth weight infants
Maternal hypoparathyroidism
Subcutaneous fat necrosis
Hypophosphatasia
Malignancy
Vitamin A intoxication
Calcium-sensing receptor defects
Benign familial hypercalcaemia with hypocalciuria
Neonatal severe hypoparathyroidism
Idiopathic infantile hypercalcaemia
Jensen syndrome (parathyroid hormone receptor mutation, hypercalcaemia and short-limbed dwarfism)

■ References

Cornblath, M, Hawdon, JM, Williams, AF, *et al.* (2000) Controversies regarding definition of neonatal hypoglycemia: suggested operational thresholds. *Pediatrics*, **105**: 1141–5.

de Rooy, L, Hawdon, J (2002) Nutritional factors that affect the postnatal metabolic adaptation of full-term small- and large-for-gestational-age infants. *Pediatrics*, **109**: e42.

Hawdon, JM (2012) Hypoglycaemia and the infant of a diabetic mother. In Rennie, JM (ed.) *Rennie & Roberton's Textbook of Neonatology*, 5th edition. Edinburgh: Elsevier, pp. 850–867.

Hawdon, JM, Ward Platt, MP, Aynsley-Green, A (1992) Patterns of metabolic adaptation for preterm and term infants in the first neonatal week. *Archives of Disease in Childhood*, **67**: 357–65.

Moore, AM, Perlman, M (1999) Symptomatic hypoglycemia in otherwise healthy, breastfed term newborns. *Pediatrics*, **103**: 837–9.

Srinivasan (1986) Plasma glucose in normal neonates. *Journal of Pediatrics*, **109**: 113–16.

Usher, R, McLean F (1969) Intrauterine growth of live-born Caucasian infants at sea level. *Journal of Pediatrics*, **76**: 901–10.

■ Further reading

Williams, AF (1997) *Hypoglycaemia of the Newborn*. Geneva: World Health Organization.

19

Endocrine disorders

Key points

■ The most common cause of ambiguous genitalia is congenital adrenal hyperplasia (CAH), causing masculinization of baby girls.
■ All cases of ambiguous genitalia require urgent investigation so that gender identity can be confirmed as soon as possible and any necessary treatment begun.
■ Consider Addisonian collapse due to CAH in any baby who presents in shock at 7–14 days with hyponatraemia, hypoglycaemia and hypotension.
■ Neonatal thyrotoxicosis can cause serious illness which requires urgent treatment if it is not to be fatal.

Endocrine disease is rare in the neonatal period. Pituitary disease may occasionally present with hypoglycaemia and diabetes mellitus can present in the first weeks of life. Think of pituitary disease in babies with midline facial defects and remember septo-optic dysplasia can take several forms and the only clue might be an absent septum pellucidum on cranial ultrasound imaging. Inappropriate (and appropriate) antidiuretic hormone secretion is common and is dealt with on p. 84. Diabetes insipidus is occasionally seen, sometimes in association with a massive intracranial haemorrhage. Parathyroid disorders are exceptionally rare in the neonatal period but the diagnosis becomes a possibility if the other, much more common, causes of hyper- or hypocalcaemia have been excluded.

■ The neonate with ambiguous genitalia

When assessing a baby with ambiguous genitalia it is essential to never guess the sex of the baby. Admit that you are in doubt and reassure the parents that the cause can be determined and the appropriate sex assigned with little delay in nearly all cases.

Ambiguous genitalia may be due to incomplete virilization of a genetic male or virilization of a genetic female or disorders of gonadal development including chromosomal abnormalities such as Turner syndrome, Klinefelter syndrome and sex chromosome mosaicism (Table 19.1).

Management of the neonate with ambiguous genitalia

Explain the situation carefully to the parents. Take a detailed family history and also note any history of maternal drug exposure during pregnancy.

Carefully examine the baby. Measure the size of any phallus and note the position of the urethral orifice. The following features are vital in helping to establish the

Table 19.1 Causes of disordered sexual development

Undervirilized male
Anti-Müllerian hormone deficiency
Testosterone deficiency
Deficient
– 20,22 desmolase
– 3β hydroxysteroid dehydrogenase
– 17α hydroxylase
– 17,20 desmolase
– 17 ketosteroid reductase
Leydig cell hypoplasia
Gonadotrophin deficiency or resistance
Impaired peripheral androgen responsiveness
5α reductase deficiency
Androgen insensitivity, partial or complete
Dysmorphic syndromes
Idiopathic
Virilized female
Virilizing congenital adrenal hyperplasia
Deficient
– 21α hydroxylase
– 11β hydroxylase
– 3β hydroxysteroid dehydrogenase
Aromatase deficiency
Maternal androgen excess
Endogenous
Exogenous
Dysmorphic syndromes

diagnosis, planning the investigations and guiding the initial discussions with the parents, but follow the advice given here (Table 19.1) and wait for an expert:

1. Are testes palpable outside the abdominal cavity? The baby is usually an under-virilized male.
2. Can a uterus be demonstrated with ultrasound? The baby is then an over-virilized female.
3. Is the baby hypertensive? This localizes the abnormality in the adrenal.

Send blood samples for urgent chromosome analysis and also send blood and urine samples for urgent analysis to establish the diagnosis of congenital adrenal hyperplasia (CAH). This is the most common cause of ambiguous genitalia and can cause fatal Addisonian collapse within the first 10–14 days, so diagnosis is urgent. If CAH is not confirmed on the basis of a clinical examination and the other investigations,

Table 19.2 Steps in establishing the diagnosis in an infant of uncertain sex

Clinical feature			
Palpable gonads	+	+	+
Uterus present[a]	+	–	–
Increased skin pigmentation	–	–	+/–
Sick baby	–	–	–/+
Clinical diagnosis	*Gonadal dysgenesis with Y chromosome*	*Partial androgen insensitivity*	*Block in testosterone synthesis*
Investigation			
Serum 17-OHP	Normal	Normal	Normal
Electrolytes	Normal	Normal	Normal
Karyotype	45, X/46, XY or other pattern	46, XY	46, XY
Testosterone response to HCG	Definite response	Good response (both testosterone and DHT)	Blunted or absent response
Gonadal biopsy	Dysgenetic gonad, +/– tumour	Normal testis (+/– Leydig cell hyperplasia)	Normal testis
Other	–	Genital skin fibroblast culture for AR assay	Measure testosterone precursors

[a] AR, androgen receptor; DHT, dihydroxytestosterone; HCG, human chorionic gonadotrophin; OHP, hydroxyprogesterone. Requires ultrasound imaging.

further radiological and biochemical investigations can be carried out in a more leisurely manner to detect the conditions listed in Table 19.2.

Congenital adrenal hyperplasia

The incidence is 1:10,000. There are two main enzyme defects: absent 21α-hydroxylase (>90%) and absent 11β-hydroxylase (<10%).

Other rare enzyme deficiencies exist (Fig. 19.1, Table 19.1). All are autosomal recessive and antenatal detection and treatment are now possible. Population screening, measuring 17-hydroxyprogesterone on the 'Guthrie' blood spots, has been carried out, but there are no plans to introduce it into the UK.

21α-hydroxylase deficiency usually presents with virilization and/or a salt-losing state, depending on the severity of the defect. 11β-hydroxylase deficiency usually presents with virilization and/or hypertension (since the block is distal to the salt-retaining deoxycorticosterone). Identifying the virilized female is easy; males may have increased pigmentation but often present either in Addisonian crisis or, if not salt losers, with precocious puberty later in life.

The genetics of this condition have been extensively studied. The gene is on chromosome 6. Prenatal diagnosis is possible and administration of dexamethasone to the mother of a female baby with CAH can reduce the virilization and the need for extensive surgery.

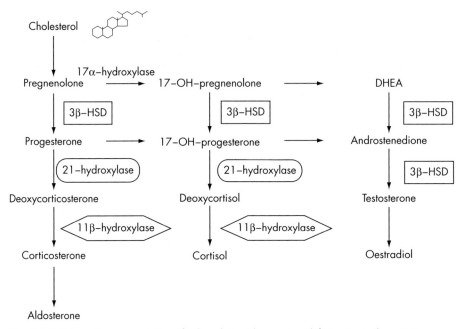

Fig. 19.1 Schematic representation of adrenal steroidogenesis – deficiencies in the activity enzymes shown leads to congenital adrenal hyperplasia. DHEA, dehydroepiandrosterone; HSD, hydroxysteroid dehydrogenase

Investigation of the child with ambiguous genitalia to establish congenital adrenal hyperplasia

1. Measure serum 17-hydroxyprogesterone and/or 11-deoxycortisol (cortisol precursors): these are raised in CAH and differentiate 21α-hydroxylase deficiency from 11β-hydroxylase deficiency (Fig. 19.1).
2. Measure adrenocorticotrophic hormone (ACTH) – a non-specific indicator of cortisol deficiency: raised in CAH.
3. Urine steroid profile can also be used to establish the diagnosis.
4. Do daily plasma and urinary electrolytes to check for salt loss.
5. Monitor the blood glucose carefully.
6. Do daily blood pressure. Salt losers may become hypotensive, but hypertension rarely presents in the newborn.
7. If CAH is confirmed, or if there are symptoms such as vomiting and weight loss, or the electrolytes suggest incipient Addisonian crisis, the initial treatment is 20–25 mg hydrocortisone/m²/day equivalent to 2.5 mg b.d. in a full-term infant; the equivalent parenteral dose can be given if the infant is vomiting. Add 25–50 μg of fludrocortisone daily with 2–4 g NaCl daily in salt losers.

The infant (often male) who presents with adrenal collapse

Any male infant who suddenly collapses with vomiting, pallor or hypotension in the first 10 days of life should be suspected of having CAH, especially if his nipples, scrotum or penis appear to be too pigmented. The infant will usually have hyponatraemia and hyperkalaemia, and is often profoundly hypoglycaemic.

Treatment

1. Give normal saline intravenously + glucose as necessary: 150 mL/kg/24 h. Plasma infusion may be necessary for resuscitation.
2. Give intravenous 50 mg hydrocortisone immediately. Oral fludrocortisone 25–50 µg can then be added.
3. Severe hyperkalaemia can be treated as outlined on p. 325.
4. Investigate as outlined above for CAH.

Other neonatal adrenal problems

Adrenal haemorrhage

This may occur in any seriously ill neonate but is characteristically associated with perinatal asphyxia. Adrenal haemorrhage may present as a loin mass or incidentally during ultrasound evaluation of the abdomen. The adrenal may calcify. Surprisingly, it rarely causes clinical problems, but if identified it is prudent to check blood glucose and do a plasma cortisol.

Perinatal steroid therapy

Repeated high-dose steroid treatment for maternal conditions such as rheumatoid arthritis can, rarely, cause fetal and neonatal Cushing syndrome. These babies have a reduced response to ACTH but few clinical problems result from it.

Babies treated with steroids for conditions such as chronic lung disease (see Chapter 14) are at risk of developing classic steroid side effects, including reduced growth, hypertension and hyperglycaemia. When steroids are withdrawn the baby usually has an essentially normally responsive hypothalamus–pituitary–adrenal axis, but if in doubt a short Synacthen test should be carried out, using 36 µg/kg of ACTH. We give steroids to cover surgery in infants who have been treated with prolonged courses of steroids.

■ Thyroid problems

Congenital hypothyroidism

The incidence of congenital hypothyroidism is about 1:3500 and is due to either thyroid dysgenesis/agenesis (usually sporadic) or goitrous cretinism (autosomal recessive or environmental). Antenatal detection is not possible; with routine neonatal hypothyroidism screening in many parts of the world, the diagnosis is now usually established before the infant presents with prolonged jaundice, lethargy, poor feeding or constipation. Most screening programmes rely on thyroid-stimulating hormone (TSH).

Infants detected on neonatal screening with TSH levels above 10 units/mL should have the diagnosis confirmed by T_3 (and T_4) measurements before starting on treatment. Since transient neonatal hypothyroidism may occur especially in preterm infants, all such patients need to be reinvestigated at 12 months of age to reconfirm the diagnosis of hypothyroidism.

In a neonate with goitre, check for maternal ingestion of goitrogens (iodides, antithyroid drugs). Unless goitrogens were the cause, or the mother comes from an area with endemic cretinism, the infant will need to be investigated for one of the rare autosomal recessive inherited forms of goitrous cretinism. However, so long as any hypothyroidism is treated, this assessment can wait until he is older.

Once neonatal hypothyroidism is suspected, after taking all the appropriate samples for investigation, start the infant on 10 µg/kg of l-thyroxine, given as a single daily dose.

Transient hypothyroidism

Small sick neonates have depressed thyroid function ($\downarrow T_4$, $\downarrow$ free T_4 and poor TSH response), and the sicker and smaller they are, the more abnormal the thyroid function. It has been suggested that this results in more severe respiratory illness and a poorer prognosis on follow-up. There is currently no justification for routine thyroxine supplementation in ill very low birth weight (VLBW) neonates, and a debate remains about replacement therapy in 'sick thyroid' syndrome.

The VLBW baby can absorb iodine from topical antiseptics through the skin. This may cause hypothyroidism as well as damage to the skin. Such preparations are no longer used in neonatal intensive care.

Neonatal thyrotoxicosis

This is due to transplacental passage of thyroid-stimulating immunoglobulin (IgG) and develops in infants born to mothers who currently have Graves' disease, or who had it in the past but are now euthyroid as a result of treatment. Only 1–3% of babies delivered to mothers with this history develop symptoms, but the disease can be life-threatening. Testing for the presence and concentration of TSH receptor antibodies during the third trimester in women with a history of Graves' disease helps to predict the babies at risk.

The neonate is usually less than 2.5 kg at birth and may develop all the signs of thyrotoxicosis, including:

1. tachycardia progressing to heart failure;
2. exophthalmos and lid lag;
3. extreme jitteriness;
4. vomiting, diarrhoea, poor weight gain;
5. sweating;
6. goitre (with a bruit) which may obstruct the trachea.

The disease may be very severe and can present at any time up to 6 weeks of age. In mild cases, symptomatic treatment with propranolol 2 mg/kg/24 h may be sufficient as the condition is transient. In more severe cases, propylthiouracil (10 mg/kg/24 h) is necessary. In very severe cases, iodides in the form of Lugol iodine solution, which prevents release of thyroid hormones, are used. The disease is usually controlled easily, and with the disappearance of maternal IgG in the neonatal plasma, antithyroid drugs can be discontinued after 4–6 months. There is a risk of recurrence in future pregnancies.

■ Further reading

Cheetham, T (2012) Neonatal endocrinology. In Rennie, JM (ed.) *Rennie & Roberton's Textbook of Neonatology*, 5th edition. Edinburgh: Elsevier, pp. 868–905.

Ogilvy-Stuart, A, Midgley, P (2006) *Practical Neonatal Endocrinology*. Cambridge: Cambridge University Press.

20

Neonatal jaundice and liver disease

Key points

- Jaundice which is present in the first 24 hours of life must be investigated and treated as an emergency.
- High bilirubin levels can cause encephalopathy, and once this develops the chance of permanent handicap is very high.
- National Institute for Health and Clinical Excellence (2010) guidelines provide advice on treatment thresholds individualized by gestational age and recommend measurement of the bilirubin level in all babies who are thought to be jaundiced on clinical inspection, which is not a reliable way to assess the severity of hyperbilirubinaemia.
- Babies who are less than 38 weeks' gestational age, have a family history of neonatal jaundice requiring treatment, or are exclusively breast fed are at higher risk of developing significant hyperbilirubinaemia and should be assessed for visible jaundice at every opportunity within the first 72 hours of life.
- Jaundice persisting after 14 days of age (21 days in preterm babies) must be investigated. The minimum recommended investigations are split bilirubin, full blood count, maternal and neonatal blood group and neonatal Coombs' test, thyroid function, urine for culture and a clinical examination. Glucose-6-phosphatase dehydrogenase deficiency should be considered in high-risk populations.
- Dark yellow urine and chalky white stools are not normal for the newborn and should be investigated.

Jaundice is one of the most common clinical signs in neonatal medicine; approximately 60% of normal healthy term babies and 80% of preterm babies develop visible jaundice in the first week of life. Jaundice is the most frequent cause of admission after early discharge from the postnatal ward. In the vast majority of these babies jaundice is harmless, although healthy babies with no underlying disease are not immune to the neurotoxic effects of unconjugated bilirubin. There are many conditions which can lead to an elevated level of unconjugated bilirubin in babies, and these can be broadly grouped into haemolytic and non-haemolytic causes. In a few babies with prolonged jaundice there is serious underlying disease such as biliary atresia, in which early diagnosis dramatically improves the chance of intact survival. Up to a third of breast-fed babies are clinically jaundiced at 2 weeks of age. Jaundice is more difficult to recognize in babies with dark skin tones and can be missed without close examination of the sclerae, gums and blanched skin. Babies from ethnic groups with dark skin tones are over-represented in kernicterus registries and population studies of hyperbilirubinaemia.

Physiology

The haem from 1 g of haemoglobin yields 600 μmol (35 μg) of unconjugated bilirubin, and the normal term baby breaks down about 0.5 g of haemoglobin every 24 hours. In the plasma, unconjugated bilirubin is mainly bound to albumin and less than 5 nmol/L per litre of free unconjugated bilirubin is normally present. Unconjugated bilirubin which is bound to albumin can be displaced by many drugs.

Unconjugated bilirubin is taken up in the liver and is then combined with glucuronic acid in the presence of the enzyme glucuronyl transferase to produce conjugated bilirubin (Fig. 20.1). This is actively transported out of the liver cell into bile and travels into the gut where some passes out of the body in stool, being converted to urobilinogen by bacteria in the colon. Within the gut, if transit time is increased, conjugated bilirubin is deconjugated again by the glucuronidases produced by bacteria in the gut lumen and present in breast milk. The unconjugated bilirubin is absorbed into the enterohepatic circulation and once more adds to the total pool of bilirubin which the liver has to metabolize. In the presence of obstruction to the biliary tree, conjugated bilirubin refluxes into the plasma and may be excreted in the urine.

All these hepatic functions are impaired in the preterm or ill term newborn compared with the normal, healthy, full-term baby and, in particular, defective conjugation cannot cope with a large postnatal bilirubin load from breakdown of red blood cells.

Bilirubin biochemistry

In most babies the majority of the bilirubin is present as the unconjugated form, with less than 20–40 μmol/L (1–2 mg%) of conjugated bilirubin. Unconjugated and conjugated bilirubin are also known as indirect-reacting and direct-reacting bilirubin, a name which reflects the chemical test for measuring bilirubin in the laboratory. If a 'split' bilirubin test is asked for, the laboratory will do tests which measure both

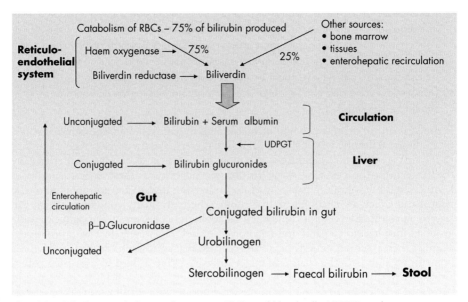

Fig. 20.1 Bilirubin metabolism and excretion. RBCs, red blood cells; UDPGT, uridine diphosphoglucuronyl transferase

conjugated and unconjugated bilirubin. In routine neonatal practice bilirubin is measured in the nursery using a bilirubinometer. This equipment uses a colorimetric method and measures total bilirubin. The result obtained includes both unconjugated and conjugated bilirubin, together with the coloured photoisomers such as lumirubin which are non-toxic. Transcutaneous bilirubinometry can be helpful (see below).

Bilirubin encephalopathy (kernicterus)

Strictly speaking, kernicterus is a pathological diagnosis describing yellow staining of the basal ganglia. The term is also used to describe the clinical features of bilirubin encephalopathy. The cells that are most prone to this type of damage, and which therefore become stained by the bilirubin to give kernicterus (literally 'yellow nuclei'), are those which are metabolically active and receive the largest blood flow. In neonates these are the cells of the basal ganglia and the mid-brain. The damage is caused by free bilirubin in the extracellular fluid binding to neuronal cell membranes, with severe and complex biochemical sequelae for the cell. The likelihood of free bilirubin leaking out of the plasma and binding to cell membranes is increased by disruption of the blood–brain barrier associated with problems such as acidosis. MRI can demonstrate abnormal signal in the globus pallidus in cases of kernicterus (Fig. 20.2). MRI and auditory-evoked potentials should be offered to babies who experience significant hyperbilirubinaemia (levels of more than 400 μmol/L).

In early bilirubin encephalopathy the baby is hypotonic and lethargic, but later the baby becomes hypertonic and irritable and may seize. If left untreated the condition is fatal, or it may cause severe brain damage in survivors, who have athetoid cerebral palsy, deafness, upgaze palsy and intellectual retardation. Immediate treatment when early signs are present can prevent sequelae, but with late or long-standing signs permanent central nervous system damage is inevitable.

Preventing bilirubin encephalopathy

We use the National Institute for Health and Clinical Excellence (NICE) guideline charts (www.nice.org.uk). A sample chart for term babies is shown in Fig. 20.3. Suitable charts for babies of different gestational ages are freely available for download.

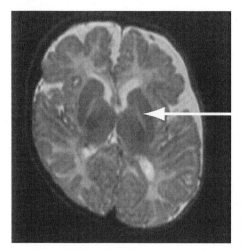

Fig. 20.2 MRI showing abnormal signal in the globus pallidus in a case of kernicterus (arrow)

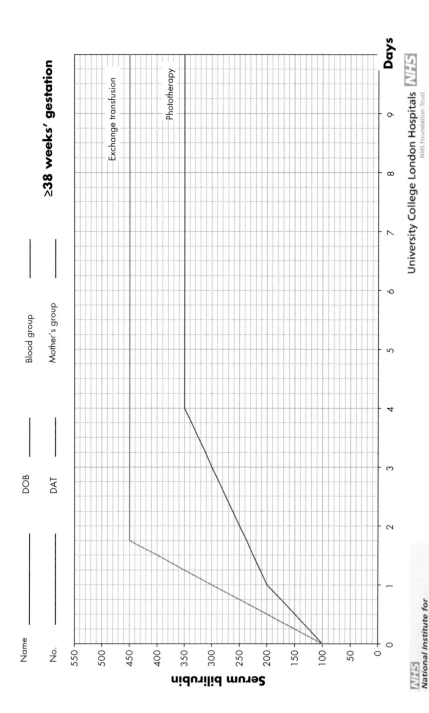

Fig. 20.3 Treatment threshold graph suitable for the management of hyperbilirubinaemia in term babies. From National Institute for Health and Clinical Excellence (2010) CG 98 Neonatal Jaundice. London: NICE; available from www.nice.org.uk/guidance/CG98; reproduced with permission; data accurate at time of going to press

The rate of rise is very important, and a bilirubin which is rising at more than 8.5 μmol/L/h suggests haemolysis and may not be controlled by phototherapy. In this situation intravenous immunoglobulin is effective if the cause is ABO or rhesus incompatibility, and a single intravenous dose of 500 mg/kg should be given.

Techniques for measuring free bilirubin or reserve albumin-binding capacity are not reliable enough for routine clinical application. The importance of the plasma albumin can be included in the assessment by measuring the bilirubin–albumin ratio (1 g albumin = 15.15 μmol albumin, thus an albumin of 45 g/L = 680 μmol/L). For term babies a bilirubin–albumin ratio of 0.8 has been suggested to be an indication for an exchange transfusion if they are well, and 0.72 if they are ill. However, this calculation is not routine in clinical practice and the use of the ratio was not supported by review of the evidence for the NICE guideline. The results of a prospective clinical trial are awaited.

■ Differential diagnosis of neonatal jaundice

The natural history and evolution of the jaundice often provides a clue to the diagnosis. The distinction between 'physiological' and 'pathological' jaundice is no longer helpful now that it is appreciated that 'physiological' jaundice can cause kernicterus. Jaundice which requires treatment (i.e. crosses the treatment thresholds suggested by the NICE guidelines) should be investigated. The minimum investigations are detailed below.

■ Causes of unconjugated hyperbilirubinaemia

Aetiology

Whether a baby develops jaundice or not is determined by the balance between the load of haem that reaches the liver from red blood cell (RBC) breakdown and the liver's capacity to produce conjugated bilirubin. The normal newborn, particularly if premature, is predisposed to jaundice because he has low levels of ligandin and glucuronyl transferase. Factors that increase the likelihood of a baby developing jaundice are listed below, and babies who become jaundiced for no other reasons than these are said to have 'physiological jaundice'. The factors include:

1. breast feeding;
2. neonatal red cells have a shortened life span, 60–70 days at term, about 40 days if premature;
3. polycythaemia increases the rate of RBC breakdown. It is often the result of a large placental transfusion; delayed clamping of the cord increases the incidence of jaundice to over 30%;
4. breakdown of bruises or RBC extravasated into tissues. This may be marked, e.g. following breech presentation, forceps delivery or with large cephalhaematomata;
5. dehydration and a hypocaloric intake (usually breast-fed babies);
6. unconjugated bilirubin recirculating via the enterohepatic route (Fig. 20.1). The slower the intestinal transit time, the more bilirubin comes from this source;
7. Gilbert syndrome is a contributory factor in some cases.

Investigation

When the bilirubin reaches treatment levels in a term baby, the following further investigations should be done as a minimum:

- full blood count, packed cell volume;
- group and direct antiglobulin test (DAT);
- blood, urine and surface swab cultures if indicated by the baby's clinical condition;
- investigate for glucose-6-phosphatase dehydrogenase deficiency where appropriate.

Measuring bilirubin

Transcutaneous bilirubin measurement has evolved to a range of accuracy that it can be used with confidence in the assessment of the degree of jaundice up to levels of 250 μmol/L in babies of 35 weeks' gestation and above. These devices measure yellow pigments including bilirubin in blanched skin by sampling from the forehead or anterior chest wall over the sternum. They provide a significant positive correlation with serum bilirubin levels in moderately jaundiced infants and reduce the requirement for blood sampling. The difference between transcutaneous bilirubin and serum bilirubin widens at levels above 250 μmol/L, and validation of the accuracy of transcutaneous bilirubinometry in preterm babies born at <35 weeks' gestation is limited. The current UK NICE guidance recommends that if a transcutaneous bilirubinometer records a bilirubin level above 250 μmol/L, a serum sample should be taken to check the bilirubin level more accurately. Phototherapy, through its bleaching effect on the skin, precludes the use of transcutaneous bilirubinometry to monitor the progress of treatment once phototherapy is in progress.

Most neonatal units (NNUs) use 'near patient testing' with a bench bilirubinometer, so that bilirubin results are available within minutes 24 hours a day on all days of the year. The convenience of this way of measuring bilirubin is not in doubt, but significant errors can arise from incorrect spectrometer use and poor maintenance. The method works by colorimetry so that a grossly lipaemic or haemolysed specimen, or one in a dirty container, will not give an accurate result. These machines are not generally accurate at very high values.

■ Breast feeding and jaundice

Breast-fed babies develop higher levels of bilirubin than formula-fed babies and their jaundice persists for longer. The healthy term breast-fed baby is not immune to kernicterus. In about 1:700 healthy term babies the serum bilirubin rises above 340 μmol/L, and most of these babies are breast-fed. The justified enthusiasm for breast feeding and early neonatal discharge means that babies can become markedly jaundiced in dimly lit bedrooms under the (sometimes) none too watchful eye of health care professionals and parents hitherto wholly lacking experience in assessing and managing neonatal jaundice. Disaster, in the form of kernicterus, can result. NNUs must ensure that those responsible for babies discharged early are trained to recognize and manage neonatal jaundice and these professionals must have ready access to rapid turnaround of bilirubin estimations at all times. According to NICE guidelines, this means access to a transcutaneous bilirubinometer or ready availability of blood testing.

In early-onset breast-feeding jaundice the small group of babies at high risk of developing potentially damaging levels of bilirubin can be predicted from an early estimation of the level (Bhutani *et al.* 1999). A bilirubin level of 137 μmol/L at 24 hours is above the 95th centile for term babies (Fig. 20.2) and babies' physiological jaundice 'track' according to their bilirubin centile. Babies with haemolysis or another reason for jaundice do not track, and clearly two estimations are required before

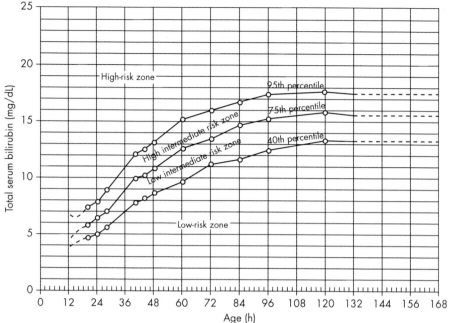

Fig. 20.4 Hour-specific bilirubin values from a group of over 13,000 healthy babies. From Bhutani *et al.* (1999) with permission. Note conversion of mg/dL to μmol/L requires multiplication by 17.1

an entirely safe assumption can be made that this is the reason for jaundice in an individual baby. Repeat bilirubin estimation and careful clinical vigilance are essential for the group who reach the 95th centile early, because phototherapy is likely to be required. An adequate milk intake should be continued and if the criteria for phototherapy are met, treatment must be arranged, breast feeding can continue and the bilirubin will fall. A failure of jaundice to respond to phototherapy is unusual and should alert the neonatologist to an alternative cause, such as haemolysis.

The persisting late (>14-day) jaundice seen in breast-fed babies is not likely to cause kernicterus. Once the diagnosis is secure on the basis of the progression of the jaundice, a bilirubin consistently below 340 μmol/L and the exclusion of serious causes of prolonged jaundice, no treatment is required. Although stopping breast feeding for 24 hours will cause a rapid decline in the bilirubin level and establish the diagnosis, this practice is not justified as it will compromise the likelihood of successful long-term lactation.

■ Some specific causes of unconjugated hyperbilirubinaemia

Haemolytic disease of the newborn

This is the most common cause of severe jaundice, which develops rapidly during the first 24 hours. Now that rhesus haemolytic disease has become rare,

ABO haemolytic disease of the newborn (HDN) is the most common form, but rhesus haemolytic disease remains the most severe. Other blood group incompatibilities (Duffy, Kell) can cause a similar picture.

Haemolytic anaemia

Many intrinsic structural or biochemical disorders of the red cell present with early-onset jaundice due to increased RBC breakdown, which may be severe enough to require phototherapy and exchange transfusion to prevent kernicterus. They include spherocytosis, glucose-6-phosphatase dehydrogenase deficiency, and the alpha-thalassaemia syndromes.

Septicaemia

See Chapter 16.

Bacterial infection causes increased RBC destruction, liberating more bilirubin, and impairs the ability of the liver to clear bilirubin from the plasma. Infection should always be suspected in any neonate with a sudden onset of jaundice not due to haemolytic disease or red cell abnormalities, but is not probable in a well baby with no clinical signs suggesting sepsis.

■ Prolonged neonatal jaundice

There are various conditions in which neonatal jaundice is prolonged beyond the first week. The minimum investigations are a total bilirubin with conjugated and unconjugated bilirubin, full blood count, urine for reducing substances and culture, thyroid function test and clinical examination (NICE 2010).

■ Prolonged unconjugated hyperbilirubinaemia

The conditions listed under group I in Table 20.1 can usually be excluded quite easily by appropriate blood tests and cultures.

Of the conditions listed in group III in Table 20.1, it is vital not to miss galactosaemia (pp. 249–250) and hypothyroidism (p. 257), since these are preventable causes of learning difficulty. The possibility of cystic fibrosis can be investigated by a search for the more common genetic deletions and by measurement of plasma immunoreactive trypsin; in most regions of the UK screening is now carried out.

■ Conjugated hyperbilirubinaemia

When conjugated hyperbilirubinaemia is recognized, appropriate biochemical and serological tests should be carried out since accurate diagnosis is important on both prognostic and therapeutic grounds (Table 20.2). Very pale stools and dark urine are not normal for babies, and this combination in a jaundiced baby should always lead to urgent investigation. Remember that many babies who develop obstructive jaundice will only have received oral vitamin K, and are at risk of late-onset haemorrhagic disease of the newborn (p. 318). Giving an extra dose of intramuscular vitamin K does no harm, and it can prevent devastating and damaging intracranial haemorrhage accompanying whatever is causing the jaundice. Bruising and bleeding are common presenting features in babies with obstructive liver disease.

Table 20.1 Causes of prolonged unconjugated hyperbilirubinaemia

Group I	Persistence of acute neonatal cause (unconjugated hyperbilirubinaemia)
	Haemolytic anaemia (immune, spherocytic or non-spherocytic)
	Chronic low-grade infection (bacterial or viral)
Group II	Breast milk jaundice (unconjugated)
Group III	Rare causes of unconjugated hyperbilirubinaemia
	Galactosaemia
	Hypothyroidism
	Aminoacidaemia (increased tyrosine, methionine)
	Pyloric stenosis
	Intestinal obstruction
	Drugs
	Fructosaemia
	Lucey–Driscoll syndrome (serum conjugation inhibition)
	Crigler–Najjar syndrome
	Gilbert's disease
	Cystic fibrosis
	Lipid storage disorders (e.g. Niemann–Pick, Gaucher's)
Group IV	Conjugated hyperbilirubinaemia
	Biliary atresia
	Other causes of obstructive jaundice

Table 20.2 Causes of obstructive jaundice

Hepatitis
A, B, C and others
Congenital infection (e.g. rubella, cytomegalovirus, toxoplasmosis)
Giant cell neonatal hepatitis
Galactosaemia
Other viral infection (e.g. echovirus, reovirus)
Inspissated bile syndrome (can occur after rhesus disease)
Cystic fibrosis
Biliary atresia
Biliary hypoplasia, e.g. intrahepatic biliary hypoplasia – Alagille syndrome
Endocrine disorders (hypothyroidism, hypopituitarism)
Inborn errors of metabolism (tyrosinosis, Gaucher's, Niemann–Pick, hypermethioninaemia)
Graft versus host disease
α_1-antitrypsin deficiency
Inherited defects (Dubin–Johnson, Rotor)
Extrinsic biliary obstruction (bands, tumour, cholodochal cyst)
Gallstones; spontaneous perforation of the bile ducts
Prolonged total parenteral nutrition

(continued)

Table 20.2 *(Continued)*

| Lipid storage disease |
| Infantile polycystic disease |
| Neonatal haemochromatosis |
| Bile acid synthetic defects |

Hepatitis syndrome of infancy

Four main pathological entities account for this syndrome:

1. Hepatocellular disease: hepatitis.
2. Inflammation and bile duct damage.
3. Disorders of the main intrahepatic bile ducts.
4. Disorders of the extrahepatic bile ducts.

The hepatitis syndrome of infancy is characterized by clinical and laboratory features of liver dysfunction, of which the most distinct is conjugated hyperbilirubinaemia. Babies usually have inflammatory changes in the liver histology – hence the name hepatitis – but the cause is only rarely infective. Hepatocellular disease may be associated with a wide range of infective, genetic, endocrine, vascular, toxic, familial, genetic or chromosomal disorders. The management of a suspected case is urgent admission and investigation for sepsis and metabolic disease. Check coagulation, and give vitamin K and fresh frozen plasma if required because intracranial bleeding is a common associated complication. Exclude galactose and fructose from the diet and arrange an early referral for specialist advice. Standard tests of liver function, such as serum bilirubin, alkaline phosphatase, aspartate transaminase, glutamyl-γ-transferase (GGT), albumin and prothrombin time, do not help to distinguish between the four main groups of disorders. All stools passed must be saved in the dark and examined for yellow or green pigment.

A skilfully interpreted percutaneous liver biopsy performed under local anaesthesia using the Menghini technique is diagnostic in up to 90% of cases. If all portal tracts show increased oedema, fibrosis and bile duct reduplication, this strongly suggests major bile duct disease, of which the most common is biliary atresia. This appearance can be found also in genetic disorders such as PiZ α_1-antitrypsin, cystic fibrosis, Alagille syndrome, total parental nutrition (TPN)-induced liver injury and endocrine disorders associated with septo-optic dysplasia. It also occurs in some infants who will ultimately develop bile duct hypoplasia and in disorders of the intrahepatic bile ducts. All of these disorders can cause complete cholestasis.

Total parenteral nutrition jaundice

In routine neonatal practice by far and away the most common cause of conjugated hyperbilirubinaemia is jaundice associated with TPN in the ill low birth weight neonate. Sepsis is undoubtedly a contributory factor. Other than stopping the TPN, no treatment is effective. Phenobarbitone, ursodeoxycholic acid and cholecystokinin have been found to reduce the level of bilirubin in some babies.

Biliary atresia

It is now clear that the earlier biliary atresia (incidence 1:14,000) is diagnosed, the better the results of surgery – usually a Kasai porto-enterostomy. All babies

Neonatal jaundice and liver disease

still jaundiced at 14 days should have a urinalysis and split bilirubin measurement. Those with marked bilirubinuria and/or a conjugated hyperbilirubinaemia should be referred at once to a paediatrician with special expertise in liver disease. Give vitamin K prior to transfer.

Treatment of neonatal jaundice

The underlying causes of the jaundice must always be sought and treated appropriately. In addition, specific therapy for the jaundice should be started if kernicterus is a threat.

Treatment of physiological jaundice

Term babies

The vast majority of babies require no treatment. Dehydration and underfeeding may be present if the weight loss exceeds 10%. We start phototherapy in term babies more than 96 hours old when the bilirubin has risen to 350 µmol/L, according to the NICE guidelines (Fig. 20.1), and use the appropriate chart for more preterm babies.

Preterm babies

In low birth weight babies who are already on the NNU, in whom kernicterus may develop at much lower bilirubin levels, give phototherapy when the total bilirubin reaches the appropriate level according to the NICE guideline charts. The plateau level is equal to the (gestational age × 10) –100, and is set at after 72 hours of age.

Treatment of severe jaundice

Phototherapy

Phototherapy, with light of wavelength 425–475 nm, reduces the amount of unconjugated bilirubin in plasma in three ways:

1. Geometrical isomerization of the bilirubin to produce water-soluble isomers which are slowly excreted; they revert to toxic isomers in the dark or when phototherapy is discontinued.
2. Intramolecular photoconversion between adjacent pyrrole rings – this produces a stable isomer called lumirubin which is rapidly excreted.
3. Photo-oxidation to colourless pyrollic and dipyrollic compounds.

The isomers produced in reactions 1 and 2 are formed immediately phototherapy starts. They are yellow and indistinguishable from natural bilirubin in the bilirubinometer, but they are polar and non-toxic. Therefore as soon as phototherapy starts, although the measured bilirubin may not fall, some is present in a considerably less toxic form. By the time equilibrium is reached after 12 hours of phototherapy, about 20% of the total bilirubin measured by the bilirubinometer is in the form of non-toxic photoisomers.

Many phototherapy devices are now available. Modern phototherapy equipment is powerful, generating spectral irradiance above 20 µW/cm^2 per nanometre of wavelength. Use can reduce bilirubin in non-haemolysing babies by more than 40% in 24 hours. Single phototherapy reduces bilirubin by about 20% of the initial value in 24 hours. Multiple phototherapy combined with fluid replacement is highly effective treatment and can avoid the need for exchange transfusion, which has now become rare. A failure to respond to phototherapy appropriately given is of concern;

the bilirubin level should fall within hours, and, if it does not, active haemolysis is likely and blood should be urgently cross matched because an exchange transfusion is likely.

Phototherapy should be used continuously until the bilirubin is falling consistently and is below the 'safe' line for gestation. A small rebound is usual after stopping treatment, but, if the bilirubin rises significantly once phototherapy is stopped, restart it and check that there is no new cause of hyperbilirubinaemia. Do *not* give phototherapy for conjugated jaundice, because the baby is likely to turn a deep brown colour, probably due to photodegradation of porphyrins which are raised in the plasma of babies with conjugated hyperbilirubinaemia

No serious long-term sequelae of phototherapy have been reported. However, phototherapy:

1. decreases gut transit time, causing diarrhoea, probably owing to the irritant effect on the bowel of the photoisomers of bilirubin;
2. increases fluid loss through the skin and gut;
3. exposes the neonate to the risks of hypo- and hyperthermia, and powerful modern lights may cause superficial burns;
4. causes erythematous rashes.

Probably the most serious adverse effect of phototherapy is the anxiety it provokes in mothers who have their babies removed, blindfolded and laid almost naked under a bright light.

When giving phototherapy, do the following:

1. Give it in the postnatal ward beside the mother if the baby is otherwise well and weighs more than 2 kg.
2. Allow breaks for breast feeding unless the level is approaching the exchange line (see NICE guidance).
3. Keep as much of the baby as unclothed as possible. Many babies are covered with nappies, hats, bootees, blindfolds and bits of sticky tape holding on various monitors, with the result that little light reaches the skin.
4. Take great care with the thermal environment. Naked babies in a cool room may become hypothermic, and preterm babies in incubators may overheat owing to the radiant heat output of the phototherapy unit.
5. Watch the baby's fluid balance. Phototherapy may double the fluid loss through a small baby's skin and gut, and appropriate increases in oral or intravenous fluid are necessary.
6. Blindfold the baby, but be careful that this does not cause conjunctivitis owing to irritation from the bandaging; alternatively use a special plastic lightproof head box.
7. Check the irradiance of the lights after every 100–200 hours of use to ensure that they are still effective.
8. Make sure that the lamps are kept cool and not used as dumping grounds for papers, towels, etc.

Exchange transfusion

This technique not only washes out bilirubin, it also removes haemolytic antibody and corrects anaemia. Exchange transfusion is the only technique which can be used when the bilirubin must be lowered urgently because it has reached potentially toxic levels or the baby is showing early clinical evidence of kernicterus.

Exchange transfusion can be used in the following situations:

1. Severe non-haemolytic anaemia from any cause.
2. Sepsis.
3. To remove drugs or accumulated toxic metabolites in depressed neonates or in those with inherited metabolic errors.

To achieve a 90–95% swap of the baby's blood, twice the blood volume (i.e. 2 × 85 mL/kg = 170 mL/kg) should be exchanged. Smaller volumes can be used when exchange transfusion is used in conditions other than HDN (such as anaemia). Various techniques have been used, but the following are the two most common approaches:

1. The serial withdrawal and injection of aliquots of blood through a central vein (usually the umbilical vein) until the required volume has been exchanged.
2. The continuous removal of blood from the umbilical or some other large artery, balanced by continuous infusion into a vein.

When using the push/pull technique, each cycle (withdrawing 5, 10 or 20 mL and then injecting 5, 10 or 20 mL) should take 4–5 minutes, taking at least 2–3 minutes for the infusion. The smaller volumes should be used in low birth weight or sick babies. A full exchange by either technique should last about 1.5–2 hours.

Throughout the exchange the baby must have continuous electrocardiograph (ECG) monitoring and be closely observed. In the very ill baby, the control of the exchange will be much better with continuous monitoring of blood pressure and frequent blood gas estimation.

Complications and hazards of exchange transfusion

- *Catheter-induced complications:* these include air emboli and aortic or portal vein thrombosis. Haemorrhage may occur from the umbilical stump or catheters. Exchange transfusion may cause necrotizing enterocolitis (see Chapter 2). All these can usually be avoided by the correct technique.
- *Haemodynamic complications:* unless great care is taken during the exchange transfusion, excess blood may be removed or injected, with disastrous consequences. In addition, too rapid an exchange by the push/pull technique can cause progressive cardiorespiratory deterioration.
- *Hypoglycaemia:* see Chapter 18.
- *Hypocalcaemia:* the ECG should always be monitored during exchange transfusion to detect hypocalcaemia. With modern blood preparations this is very rare, and routine calcium supplementation is not necessary; if cardiac arrhythmias occur, give 1 mL of intravenous 10% calcium gluconate slowly and repeat it if necessary.
- *Hyperkalaemia:* in bank blood preserved in CPD-A, the 'plasma' potassium increases steadily, by about 0.5 mmol/day. Hyperkalaemia may therefore develop if blood older than 2–3 days is used. Its treatment is outlined on p. 325.
- *Acidaemia:* bank blood less than 24 hours old stored in citrate-phosphate-dextrose-adenine CPD-A has a H$^+$ of 80 nmol/L (pH 7.1). Therefore, during exchange transfusion in sick babies, check the blood gases once or twice and correct any metabolic acidaemia which develops.
- *Tissue hypoxia:* the 2,3-diphosphatidylglycerol (DPG) levels are sustained reasonably well in CPD-A blood.

Age of blood

The quality of blood, even when stored in CPD-A, deteriorates rapidly. The PH falls, the PCO_2 rises, the potassium concentration rises and the DPG falls steadily. It is hyperosmolar, hypernatraemic, free of calcium and contains citrate which babies may find difficult to metabolize. For exchange transfusion in sick babies, particularly those who are very low birth weight, blood less than 48 hours old should be used; blood older than this poses an unacceptable metabolic stress.

■ References

Bhutani, VK, Johnson, L, Sivieri, EM (1999) Predictive ability of a predischarge hour-specific serum bilirubin for subsequent significant hyperbilirubinemia in healthy term and near-term newborns. *Pediatrics*, **103**: 6–14.

National Institute for Health and Clinical Excellence (2010) Clinical Guidance 98 (www.nice.org).

■ Further reading

Ives, NK (2012) Neonatal jaundice. In Rennie, JM (ed.) *Rennie & Roberton's Textbook of Neonatology*, 5th edition. Edinburgh: Elsevier, pp. 672–92.

Mieli-Vergani, G, Hadzic N (2012) Liver disease. In Rennie, JM (ed.) *Rennie & Robertson's Textbook of Neonatology*, 5th edition. Edinburgh: Elsevier, pp. 697–706.

21

Gastroenterological problems

Key points

- The gut is an organ of immunoprotection (gut-associated lymphoid tissue), an endocrine organ, and a reservoir for bacterial organisms (which can translocate to cause septicaemia).
- The aetiology of necrotizing enterocolitis (NEC) is complex. Most cases occur in preterm babies who have been fed milk, especially formula milk.
- Treatment of NEC involves resting the gut for 7–10 days, using total parenteral nutrition, antibiotics and full intensive care.
- Perforation or failure to improve within 7–10 days is usually an indication for a laparotomy in NEC.
- Bilious or faeculent vomiting and bleeding per rectum in babies must always be investigated, but not all causes are serious.
- Bile-stained vomiting in babies indicates a surgical condition until proved otherwise.

Basic physiology of the fetal and neonatal gut

The gastrointestinal tract develops from the primitive digestive tube and by the sixth week it is elongating so fast that a loop projects beyond the embryonic body. This loop rotates and begins to return to the abdominal cavity at around 10 weeks. Failure of this process can lead to exomphalos, or malrotation. Other problems which arise from abnormal embryological development of the gut are duplication cysts, areas of atresia (often thought to be due to vascular infarcts) and annular pancreas causing duodenal obstruction. Hirschsprung's disease is caused by the absence of neural crest-derived enteric ganglia to populate the terminal hindgut. The resulting lack of gut motility results in partial or complete gut obstruction. The gut lengthens considerably during development, so that by term the length of the small intestine is about 200 cm, half of the growth having occurred in the last trimester.

The fetus swallows amniotic fluid, and absorbs proteins from it, from about 16 weeks, but does not develop a coordinated suck–swallow mechanism until much later. Inability to swallow can lead to polyhydramnios in pregnancy, and this may be a marker of a muscle disorder or oesophageal atresia. During fetal life, transfer of important proteins takes place this way and for a few days after birth all newborns can absorb intact proteins. This is thought to be very important in allowing passive immunity by facilitating the absorption of immunoglobulins from colostrum, and in the animal kingdom some species die from infection if this transfer does not occur.

By 34–36 weeks a preterm baby can usually coordinate suck–swallow bursts sufficiently well to maintain milk intake without a gastric tube. Before this, remarkably,

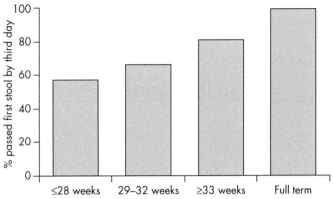

Fig. 21.1 The percentage of babies at different gestations who have passed stool by the third day of life

even a baby of 25 weeks' gestation can digest and absorb nutrients from the gut if given milk via a nasogastric tube. The transit time of a baby of 32 weeks is around 9 hours, twice as long as a term baby, and the gut motility at 26 weeks is even slower. Very preterm babies often do not pass stool for the first 3 days whereas at term 98% have passed stool in the first 36–48 hours (Fig. 21.1).

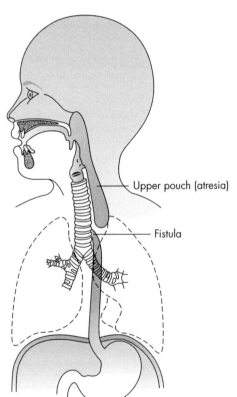

Upper pouch (atresia)

Fistula

Fig. 21.2 Oesophageal atresia with fistula. From Rennie and Robertson. (2012) with permission

■ Cleft lip and palate

The diagnosis may have been suspected antenatally, but small clefts of the soft palate are easily missed at routine neonatal examinations only to present later on with feeding problems. Expert advice should be sought as early as possible, particularly regarding feeding. Long-term results are excellent and parents are helped and encouraged by photographs showing the eventual appearance provided by support groups.

■ Oesophageal atresia and tracheo-oesophageal fistula

There may have been polyhydramnios during the pregnancy. After birth affected babies have a lot of frothy saliva which they cannot swallow, and they are prone to coughing, choking and cyanotic episodes. Most cases (85%) have a blind-ending upper pouch, with a fistula between the lower pouch and the trachea (Fig. 21.2).

The cornerstone of diagnosis is a chest and abdominal X-ray with a large-bore nasogastric or orogastric tube in situ. The X-ray confirms that the tip of the tube lies at around the T2–4 level (Fig. 21.3). If the tube lies at a lower level and the aspirate is blood-stained, think of oesophageal perforation (particularly if the baby has been intubated). The abdominal X-ray, if the gut contains gas, confirms that a fistula must exist. Contrast studies are not necessary and carry a risk of aspiration of contrast medium into the lungs. Remember that many of these babies have other abnormalities such as imperforate anus, cardiac, vertebral or genitourinary abnormalities.

If the diagnosis is confirmed, arrangements must be made to transfer the baby urgently to a paediatric surgical centre. During transfer the upper pouch must be kept as empty as possible, by frequent or continuous suction on a large-bore tube (a Replogle tube), nursing the baby head-up and prone. In most babies a primary anastomosis can be achieved, but in some there is a large gap between the ends of the oesophagus and a long course of treatment is required, sometimes with colon interposition. The prospects

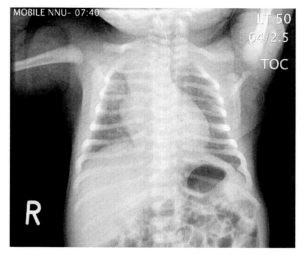

Fig. 21.3 X-ray showing nasogastric tube held up in the oesophagus

of a good outcome are excellent for babies of more than 1500 g, without associated major congenital heart disease. Gastro-oesophageal reflux, stricture and a tracheo-oesophageal fistula cough ('TOF cough') related to tracheomalacia are all common childhood problems after repair.

■ Congenital diaphragmatic hernia

The incidence is around 1 in 2000–5000 births, and most congenital diaphragmatic hernias (CDHs; 80–90%) occur in the left side through the foramen of Bochdalek. In a left-sided hernia, the bowel, stomach, spleen and often part of the left lobe of the liver are contained within the left hemithorax. Bilateral CDH is very rare and the prognosis is poor. Most cases are now diagnosed antenatally, although the combination of clinical signs including a displaced mediastinum, scaphoid abdomen and poor oxygenation should still raise suspicion as the occasional case is missed on prenatal scanning.

The major determinant of outcome is the degree of pulmonary hypoplasia, which is present to some extent in virtually all babies with CDH. The hypoplasia is worse on the ipsilateral side, where sometimes there is only a small piece of lung, but there is an alteration in lung volume and structure on both sides, with reduced alveolar numbers and abnormal medial muscular hypertrophy. There is often an additional effect on development of the ventricle of the heart on the affected side. The earlier the diagnosis is made antenatally the worse the prognosis, and if the liver is in the chest (in left-sided CDH) this is a further marker of adverse outcome. The other indicator of severe pulmonary hypoplasia is a low lung–head ratio, and a fetus with a ratio of ≤1 has a poor prognosis. The combination of a lung–head ratio ≤1 and 'liver up' is used to offer fetal intervention in some centres, because the predicted survival is less than 10%. The most frequently used intervention is fetal endoscopic tracheal occlusion (FETO). In this technique a balloon is inserted into the fetal trachea using a minimally invasive technique at 26–28 weeks with removal by puncture or fetoscopy at about 34 weeks.

Antenatal diagnosis offers the possibility of delivery in a regional centre. When attending the delivery of such a baby, bagging with a facemask should be avoided because the gut fills with air and further displaces the mediastinum. Babies should be intubated, ventilated and muscle relaxed as soon as possible. A large-bore nasogastric tube should be passed to decompress the stomach and small bowel. Ventilatory management is then along the lines of 'gentle ventilation', in order to minimize volutrauma and avoid pneumothorax – an ever-present risk given the abnormal lung structure. We give surfactant to babies with CDH, although not all centres agree with this.

Many babies with CDH have an initial 'honeymoon' period shortly after birth, with acceptable blood gases, before entering a phase of instability due to pulmonary hypertension with hypoxia, acidosis and hypercarbia. Surgery has no place in the management at this stage, which is entirely medical and along the lines suggested for pulmonary hypertension in Chapter 13 – namely, optimizing homeostasis, oscillatory ventilation and iNO. Monitor the oxygenation index (Appendix 2). Some have suggested that if the best oxygenation index on the first day is below 82 survival is improved to above 90%, whereas it was only 18% in those with an oxygenation index above 82 (Sinha *et al.* 2009). The role of extracorporeal membrane oxygenation (ECMO) is controversial, with some centres offering repair on ECMO and others considering that if the pulmonary hypoplasia is severe enough that ECMO is required then the prognosis is too poor to justify the use of such an aggressive approach. Surgery is delayed until the baby is stable, and involves reducing the abdominal viscera into the abdomen, repairing the diaphragm (quite often with a patch) and fixing the inevitable malrotation of the gut.

Most modern series of the outcome of CDH report survival of around 50–60% without FETO or ECMO. Survivors do not have normal lung function, and 16% are discharged in oxygen. Chest asymmetry, pectus excavatum and scoliosis can occur. Recurrence can occur, particularly if a patch repair was required, owing to the inability of the patch to expand with growth. Gastro-oesophageal reflux is a major problem and can cause recurrent aspiration. Sensorineural deafness seems to be a particular problem in CDH, persistent pulmonary hypertension of the newborn and ECMO survivors.

Intestinal obstruction

Bile-stained vomiting is surgical until proved otherwise. Although intestinal obstruction is not invariable, the finding of genuinely green vomit mandates further investigation for intestinal obstruction, caused by atresia or malrotation. The main practical problem lies in determining the difference between genuinely green vomit and pale yellow vomit. Bile is a golden yellow colour but turns green on contact with gastric acid. In clinical practice and if in doubt, it is safer to investigate. Remember that mechanical obstruction to the gut may be associated with impairment of the gut blood supply that can cause gut necrosis with loss of gut length, peritonitis and bacteraemia.

Duodenal atresia

In about two-thirds of cases the atresia is distal to the opening of the bile duct so that the baby presents with bile-stained vomiting and passage of only small amounts of meconium. The remaining third present with vomiting which is not bile-stained. Abdominal distension is absent, but visible gastric peristalsis may be seen. Abdominal X-ray shows the classic 'double bubble' appearance. The baby should be examined carefully for evidence of other syndromes, particularly Down syndrome. The stomach should be kept empty with a large-bore tube on free drainage and hourly aspiration, and any electrolyte disturbances corrected while transfer to a paediatric surgical centre is arranged. The results of surgery are good, but feed tolerance can be slow because of poor propulsion of feed.

Malrotation, incomplete obstruction and volvulus

This can be a difficult diagnosis to make because the obstruction is not complete and hence the onset of signs can be delayed, and the signs are less obvious than in a complete obstruction. The usual cause is Ladd's bands causing a partial duodenal obstruction, but there can be obstruction from an annular pancreas, mucosal webs or duodenal stenosis. The risk of missing a baby with malrotation is that the vascular supply to the midgut (which runs through a narrow pedicle of mesentery in this condition) will become obstructed by twisting (volvulus), resulting in ischaemia and loss of gut. Plain abdominal X-rays can be normal and the diagnosis can reliably be made only with a contrast study. Doppler studies of the position of the superior mesenteric axis can provide helpful information, but not all hospitals can provide a radiologist with the skill to perform this test.

Small bowel atresia

Atresia of the small bowel also presents with bile-stained vomiting and abdominal distension. Distended loops of bowel are often visible and palpable. X-rays show loops of bowel, often with fluid levels. Intra-abdominal calcification suggests meconium peritonitis secondary to intra-uterine bowel perforation. Again, the management is 'drip and suck' while awaiting surgery. Some babies lose considerable amounts of bowel, and sometimes there is more than one area of atresia. Investigations for cystic fibrosis should be performed.

Meconium ileus

Between 10% and 20% of babies with cystic fibrosis present with meconium ileus. The underlying problem is inspissated mucus forming a plug in the colon and ileum and producing an intraluminal obstruction. The clinical presentation is abdominal distension, bile-stained vomiting and failure to pass meconium. X-rays usually show bowel distension with a coarse granular appearance produced by bubbles of air in the trapped meconium, although this is not specific.

Initial management is 'drip and suck' with nil by mouth. The obstruction can often be cleared using a Gastrografin enema, but this treatment needs to be done by an experienced radiologist. Laparotomy is sometimes required.

Imperforate anus, anorectal malformation

If the anal opening is wholly absent, obstruction will clearly occur. It is therefore vital to check the anus in any baby with obstruction. Even if the anus is present there may be stenosis. If there is no anal opening there is often a fistula, leading to the passage of meconium into the vagina in a girl or at some point on the perineum (or via the penis) in a boy.

Exomphalos

Exomphalos is more common than gastroschisis. The diagnosis is often made prenatally with ultrasound. Exomphalos is frequently associated with chromosome abnormalities or congenital heart defects. The condition may be a marker for Beckwith–Wiedemann syndrome. The term encompasses a range of defects, including a small umbilical defect with gut prolapsing into the cord, through to giant defects containing bowel and liver. The prognosis is generally good, although large defects may require a staged repair.

Gastroschisis

In gastroschisis the bowel is extruded from the abdominal cavity through a defect that is usually just to the right of the umbilicus. Babies with gastroschisis are often born to young mothers and are of low birth weight. They do not usually have other conditions. The bowel is exposed and the baby loses heat and fluid very quickly after birth, with a danger of shock developing. The emergency treatment consists of wrapping the abdomen in cling-film, maintaining temperature and replacing fluid losses. Surgical treatment involves either a primary repair with return to the abdomen or the application of a 'silo' which is gradually reduced in size over a period of days. Over 90% of babies survive, although enteral feeding can take weeks or months and some have associated atresia or short gut syndrome.

Necrotizing enterocolitis

Necrotizing enterocolitis (NEC) is a serious disease that primarily affects preterm or small for gestational age babies and occurs almost exclusively in neonatal units (NNUs). The disease usually involves the terminal ileum and the colon, but lesions

Gastroenterological problems

can occur anywhere from the stomach to the rectum, and multiple areas may be involved. The incidence varies, but is around 2–5% in very low birth weight (VLBW) babies. Clusters of cases are relatively common and the disease can affect term babies.

Signs

NEC should always be suspected in babies with abdominal distension, bilious aspirate or vomiting, blood in the stool and signs of infection. NEC is most common in the second week of life, but late cases can occur. The staging of NEC is shown in Table 21.1. Histological proof may be obtained at laparotomy or autopsy.

Some babies have a slow insidious onset of NEC and do not progress beyond the 'suspect' stage with abdominal distension and mild systemic illness. In others, the disease progresses and the baby becomes pale and mottled, the abdominal distension increases, the stools are bloodier and the baby may vomit. Eventually an ileus develops, no stools are passed, and the vomit becomes bilious or faeculent. Bowel sounds are

Table 21.1 Staging of disease in necrotizing enterocolitis (NEC) (modified Bell's staging)

	Systemic signs	Intestinal signs	Radiographic signs
Stage IA – 'suspect' NEC	Temperature instability, apnoea, bradycardia, lethargy	Elevated pre-gavage residuals, mild abdominal distension, emesis, haem-positive stools	Normal or intestinal dilatation, mild ileus
Stage IB – suspect NEC	Same as IA	Same as IA plus bright red blood per rectum[a]	Same as stage IA
Stage IIA – definite NEC – mildly ill	Same as stage IA	Same as stage IA, plus absent bowel sounds, +/− abdominal tenderness, bloody stools	Intestinal dilatation, ileus, pneumatosis intestinalis
Stage IIB – moderately ill	Same as stage IIA, plus mild metabolic acidosis, mild thrombocytopenia	Same as stage IIA, plus absent bowel sounds, definite abdominal tenderness, +/− abdominal cellulitis or right lower quadrant mass, bloody stools	Same as stage IIA plus portal vein gas, +/− ascites
Stage IIIA – advanced NEC; bowel intact	Same as stage IIB, plus hypotension, bradycardia, severe apnoea, combined respiratory and metabolic acidosis, disseminated intravascular cogulation, neutropenia	Same as stage IIB, plus signs of generalized peritonitis, marked tenderness, and distension of abdomen	Same as stage IIB, plus definite ascites
Stage IIIB – advanced NEC; bowel perforated	Same as stage IIIA	Same as stage IIIA	Same as stage IIB, plus pneumoperitoneum

[a] Some state this makes the case IIB, and in our view bloody stool on more than one occasion certainly justifies classification as IIB

279

absent and the distended abdomen is tender. At this stage ascites may develop, and bowel perforation occurs in some cases. There may be redness and induration of the abdominal wall overlying areas of involved gut, and flank lividity appears in advanced cases. This progression may take several days or there may be a fulminant course leading to death within a few hours. In babies with severe disease apnoea, hypotension and jaundice occur early in the course of the illness.

Investigation

In addition to the usual tests which are indicated for suspected infection (p. 192), request a plain X-ray of the abdomen. If there is any suspicion of a perforation, ask for a lateral 'shoot through' horizontal film taken with the baby lying on his left side, to detect fluid levels and free intraperitoneal gas. Remember, gas collects round the liver in babies who are lying down, and can also appear in the lesser sac. In mild cases the X-rays will be normal, though occasional fluid levels may be seen; there may be some dilated bowel loops and the gut wall may be rather thicker than usual. A fixed dilated loop of gut may remain in the same position in different X-ray views, and for several days, and this is an abnormal finding. Oedema of the gut wall can give rise to an abnormal shadow from the junction between it and the peritoneal fat. Air outlining both sides of the bowel wall can give a 'barium enema-like' appearance (Rigler's sign; Fig. 21.4a), and if this is present free air is confirmed. As the disease progresses, gas bubbles (the pathognomonic feature of NEC) appear first in the bowel wall and eventually in the liver, where they are sometimes seen within the biliary tree (Fig. 21.4b). Ascites may be present, and, when an intestinal perforation occurs, free gas will be seen within the abdomen. Barium studies or diagnostic paracentesis are rarely necessary for the diagnosis.

Differential diagnosis

The history, clinical examination and X-ray findings are very characteristic. Babies with other causes of intestinal obstruction – including congenital malformation –

(b)

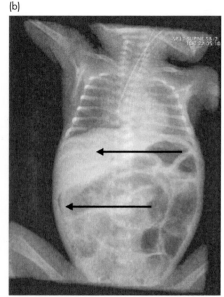

(a)

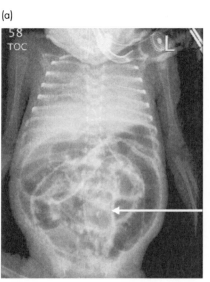

Fig. 21.4 X-rays showing (a) Rigler's sign (arrow) and (b) intramural gas with air in the biliary system

never show intramural gas and rarely pass bloody stools. A pneumoperitoneum from air tracking down from the mediastinum is usually associated with high-pressure intermittent positive pressure ventilation (IPPV) for lung disease, and there are none of the other signs of intra-abdominal sepsis. Bleeding per rectum from some local cause such as fissure-in-ano must be excluded.

Aetiology

NEC begins in the mucosa with oedema, haemorrhage and microvascular sludging. The disease is multifactorial (Fig. 21.5), with the most important risk factors being prematurity and its complications, intra-uterine growth restriction (particularly with reversed flow in the fetal umbilical artery) and oral feeding. Some hospitals have reported a temporal association between 'top-up' blood transfusions and NEC, leading others to withhold feeds during blood transfusions. This is not a practice we currently endorse.

Recent interest has focused on the importance of the role of an excessive immature inflammatory response associated with abnormal intestinal organisms (Neu and Walker 2011). The preterm mucosa is very susceptible to gut infection with gas-forming organisms, and the presence of milk in the gut probably provides a substrate for these organisms. In all babies there is a tendency for undigested carbohydrate to pass into the colon, where bacterial fermentation lowers the intraluminal pH. Carbohydrate fermentation explains the high breath hydrogen levels that are found in these babies.

Prevention

NEC is not a totally preventable disease. The disease is virtually unknown in babies who have not been fed. Some neonatologists interpreted this as an indication to avoid enteral feeds entirely until IPPV was discontinued, umbilical artery catheters (UACs) were removed, and blood gases were normal. In our view, this approach is no longer justified. The best approach is to start low-volume 'minimal' or 'trophic' enteral feeds early with breast milk and to increase feed cautiously, particularly in babies at high risk. Feeds should be discontinued at the earliest signs of excessive volumes of milk being retained in the stomach (gastric residual more than 50% of feed volume and/or 'dirty' aspirates), or abdominal distension.

Breast milk should be used to start feeding if at all possible, and in babies who are at very high risk of NEC consideration should be given to starting enteral feed with donor breast milk. In high-risk babies milk feeds should be increased at the rate of about 20 mL/kg/day; this often means increasing the feed volume by as little as 1 mL each day. Prophylactic oral administration of immunoglobulins, colonizing the gut with the 'right' sort of bacteria (probiotics), prebiotics (nutrients which enhance the growth of potentially beneficial microbes) and non-absorbable antibiotics have all been suggested, but none of them is of proven benefit, although several trials of probiotics are under way. Some consider that the case for probiotics has already been made, whereas others remain in equipoise (Tarnow-Mordi *et al.* 2010).

Treatment

Once the diagnosis has been made, a 'drip and suck' regimen must be started to rest the baby's gut. Remove all umbilical catheters unless the balance of risk suggests they must remain, and give total parenteral nutrition (TPN) through a central venous catheter (Chapter 12). Treat hypotension, anaemia and respiratory failure. These babies lose a lot of protein-rich fluid as ascites and may require blood or blood products; the serum sodium often falls. Ampicillin, gentamicin and metronidazole should be given intravenously.

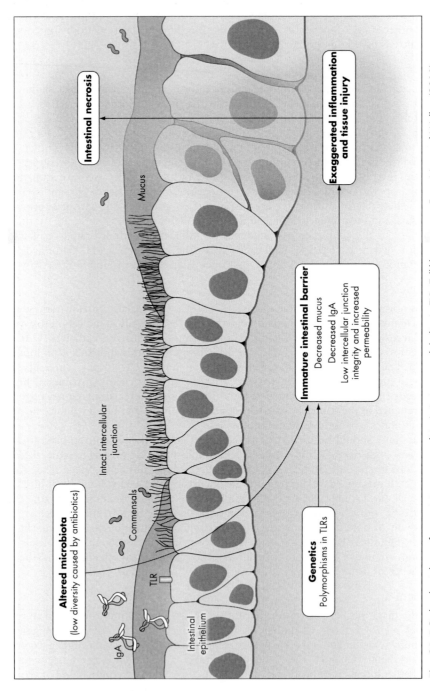

Fig. 21.5 Pathophysiology of necrotizing enterocolitis. IgA, immunoglobulin A; TLR, Toll-like receptor. From Neu and Walker (2011), reproduced with permission from Massachusetts Medical Society.

In babies with stage I disease the regimen should be reviewed after 2–3 days. If the diagnosis of true NEC is not confirmed and the baby has remained well, enteral feeds can be cautiously reintroduced at that stage. In babies with stage II disease or worse, treatment must be continued for at least 7–10 days. It is wise to seek a surgical opinion early in these cases. Abdominal X-rays should be taken frequently, including following any clinical deterioration, in order to detect bowel perforation as soon as possible, in which case laparotomy is likely to be necessary. Laparotomy should also be considered in babies who show no response to conservative treatment and in whom ileus and ascites persist for more than 4–5 days.

At laparotomy, involved segments of gut will usually be resected. If the baby is in good condition, primary anastomosis can often be performed, but many babies require a defunctioning proximal 'ostomy', which is temporary. Multiple areas of affected gut can be resected with many anastomoses, or the segments can be isolated with 'clip and drop' and returned to the abdomen in the hope that they will retain viability and allow gut continuity to be established at a later date. Sometimes there is so much gut affected that the situation is clearly hopeless. In very unstable babies, an alternative to laparotomy is to insert soft peritoneal drains and wait. Surgery is almost always needed eventually if these babies survive.

Sequelae

The mortality is about 20% among those babies who perforate, but should be less than 10% in those who do not. About 10% of babies develop a further typical attack of NEC. In a further 5–10%, particularly if they did not come to laparotomy, the area of gut involved becomes stenosed. These cases develop signs of intestinal obstruction without enterocolitis 2–6 weeks after the original illness. Barium studies at this stage demonstrate the stricture which may need to be resected with primary reanastomosis of the bowel. VLBW babies who survive NEC have a higher incidence of neurological sequelae at follow-up than control babies of similar gestation, and there is a particularly high risk of periventricular leukomalacia in those who require surgery, perhaps because of cytokine release.

Isolated bowel perforation

Various parts of the bowel may perforate spontaneously during neonatal intensive care. Gastric perforation may occur spontaneously, as a result of a nasogastric tube, or in association with face mask ventilation. Isolated ileal or colonic perforations without NEC may be the result of ischaemia due to drugs such as indometacin or emboli from UACs. It is not unknown for the bowel to be perforated by paracentesis tubes inserted to drain a pneumoperitoneum or ascites.

In all these situations the baby will develop peritonitis as bowel contents leak out and he will have abdominal distension. Plain X-ray of the abdomen will confirm free intraperitoneal air.

The treatment is laparotomy and closure of the perforation or resection of the localized area of bowel.

Short bowel syndrome

This is likely to occur after surgery for NEC, volvulus or other gut malformations if less than 40 cm of small bowel is left, particularly if the ileocaecal valve has been resected, and short bowel syndrome may occur (but with a much better long-term prognosis) with 50–100 cm of residual small bowel.

Survival has been achieved with as little as 10–15 cm of jejunum and an intact ileocaecal valve, or 25–40 cm without it. The prognosis has improved over the last 20 years, and the cornerstone of management is careful TPN. TPN is maintained while providing some enteral nutrition ('feeding the gut' or 'trophic feeding') and waiting for the bowel to grow and adapt. It cannot be stressed enough that the bowel will never adapt if enteral feeds are not given; far better to continue at a slow rate than to keep stopping and starting. Enteral feeds need to be started and increased at an extremely slow rate. Milks which are easily digested and absorbed such as Pregestimil or Nutramigen are usually used. Stool output can increase dramatically as feeds are increased and needs to be watched carefully. Agents such as H_2 antagonists (ranitidine), antimotility agents (loperamide) and bile acid binders (cholestyramine) can be helpful. A paediatric gastroenterologist must supervise difficult cases. Small bowel transplantation is possible, but is a last resort.

Gastro-oesophageal reflux

This may be a problem in babies with persistent apnoeic attacks and may complicate chronic lung disease. Reflux is also frequent in children who are brain damaged after hypoxic ischaemic encephalopathy. The diagnosis can be made clinically, on the basis of oesophageal pH studies, or a barium swallow. Therapy involves nursing the baby head-up and thickening the feed with a commercial agent such as Carobel or Thick-and-Easy. The Committee on the Safety of Medicine in the UK currently blacklists cisapride. There have been few trials to confirm the efficacy of cisapride, and it has been shown to increase the QT interval in some babies, particularly those who are being treated simultaneously with macrolide antibiotics or antifungals or who are hypokalaemic.

The baby with persistent vomiting

All babies can be expected to vomit once or twice a day. Only if the vomiting is bile-stained, faeculent, bloody or becomes persistent is investigation required. Haematemesis is considered below.

The serious causes of persistent vomiting in the neonate include the following:

1. Neonatal intestinal obstruction from any cause (see above).
2. Ileus in association with severe illness, e.g. birth asphyxia or respiratory distress syndrome.
3. Septicaemia, including meningitis.
4. NEC (see above).
5. Rare metabolic causes, e.g. galactosaemia and congenital adrenal hyperplasia (Chapter 19).
6. Raised intracranial pressure, e.g. hydrocephalus, intracranial haemorrhage.

The first four are usually associated with bilious vomiting and the diagnosis is generally easy to establish by simple clinical, laboratory and X-ray methods.

It is also important not to forget the common causes of vomiting in older babies. These include:

1. gastroenteritis;
2. upper respiratory tract infections and otitis media;
3. urinary infection;
4. pyloric stenosis.

These can present during the neonatal period, particularly in VLBW babies who remain in the NNU for several weeks. It is important to exclude urinary tract infection in this situation.

A large number of entirely normal newborn babies, however, just vomit – and it may be bilious. Immediately after birth this is often ascribed to having swallowed blood or meconium-stained amniotic fluid, or to the baby being 'mucousy'. In our view there is no longer any place for stomach washouts in babies. If the baby has a problem this will only serve to delay diagnosis and treatment, and if he is normal he should not be subjected to this unpleasant procedure.

If a baby continues to vomit in the absence of clinical abnormalities, it is safest to set up an intravenous infusion, give nothing orally and aspirate the stomach regularly for 24–48 hours before trying oral feeds again. If these are still vomited a barium meal is indicated.

Persisting diarrhoea

In the baby with frequent loose stools and failure to thrive without gastroenteritis, consider the following:

1. cow's milk protein intolerance;
2. cystic fibrosis;
3. immune deficiency syndromes (e.g. Schwachman syndrome);
4. congenital monosaccharide or disaccharide deficiency;
5. congenital chloride or sodium diarrhoea;
6. congenital microvillous atrophy;
7. autoimmune enteropathies.

Conditions 2–6 can be autosomal recessive conditions so a family history may help. The first two conditions can be evaluated in any neonatal service, but the last five require specialist referral for diagnosis and management.

Haematemesis, melaena and bloody stools in the newborn

Minor degrees of these disorders are very common, and the following conditions should be excluded before embarking on complex studies of the clotting system or diagnosing serious intra-abdominal disease:

1. swallowed maternal/placental blood at delivery;
2. swallowed maternal blood from a cracked nipple;
3. local trauma (e.g. from a nasogastric tube, laryngoscopy, overvigorous laryngeal suction);
4. fissure-in-ano.

It is important to test whether the blood is maternal (swallowed) or fetal, and this can be done using Apt's test for fetal haemoglobin. When 1% sodium hydroxide is added to a dilute solution of the bloody effluent in water, fetal haemoglobin remains pink, whereas adult haemoglobin denatures and goes brown.

The serious differential diagnoses for haematemesis or blood in the stools are as follows:

1. NEC (see above);
2. haemorrhagic diatheses of various types, including haemorrhagic disease of the newborn, and disseminated intravascular coagulation (see Chapter 23);

3. rare causes:
   (a) trauma;
   (b) Meckel's diverticulum;
   (c) malrotation;
   (d) peptic ulceration;
   (e) rectal polyps/haemangiomas;
   (f) colitis;
   (g) intussusception;
   (h) gut reduplication.

These should be sought only if the other much more common conditions have already been excluded and bleeding persists.

Hirschsprung's disease

This disorder is caused by the absence of ganglion cells from Auerbach's and Meissner's plexuses and in 70% of cases the absence is confined to the sigmoid and rectum, including the internal sphincter. Involvement of the entire colon and a variable length of small intestine occurs in 10% of cases. Hirschsprung's disease is a genetic disorder, with mutations in the *RET* proto-oncogene region of chromosome 10 known to account for many cases; others are due to a mutation on chromosome 13.

The cardinal sign is failure to pass meconium within 48 hours. Vomiting is not usually a prominent early sign, but may occur. Most babies with Hirschsprung's disease remain well, but some develop enterocolitis, a serious complication with offensive watery stool requiring urgent treatment with antibiotics and fluid replacement.

A plain X-ray of the abdomen should be done before any attempt at rectal examination, which can be followed by an explosive release of stool and gas. Rectal examination can alter the classic appearance of a 'cone' on barium enema and this investigation should be delayed for a day if a rectal examination has been done. The definitive diagnosis is made by rectal biopsy. Management depends on the length of affected bowel and often involves rectal washouts, sometimes with the formation of a colostomy in the short term followed by a 'pull-through' at a later date. About 75% of affected children will achieve rectal continence in adulthood.

References

Neu, J, Walker, AJ (2011) Necrotizing enterocolitis. *New England Journal of Medicine*, **364**: 255–64.

Sinha, CK, Islam, S, Patet, S, *et al.* (2009) Congenital diaphragmatic hernia: prognostic indices in the fetal endoluminal tracheal occlusion era. *Journal of Pediatric Surgery*, **44**: 312–16.

Tarnow-Mordi, W, Wilkinson, D, Trivedi, A, Brock, J (2010) Probiotics reduce all cause mortality and necrotizing enterocolitis: is it time to change practice? *Pediatrics*, **125**: 1068–70.

Sugarman, I, Stringer, M, Smyth AG (2012) Congenital defects and surgical problems in *Rennie & Robertson's Textbook of Neonatology*, 5th edition. Ch. 29. 4 pp. 724–754. Edinburgh: Elsevier.

Further reading

Bell, MJ, Ternberg, JL, Feigin, RD, *et al.* (1978) Neonatal necrotising enterocolitis: therapeutic decisions based upon clinical staging. *Annals of Surgery* **187**: 1–7.

Wilkinson, AR, Tam, PKH (eds) (1997) Necrotizing enterocolitis. In *Seminars in Neonatology*, vol. 2, issue 4. London: WB Saunders.

Gastroenterological problems

22

Congenital heart disease in the neonatal period

Key points

- Innocent murmurs are very common in babies.
- The features of an innocent murmur are that the baby is well, the murmur is soft systolic with normal heart sounds and does not radiate, and the pulses are normal.
- Many babies with significant cardiac disease have no murmur.
- The investigation of choice is an echocardiogram.
- Babies who present in shock with acidosis and mottled peripheries can have left heart outflow problems such as coarctation of the aorta or aortic atresia.

The incidence of congenital heart disease (CHD) is slightly less than 1:100 live births. One-third of these babies have severe defects which present in the neonatal period with cyanosis, cardiac failure, low-output shock or an arrhythmia. The risk of CHD is increased in the following situations:

- A parent or sibling has CHD.
- The baby has a syndrome or malformation known to be linked with CHD (e.g. Down syndrome, Turner syndrome, Di George syndrome, exomphalos, thrombocytopenia/absent radius).
- The mother has diabetes, or collagen vascular disease, or has exposed the fetus to teratogens (e.g. alcohol, phenytoin, lithium).
- The fetus is found to be hydropic or to have an arrhythmia.

Increasingly the diagnosis of CHD is made antenatally by specialized detailed ultrasonography, but the detection rate of the routine 18–20-week fetal anomaly scan remains poor. The four-chamber view obtained detects less than 50% of CHD and a 'normal' result cannot provide total reassurance. Coarctation and ventricular septal defect (VSD) are easily missed. Early diagnosis of CHD is vital because the outlook for these children has improved dramatically since the first ductal ligation was performed almost 60 years ago.

The fetal circulation

There are key differences between the fetal and the neonatal circulation:

- At birth, there is a shift from a circulation in parallel to one in series.
- During fetal life only 10% of the cardiac output goes to the lungs, and the pulmonary vascular bed is a relatively high-resistance, low-flow circuit.

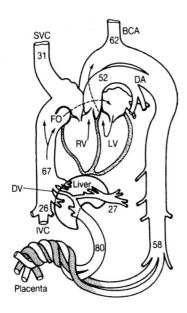

Fig. 22.1 The fetal circulation. BCA, brachiocephalic artery; DV, ductus venosus; FO, foramen ovale; IVC, inferior vena cava; LV, left ventricle; RV, right ventricle; SVC, superior vena cava.

There are three vascular structures which close soon after birth. These are:

- *the ductus venosus*, which channels some of the returning oxygenated blood travelling in the umbilical vein from the placenta through the liver, into the inferior vena cava (IVC) and hence into the right atrium (Fig. 22.1);
- *the foramen ovale*, which is a flap valve opening between the atria, which allows 33% of the blood returning to the right heart to be diverted to the left atrium and hence to the aorta;
- *the ductus arteriosus*, which in fetal life has right-to-left flow and diverts blood from the pulmonary artery into the descending aorta before it reaches the lungs.

Oxygenated blood returns from the placenta via the umbilical vein to the fetus. Once it reaches the fetal body, some blood passes through the liver to the hepatic vein and IVC, and the remainder bypasses the liver by travelling through the ductus venosus to enter the IVC. Within the right atrium blood flowing from the IVC is separated into two parts. Approximately 33% passes through the foramen ovale, into the left atrium, left ventricle (LV) and ascending aorta (Fig. 22.1). This ensures that the coronary arteries and the brain receive blood with the highest PaO_2. The remainder of the IVC flow passes into the right ventricle (RV) and pulmonary artery.

Deoxygenated blood returning from the upper part of the fetal body returns through the superior vena cava (SVC) into the right atrium and almost all of it passes into the RV. Most of the output of the RV passes from the pulmonary artery through the ductus arteriosus into the descending aorta, where it is joined by blood ejected from the LV. The ductus is kept patent *in utero* by circulating and locally produced prostaglandins.

■ Changes in the circulation at birth

At birth, the site of oxygen uptake changes from the placenta to the lungs. This occurs as follows:

1. The baby takes his first breath, pulmonary vascular resistance falls and pulmonary blood flow increases. Delay in this normal fall results in persistent pulmonary hypertension of the newborn (PPHN) (p. 162).

2. The umbilical cord is clamped and the ductus venosus begins to close (closure is complete in 76% of normal newborns by the seventh day (Fugelseth *et al.* 1997). The IVC flow falls and the systemic vascular resistance rises.
3. The increased pulmonary blood flow increases the pulmonary venous return and raises the left atrial pressure. The differential pressure between the left and right atria tends to close the foramen ovale, though bidirectional shunting across the foramen ovale is common in the normal neonate. Right-to-left shunting can become evident clinically if the right atrial pressure is higher than normal.
4. The ductus arteriosus closes owing to the rise in PaO_2 and a fall in circulating prostaglandin levels. By about 12 hours of age the ductus arteriosus is functionally closed in 90% of normal neonates. Closure may be delayed in conditions associated with hypoxaemia (e.g. respiratory distress syndrome (RDS) (pp. 127–148); cyanotic CHD (see below); PPHN (p. 162)).

■ Presentation of heart disease

Symptomatic heart disease in the neonate presents as cyanosis, shock or heart failure, or less commonly as a combination of two of these. Asymptomatic heart disease may come to light because of the incidental finding of a murmur or weak pulses, or because of the association with another diagnosis, for instance Down syndrome.

Precise diagnosis of anatomical lesions depends upon specialist investigations. The initial clinical assessment will often not point to a definite diagnosis. Rather it should be directed at answering the following specific questions:

1. Does the baby have heart disease?
2. How seriously ill is he?
3. Does he need immediate treatment?
4. Does he need referral for further investigation?

History

The history is of limited value in the diagnosis of CHD in the neonate, but it should be determined whether there is a family history of CHD, or a maternal history of diabetes mellitus or other maternal conditions that might affect the neonate's heart (e.g. systemic lupus erythematosus). Any maternal illness and/or drug ingestion during pregnancy should also be noted. There may be poor feeding, excess weight gain, or sweating in the baby.

Examination

The most important part of the examination of neonates with suspected heart disease is observation. If possible, the examination should be when the baby is quiet and settled.
Look for:

1. Cyanosis: this is surprisingly easy to miss, especially in neonates with dark skin pigmentation. Look carefully at the tongue and mucous membranes. Use a pulse oximeter if in any doubt. Remember that cyanosis depends on the presence of more than 5 g% deoxygenated haemoglobin, so it is more obvious in plethoric babies and may not be detectable in anaemic babies. Normal babies can become cyanosed around the mouth while crying, but the colour does not persist.
2. Dyspnoea: count the respiratory rate, but what is more important is to observe the pattern of breathing. Look for recession and grunting. Tachypnoea with no or moderate recession is the common pattern of breathlessness due to heart failure.

3. Look for the apex beat: is there a hyperdynamic praecordium?
4. Note dysmorphic features that would indicate a syndrome of which heart disease could be part (e.g. Down, Turner, Noonan syndromes).

Feel for:

1. The heart rate, from either a peripheral pulse or the cardiac impulse. Heart failure may be due to a paroxysmal tachycardia, or less commonly a bradycardia. Fast heart rates can be difficult to count accurately, so if necessary run off an electrocardiogram (ECG) rhythm strip to confirm the rate.
2. The strength of the pulses in all four limbs and the carotids. If the baby is quiet, the brachial, femoral and axillary pulses can all be felt. If all of the pulses are weak or absent, there may be severe left heart disease with a poor cardiac output. Weak femoral pulses with good volume upper limb pulses suggest an abnormality of the aortic arch such as a coarctation or interruption. If there is any doubt about the pulses it is important to measure the systolic blood pressure in all four limbs. Care needs to be taken to obtain accurate blood pressure measurements. It is important that the baby is quiet. Use a cuff which covers 75% of the distance from the axilla to the elbow. Make sure that the measurements are reproducible before you accept them. See Appendix 3 for normal values. A difference in systolic blood pressure of more than 20 mmHg between arm and leg suggests coarctation.
3. Peripheral perfusion. Test capillary refill, which should be <3 seconds. Note clammy, mottled skin, which is often a sign of significant heart disease in a neonate.
4. The size of the liver. Oedema is rare in neonates, but hepatic enlargement is commonly seen. Measure, in centimetres, how far the liver edge extends below the costal margin at the mid-clavicular line.
5. Thrills: praecordial thrills are nothing more than loud murmurs. They always indicate heart disease, although the degree of loudness is not a measure of the severity of the defect.

Listen for:

1. Murmurs: transient (innocent) systolic murmurs in the neonatal period are common. The most common cause is a mild degree of branch pulmonary artery narrowing which resolves with growth and disappears by the age of 6 months (Arlettaz *et al.* 1998). Innocent murmurs are not associated with any other signs of heart disease. The murmurs of VSDs are often heard only after the neonatal period, when the drop in pulmonary vascular resistance has caused sufficient shunt across the defect to cause turbulence. *Serious heart disease may exist without any murmurs being detected in the first weeks of life.*
2. The heart sounds: splitting of the second heart sound is said to be detectable in 50% of neonates by 4 hours and in 80% by 48 hours. In practice, clinical determination of the splitting of the second sound in neonates is often unreliable.
3. Any other added sounds or ejection clicks. A gallop rhythm is frequently heard in babies with heart failure.

◼ Investigations

Echocardiography

Echocardiography has revolutionized the ability to diagnose and manage CHD. Consequently, the chest X-ray (CXR) and ECG have become less important.

Echocardiography is readily available and non-invasive. If there is any doubt about whether or not a neonate has significant CHD, an echocardiogram should be carried out without delay.

Echocardiography is usually the definitive investigation in structural heart disease in the neonate. Babies have excellent echocardiographic 'windows', so that detailed anatomical views can be obtained of the whole of the heart and most of the major vessels. The main exceptions are the aortic arch, which cannot be imaged very well in a minority of cases, and the peripheral pulmonary arteries, which are hidden by the surrounding lung tissue. Cross-sectional echocardiography is supplemented by Doppler measurements of blood flows within the heart and great vessels and by direct colour Doppler imaging of blood flows. Diagnosis is now so precise that it is rarely necessary to perform any additional imaging studies in neonates before undertaking treatment by surgery or transcatheter procedures.

Pulse oximetry

Pulse oximetry is gaining ground as a potential screening tool for the detection of CHD in the newborn because the newborn examination performs poorly in this regard. A post-ductal saturation value of less than 95% in a baby breathing air is generally considered abnormal, and is found in about 5% of babies. Many babies with a low pulse oximetry reading are found to have significant cardiac disease, and others with low readings have systemic illness such as sepsis or pneumonia (Ewer *et al.* 2011).

Chest X-ray

The CXR is seldom diagnostic in CHD. Nevertheless, it is still an essential baseline investigation. The position of the heart, abdominal situs, the heart size and pulmonary vascularity should be assessed. On some films it is possible to determine the side of the aortic arch and the bronchial situs. A cardiothoracic ratio of more than 60% is outside the normal range in the neonatal period.

Electrocardiogram

For information on how to interpret the neonatal ECG, including the criteria for ventricular hypertrophy and the axis, see Appendix 7.

Differential diagnosis

An approach to the differential diagnosis of babies with probable heart disease is given in Figs 22.2–22.4.

▇ Heart murmurs in asymptomatic babies

Heart murmurs are commonly heard during the neonatal examination. The exact prevalence varies widely and depends on the postnatal age and skill of the examiner. The incidence of murmurs detected ranges from six to 759 per 1000 neonatal examinations (Ainsworth *et al.* 1999 (6:1000); Arlettaz *et al.* 1998 (21:1000); Braudo and Rowe 1961 (750:1000)).

The most helpful 'further investigation' of a baby with a murmur is an examination by an experienced observer. A CXR and ECG were traditionally performed, but add

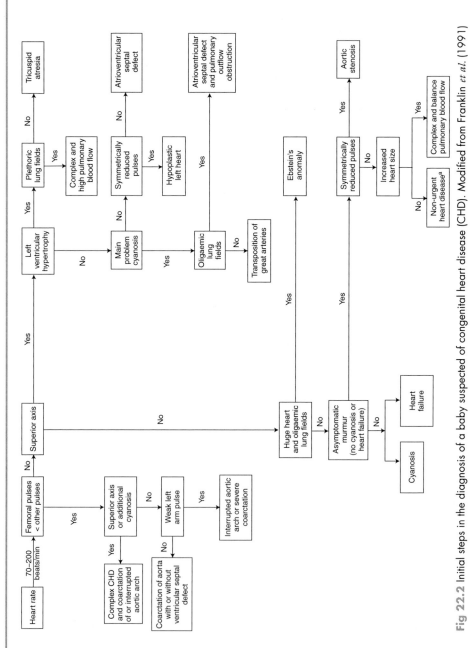

Fig 22.2 Initial steps in the diagnosis of a baby suspected of congenital heart disease (CHD). Modified from Franklin *et al.* (1991)

* Franklin, RCG, Spiegelhalter, DJ, McCartney, FJ, Bull, K (1991) Evaluation of a diagnostic algorithm for heart disease in neonates. *BMJ* 203:935–939.

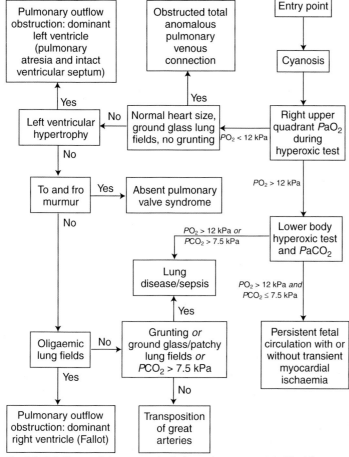

Fig 22.3 Differential diagnosis of a baby with cyanosis. Modified from Franklin *et al.* (1991)

little to this clinical assessment in distinguishing those babies with significant CHD. Pulse oximetry (see above) is quick and easy to perform and should be considered prior to discharge in an apparently well baby with a murmur.

Innocent murmurs have several positive features (Arlettaz *et al.* 1998):

- The murmur is grade 1–2/6 and heard at the left sternal edge without radiation.
- There are no audible clicks.
- The pulses are normal.
- The baby is otherwise well.

Suspicious features on examination such as:

- murmur grade 3/6 or more, radiating to the back or upper left sternal edge;
- pansystolic murmur;
- murmur extending into diastole;
- harsh quality;
- abnormal second heart sound;
- early or mid-systolic click.

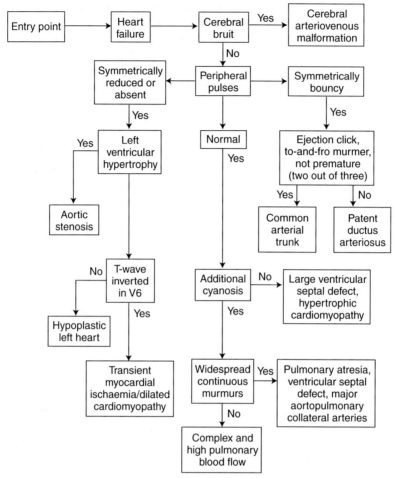

Fig 22.4 Differential diagnosis of congenital heart disease where heart failure is present. Modified from Franklin *et al.* (1991)

Suspicious features mean that the baby should remain in hospital, pulse oximetry should be performed, a CXR and ECG should be obtained, and an early cardiological opinion with echocardiography sought (Figs 22.2–22.4). Otherwise the baby can go home to be reviewed in the outpatient department in a few weeks. Give general advice to the parents with instructions to return early if the baby feeds poorly, fails to gain weight or is breathless or sweaty with feeds.

■ Congenital heart disease presenting as shock with acidosis

Babies with poor left heart function (hypoplastic left heart syndrome (p. 298); interrupted aortic arch; severe coarctation of the aorta (p. 297)) frequently present with shock during the first few days of life. The baby feeds poorly, grunts, has cold peripheries and progresses to become mottled with a generally low-volume pulse. Investigation reveals a profound metabolic acidosis and there can be confusion with a diagnosis of inborn error of metabolism (p. 245) or sepsis. It is important to exclude treatable CHD as early as possible in this situation because some of these babies have an excellent chance of intact survival with surgery.

■ Congenital heart disease presenting as heart failure

Signs of heart failure

Neonates with heart failure usually present with breathlessness on feeding, and increasing lethargy. Weight gain is poor. The babies may be cold, pale and sweaty, with grunting, indrawing and possibly cyanosis. The respiratory rate will be increased to >60 breaths/min; tachypnoea may be the only sign of mild heart failure. There may be pulmonary crepitations, and a tachycardia of at least 150 beats/min. The severity of heart failure can be assessed by the degree of hepatomegaly. Weight gain in excess of 30 g/kg/day suggests fluid retention (Table 22.1).

Feel the peripheral pulses and listen to the heart to see if there is a gallop rhythm, as well as the signs that are characteristic of the individual defect. The CXR will show an increased cardiothoracic ratio, and may show increased pulmonary vascular markings, possibly pulmonary oedema.

Causes of heart failure

In premature babies, heart failure can be caused by the following:

1. Patent ductus arteriosus (PDA)
2. VSD;
3. metabolic causes – hypoxia, hypoglycaemia, hypocalcaemia, hypomagnesaemia.

In full-term babies from birth to 1 week, one of the following is likely to be the cause of the heart failure. These are predominantly diseases of the left side of the heart:

1. aortic atresia;
2. severe aortic valve stenosis;
3. coarctation of the aorta;
4. interrupted aortic arch;
5. transient myocardial ischaemia of the newborn;

Table 22.1 Signs of congestive cardiac failure in neonates

■ Tachypnoea over 60 breaths/min with or without a grunt
■ Pallor and sweating during feeds
■ Taking more than 30 minutes to feed
■ Tachycardia over 150 beats/min (unless the cause is heart block)
■ Hepatomegaly
■ Cardiomegaly, cardiothoracic ratio greater than 60% on chest X-ray
■ Gallop rhythm
■ Weight gain in excess of 30 g/kg/24 h
■ Failure to thrive

6. cardiomyopathies (e.g. coxsackie B myocarditis);
7. arrhythmias (tachycardias or bradycardias);
8. arteriovenous fistulae (e.g. cerebral or hepatic);
9. atrioventricular valve incompetence;
10. arterial valve incompetence;
11. obstructed anomalous pulmonary venous drainage;
12. combined complex lesions;

After the first week, as the pulmonary vascular resistance falls, left-to-right shunts become an important cause of heart failure. These include the following:

1. VSD;
2. PDA;
3. truncus arteriosus;
4. non-obstructed anomalous pulmonary venous drainage;
5. atrioventricular septal defect.

■ Treatment of heart failure in the newborn

1. Correct all associated metabolic problems and apply the routines of neonatal cardiorespiratory care described in Chapter 13.
2. Make sure that the baby has an adequate calorie intake; use nasogastric feeding if he cannot take an adequate volume for himself. Additives to milk are often needed.
3. Nurse the baby in the neutral temperature range (see Chapter 7).
4. Administer diuretics: give furosemide first. If more than once daily furosemide is required, add spironolactone in the same dose as furosemide. A check should be kept on the electrolytes, particularly in premature babies.
5. Consider angiotensin-converting enzyme inhibitors (e.g. captopril): these reduce the work of the heart and may reduce the size of a left-to-right shunt. Do not consider drugs apart from diuretics without expert cardiological assessment and advice.
6. If heart failure cannot be controlled medically, surgical correction of the lesion offers the baby the only hope of survival. It is essential that the anatomical diagnosis be obtained in all babies presenting in heart failure. If the heart failure is severe, arrange early transfer to a specialist centre.

■ Individual conditions which can cause heart failure or shock

See Fig. 22.4

Patent ductus arteriosus

In premature babies usually recovering from RDS, a symptomatic PDA presents with a progressive increase in $PaCO_2$, an increasing inspired oxygen requirement and the need for more vigorous intermittent positive pressure ventilation (IPPV). In babies who are not on IPPV, PDA presents with increasing dyspnoea, increasing oxygen requirements or apnoeic episodes.

On examination, the pulses are bounding with a hyperactive praecordium, tachycardia and often a gallop rhythm. A systolic, or continuous, murmur is maximal at the first left intercostal space and a mid-diastolic murmur at the apex may be audible. The CXR may show an increased heart size and pulmonary plethora, but the ECG is not helpful.

Echocardiography has shown that the ductus is patent in many preterm babies whether or not they are symptomatic. In symptomatic babies, echocardiography shows normal anatomy, but an enlarged left atrium and LV indicative of a left-to-right shunt. It is usually possible to see the ductus in suprasternal notch views and to demonstrate flow across it with colour Doppler. The significance of a PDA detected with echocardiography must be assessed in the light of the clinical picture. Treatment of the PDA in preterm babies remains controversial, with wide inter-unit variation in practice (Benitz 2010).

Treatment consists of controlling pulmonary oedema by respiratory support with continuous positive airways pressure or IPPV plus positive end expiratory pressure, and fluid restriction initially to 60–90 mL/kg. Fluids can be increased by 10 mL/kg day, provided that there is no oedema and the urine osmolarity is in excess of 200 mosmol/kg, until a slow but steady weight gain is attained. Furosemide can be given, but there are theoretical reasons and some clinical evidence to suggest that furosemide promotes ductal patency. Indometacin in a dose of 0.1 mg/kg day for 6 days or 0.2 mg/kg, 8–12 hourly for three doses can achieve closure, but to be effective it needs to be given early – preferably less than 8 days after birth. In these circumstances indometacin has a response rate of nearly 80%. Ibuprofen is a suitable alternative. Indometacin is contraindicated if the platelet count is low, there is renal impairment, ductal-dependent CHD or a gut abnormality. The risk of gut perforation is increased when indometacin and steroids are used together. A third of babies relapse. Often when they relapse no further treatment is required because they have been successfully weaned from ventilation, but in babies who are still ventilator-dependent a further course can be tried. Indometacin is less effective in babies who, irrespective of gestation, are more than 3 weeks old. Surgical closure should be considered in babies who remain ventilator-dependent and who prove to be unresponsive to indometacin. Indometacin or ibuprofen should always be used first, unless it is contraindicated.

Coarctation of the aorta

Severe forms of coarctation, often with marked tubular hypoplasia of the aortic isthmus, present with heart failure. The symptoms arise when the ductus begins to close, and this can occur on the first day or during the first week of life. Less severe forms may be detected because of weak or absent peripheral pulses in an asymptomatic baby.

The abnormality of the peripheral pulses may be masked by persistence of the ductus arteriosus. However, Doppler measurements of blood pressure usually show more than a 20 mmHg difference between the upper and lower limbs. The upper limb hypertension may not be present if there is a large VSD giving a low-resistance run-off into the pulmonary circulation. There may be a gallop rhythm and either no murmur or the systolic murmur of a VSD, atrioventricular valve incompetence or aortic stenosis. Differential pulses between the two arms suggest an aberrant origin of one subclavian artery.

CXR shows a large heart with pulmonary venous congestion. The ECG shows either biventricular or right ventricular hypertrophy. Cross-sectional echocardiography will demonstrate the associated lesions and shows narrowing of the aortic arch in the isthmal area, often with a shelf projecting from the posterior wall of the aorta. The coarctation shelf is usually preceded by a hypoplastic segment, and the transverse aorta may be hypoplastic, too. Aortic valve abnormalities are present in 25% of cases.

Urgent transfer to a cardiac centre is required. Pending transfer, treatment for heart failure should be started and the baby should be ventilated for transfer. Start an infusion of prostaglandin E$_2$ to maintain ductal patency. Consider starting an infusion of dopamine (5 µg/kg/min) to improve renal perfusion.

Early surgical repair of the coarctation is performed. This may be combined with repair of any associated lesions, such as a VSD. Coarctation repair can be combined with pulmonary artery banding for complex defects with an unrestricted pulmonary blood flow.

Repair of the coarctation leads to a rapid improvement of the heart failure. Recurrence of the coarctation is not uncommon, so careful surveillance of these babies is essential. Repair often leads to a reduced pulse in the left arm. This can cause difficulties with subsequent blood pressure measurements.

Aortic atresia (hypoplastic left heart)

Babies with this condition are of normal birth weight and gestational age, but cardiac failure with shock and varying degrees of cyanosis appear soon after birth. Poor or absent peripheral pulses in all areas and mottled peripheries are characteristic. There is a marked metabolic acidosis. Auscultation reveals a loud single second heart sound. A soft ductal murmur may be present. Chest radiography shows marked cardiomegaly, with pulmonary congestion – a 'globular heart'. The ECG shows right axis deviation, right atrial hypertrophy, right ventricular hypertrophy, with a qR pattern over the right primordial leads. If this condition is suspected it is essential that an early echocardiogram is obtained so that the parents can be advised of the diagnosis. If necessary, the baby's condition can be improved by a prostaglandin infusion pending definitive diagnosis. Developmental abnormalities of the brain occur in up to 30% of cases, so brain MRI is indicated.

Cross-sectional echocardiography will confirm the diagnosis. The mitral valve is small or imperforate, and the left ventricular cavity small, often with a thick wall with endocardial fibroelastosis. The aortic valve is an imperforate membrane, with a small valve ring and a small ascending aorta that may be little larger than a coronary artery, and nearly always is less than 6 mm in diameter. There is coarctation in 60–70% of cases. A large patent ductus connecting the main pulmonary artery with the descending aorta is the only source of systemic blood flow.

Management involves staged palliative surgery (the Norwood approach), or palliative comfort care. Although survival of the first stage of the Norwood procedure is good, fewer infants survive the further stages and the neurodevelopmental outcome is not normal (Wernovsky and Newburger 2003). Without treatment the condition is fatal, usually within a few days.

Aortic valve stenosis

When this is severe ('critical' aortic stenosis), it presents with cardiac failure and a low output state. There may be hypotension and acidosis, which are more severe the tighter the stenosis. The pulses are all of small volume. There is an ejection systolic murmur at the second right intercostal space, conducted to the carotid vessels. The lack of an ejection click reflects the severe obstruction in this age group. The second heart sound is closely split or often single. Critical aortic stenosis lies at one end of a spectrum, the mildest of which may not present until adult life. Symptomatic aortic stenosis at sub- or supravalvular level is rare in the newborn.

CXR shows a large heart with pulmonary venous congestion. The ECG shows left ventricular hypertrophy – differentiating it from aortic atresia – occasionally with ST segment depression, and T-wave inversion. Cross-sectional echocardiography shows a thickened, usually dysplastic, aortic valve that may be bicuspid. The ascending aorta may be smaller than usual but is more than 6 mm in diameter. There is usually post-stenotic dilatation. The LV is thick walled, often with endocardial fibroelastosis, and may show reduced contractility. Doppler can be used to measure the gradient across the aortic valve, but at this age gradient is not an indication of severity as low velocity may reflect poor ventricular function and reduced cardiac output.

The prognosis for this condition is critically dependent on the function of the LV, which can deteriorate during fetal life. Overall, when aortic stenosis presents in the neonatal period there is a mortality of about 50%. Early referral to a specialist centre is essential. Treatment is usually by balloon dilation of the aortic valve. Pending transfer, treat the heart failure and acidosis appropriately. If the failure and low-output state are severe, an attempt to reopen the ductus with a prostaglandin infusion is indicated. Ventilate the baby for transfer and consider starting a dopamine infusion.

Ventricular septal defect

This is the most common form of CHD and a large defect can cause heart failure in the first weeks of life. Most VSDs do not present at this time, and the murmur appears later as the right heart pressure falls. There is a harsh systolic murmur and the CXR shows a large heart with pulmonary plethora. The ECG may show biventricular hypertrophy. Medical treatment for heart failure should be tried, but babies who do not respond need early surgery.

Atrioventricular canal defect

This condition is associated with Down syndrome. There is a complex intra-atrial septal defect and VSD.

Pulmonary atresia with ventricular septal defect and major aortopulmonary collateral arteries

In this condition the pulmonary circulation is usually supplied by a PDA with or without major aortopulmonary collateral arteries (MAPCAs). The pulmonary arteries are often underdeveloped. Pulmonary atresia with a VSD presents in a similar fashion to tetralogy of Fallot. There will be no murmur from the right ventricular outflow tract, but continuous murmurs from major pulmonary collateral arteries may be present. Pulmonary atresia with a VSD and MAPCAs is usually treated like severe tetralogy. The prognosis depends upon the presence and size of the pulmonary arteries. If central pulmonary arteries are present, the first step is usually an aortopulmonary shunt. The condition is associated with deletions of chromosome 22.

Truncus arteriosus (can present with cyanosis and heart failure)

This defect consists of a single arterial trunk that leaves the heart through a single semilunar valve and supplies the aorta, the pulmonary trunk and the coronary arteries. A subarterial VSD is always present. The baby is usually not obviously cyanosed, but a hyperoxia test is abnormal. The pulses are bounding because of the run-off to the lungs through the pulmonary arteries. The first heart sound is normal. There is an ejection click in 50% of cases, an ejection systolic murmur is heard at the upper left sternal border but may be very quiet, and there is a loud single second sound, which represents truncal closure. An early diastolic murmur of truncal valve insufficiency, which is diagnostic if present, is a bad prognostic sign. There is tachypnoea, and heart failure develops usually in the third or fourth week.

Initial management consists of vigorous treatment of heart failure.

Heart muscle disease

Several forms of cardiomyopathy can produce heart failure in the neonatal period. These include the following:

- hypoxic ischaemic encephalopathy;
- anomalous origin of the left coronary artery;
- viral myocarditis (p. 206);
- hypertrophic cardiomyopathy.

The most common conditions that cause neonatal hypertrophic cardiomyopathy are maternal diabetes and steroid treatment for chronic lung disease. These two conditions do not usually give rise to symptoms and need no treatment. Hypertrophic cardiomyopathy of the autosomal dominant variety, or in association with Noonan syndrome, may be progressive and give rise to symptoms because of outflow tract obstruction and poor ventricular compliance or serious arrhythmias. More rarely, the cause is a glycogen storage disease or a mitochondrial abnormality. The management is difficult and controversial. Inotropes and vasodilators may be detrimental as they can accentuate the left ventricular outflow obstruction. There may be a role for beta-blockade in some cases, under supervision of a paediatric cardiologist.

■ Cyanotic heart disease

See Figs 22.2 and 22.3 for differential diagnosis.

Diagnosis

Cyanosis with minimal dyspnoea in a baby should suggest the possibility of cardiac disease, particularly if the CXR does not show the evidence of respiratory disease (Table 13.5). In some forms of CHD there may be no murmur. Furthermore, because of the high oxygen affinity of fetal haemoglobin, babies with cyanotic heart disease involving common mixing of systemic and pulmonary venous return within the heart are often not cyanosed in early life. If there is a suspicion of cyanosis, the presence of hypoxaemia must be confirmed by pulse oximetry and arterial blood gas analysis.

Hyperoxia test

This test was described before echocardiography was widely available, but it still has a place in the assessment of a baby with suspected CHD, especially if echocardiographic skills are a long ambulance journey away.

A PaO_2 of less than 20 kPa (150 mmHg) when the baby is breathing 100% oxygen is very suggestive of cyanotic CHD unless there is severe lung pathology. A PaO_2 greater than 33 kPa (250 mmHg) excludes virtually all types of cyanotic CHD. Pulse oximetry will not provide the same assurance because a baby can achieve 100%

saturation at PaO_2 levels well below 20 kPa. A very low PaO_2 with a normal $PaCO_2$ suggests a cardiac cause of right-to-left shunting. An elevated $PaCO_2$ strongly suggests lung disease (Chapter 13). Always consider the possibility of septicaemia, particularly in a hypotensive baby or if there are apnoeic episodes.

Right-to-left shunts in neonates with normal hearts

There are two related conditions that can cause right-to-left shunts and therefore cyanosis in neonates with structurally normal hearts:

- persistent pulmonary hypertension of the newborn (see pp. 162–163);
- transient myocardial ischaemia.

Right-to-left shunt caused by structural heart defects (See Fig. 22.3)

Transposition of the great arteries

The incidence is 1:3000 live births. The aorta arises from the RV and the pulmonary trunk from the left, which produces persistent hypoxia, the severity of which is dependent on whether there are associated shunts through the foramen ovale, the ductus arteriosus or septal defects.

The predominant physical sign is cyanosis. In uncomplicated cases there are often no murmurs. A VSD is the most common associated abnormality, followed by pulmonary stenosis. The ECG is normal during the first few days but later shows moderate right ventricular hypertrophy with upright T waves in V_1. At birth the CXR is usually normal. The classic CXR of an 'egg-shaped' heart with a narrow vascular pedicle is seen rarely and is a relatively late finding. Pulmonary plethora is observed when a large ductus or a VSD is present.

Cross-sectional echocardiography shows the posterior great artery arising from the LV to be the pulmonary trunk. The aorta arises in parallel with it anteriorly from the RV. During the first few days of life, the ductus arteriosus closes and the baby becomes lethargic, mottled and tachypnoeic, with severe hypoxia and acidosis, rapid deterioration and death. The severity of hypoxia depends upon the potential for mixing across the foramen ovale and the presence and size of any VSD. When the diagnosis is suspected, a prostaglandin infusion should be commenced and the baby must be referred to a specialist centre. Nowadays, most centres undertake an arterial switch operation within a few days of diagnosis. Balloon septostomy enlarges the foramen ovale and helps to stabilize the situation by mixing the circulations and is still likely to be needed if there is a poor response to prostaglandins or if early surgery cannot be done.

Tetralogy of Fallot

In this defect there is a large VSD and infundibular pulmonary stenosis, often associated with pulmonary valve and pulmonary arterial stenosis. Cyanosis is present from birth in about 20% of cases and deepens with crying. Those that present as newborns tend to have pulmonary atresia or a very narrow right ventricular outflow tract. Those with pulmonary atresia will be duct-dependent. Tetralogy without cyanosis ('pink Tet' cases) presents with a pulmonary outflow murmur; the harsh ejection systolic murmur of infundibular stenosis tends to diminish with severe narrowing and may disappear completely during 'cyanotic spells'. Splitting of the second heart sound may be heard if the obstruction is mild, but it becomes single with progressive narrowing.

The chest film is often diagnostic in that there is a normal cardiothoracic ratio with a decrease in pulmonary vascularity and a small or absent pulmonary trunk contour giving a 'pulmonary artery bay' or 'boot-shaped heart'. A right-sided aortic arch is seen in 30% of cases.

Cross-sectional echocardiography shows a large aortic root over-riding a subaortic VSD and the interventricular septum. The infundibular part of the septum deviates anteriorly into the right ventricular outflow tract, creating infundibular pulmonary stenosis. The severity of the pulmonary stenosis can be estimated with Doppler. The pulmonary valve ring and pulmonary arteries are reduced in size to a variable degree. With severe infundibular and valve narrowing, echocardiographic differentiation from pulmonary atresia with a VSD is difficult, but, in tetralogy, colour Doppler will usually show the anterograde flow across the right ventricular outflow tract.

If arterial hypoxia is severe, a prostaglandin infusion may be required, pending transfer to a specialist centre. Treatment there is governed by the size of the pulmonary arteries. If they are large, complete correction with VSD closure and resection of infundibular stenosis is possible. Some centres prefer initial management with a Blalock shunt to encourage growth of the pulmonary arteries before total correction at a later stage. Hypercyanotic spells are uncommon in neonates. If they occur, they should be treated with facial oxygen and intravenous morphine. It is rare to need to progress to intravenous propranolol, followed by ventilation and sedation, and if this is required an immediate referral for surgery should be made.

Pulmonary atresia with intact ventricular septum

This condition is sometimes referred to as 'hypoplastic right heart', since a characteristic feature is a small, dysplastic RV. These babies all present with cyanosis in the newborn period. The pulmonary blood flow is always dependent upon flow through the ductus. There is usually persistent cyanosis from birth, which deepens as the ductus flow diminishes. The outflow of venous blood from the right atrium is obstructed, which can lead to marked hepatic enlargement. Auscultation reveals a single second sound and no murmur, or a ductus, or a tricuspid regurgitation murmur.

The ECG usually shows a QRS axis between +120° and −30°, right atrial hypertrophy and paucity of right ventricular forces with a dominant S in V_1. The CXR shows a normal-sized or large heart depending on the degree of right atrial dilation secondary to tricuspid incompetence. There is decreased vascularity and an absent main pulmonary artery shadow, creating a pulmonary artery bay. The aortic arch is usually on the left side.

Cross-sectional echocardiography shows an enlarged right atrium. In 85% of babies the RV is very small but thick walled, often with endocardial fibroelastosis. The tricuspid valve is often small and dysplastic. The pulmonary valve is usually an imperforate membrane with a good-sized main pulmonary artery, but at the other extreme there may be absence of the outlet portion of the RV and of most of the pulmonary trunk. Colour Doppler often shows marked tricuspid incompetence. The absence of flow across the pulmonary valve differentiates the condition from severe pulmonary valve stenosis. Immediate transfer to a specialist centre, with prostaglandin infusion to maintain duct patency, is essential.

Surgical treatment involves an aortopulmonary shunt, with valvotomy if possible, and atrial septostomy may be necessary. The prognosis is proportional to right ventricular size and the size of the central pulmonary arteries, but is often poor.

Pulmonary valve stenosis

When this is severe, it often presents with a loud systolic murmur along the upper left sternal edge and radiating to the back. The second sound is single and a pulmonary ejection click is usually absent. Cyanosis and hepatic enlargement appear with right ventricular failure, often associated with tricuspid regurgitation. This usually occurs during the first week of life. Sinus tachycardia and a low output state may be present.

The ECG shows right atrial and right ventricular hypertrophy, with ST segment depression over the RV suggesting suprasystemic pressure in the RV. The CXR shows a normal-sized or large heart depending on the degree of right atrial enlargement, and reduced or normal pulmonary vascularity. Poststenotic dilatation of the main pulmonary artery is not seen in the neonatal period.

Cross-sectional echocardiography reveals right atrial enlargement and a thick-walled RV that may be normal sized or small, often with bright subendocardial echoes suggesting endocardial fibroelastosis. The pulmonary valve is often a thick, dysplastic membrane but may be thin and doming. Pulmonary arteries are normal sized or small. Colour Doppler reveals a high-velocity jet across the pulmonary valve and possibly tricuspid regurgitation. The gradient across the pulmonary valve can be estimated from the Doppler trace, but this is not a reliable measurement of severity, especially if the ductus is open.

Anti-failure treatment should be instituted. In a neonate the circulation may be duct-dependent and a prostaglandin infusion should be considered. Urgent referral for surgery or transcatheter balloon dilation of the pulmonary valve is essential.

Tricuspid atresia

Tricuspid atresia generally presents with cyanosis from birth, unless the pulmonary blood flow is increased. The high right atrial pressure causes an enlarged liver. Approximately 50% of cases have a systolic murmur at the lower left sternal edge, but 25% have no murmurs. The second sound is single.

CXR shows a square heart with cardiac enlargement in proportion to the pulmonary blood flow. There is a prominent SVC and right atrium, and the pulmonary artery segment may be absent. Lung fields are usually oligaemic. The ECG usually shows left axis deviation (usually $-30°$ to $-60°$) and extreme paucity of right ventricular forces (more pronounced than pulmonary atresia). Right atrial hypertrophy is usually present.

Cross-sectional echocardiography most commonly shows a total absence of the valve, with the right atrium separated from the ventricles by a wedge of atrioventricular sulcus tissue, and rarely a thin imperforate membrane is seen. The blood reaches the left side of the heart through an atrial septal defect (ASD), with the atrial septum bulging from right to left. If the ASD is small (restrictive), there is marked dilatation of the IVC and hepatic veins. The right ventricular cavity is diminutive or absent in 70% of cases. There may be associated pulmonary atresia, in which case pulmonary blood flow is dependent on the ductus arteriosus. In 70% of babies the pulmonary artery arises from the small RV and the aorta from the LV. In these cases the pulmonary blood flow is usually reduced, because of obstruction at the level of the VSD or within the cavity of the small RV. In contrast, in a minority of cases, there is ventriculo-arterial discordance (transposition of the great arteries) in association with tricuspid atresia. The pulmonary artery arises from the LV, causing excessive pulmonary blood flow. The aorta arises from the RV and this may be associated with subaortic stenosis and coarctation.

If the baby is severely hypoxic, start a prostaglandin infusion. Treatment with diuretics is unwise until the degree of obstruction at the level of the atrial septum has been determined. If there is a restrictive ASD, an atrial septostomy must be performed.

The surgical approach depends upon the anatomy. Reduced pulmonary blood flow is managed with an aortopulmonary shunt. If the pulmonary blood flow is high, pulmonary artery banding may be required. In the older child definitive treatment by a Fontan procedure (right atrial to pulmonary artery conduit) may be possible. In reality, only about 50% of patients survive to have a Fontan procedure, and the long-term prognosis for survivors of surgery is uncertain.

Ebstein's malformation

This is a rare cause of cyanosis in the newborn, but milder, often asymptomatic, cases are not rare. The tricuspid valve is dysplastic and may be both stenotic and incompetent. The right atrium is often markedly dilated. This can lead to pulmonary hypoplasia and it is upon this that the prognosis of neonates presenting with this condition chiefly depends. The CXR shows a very large heart and reduced pulmonary perfusion. The ECG shows paucity of RV forces with a dominant S wave in V_1; the malformation predisposes to supraventricular tachycardias (SVTs) and the delta waves of Wolff–Parkinson–White (WPW) syndrome may be seen. Echocardiography confirms the diagnosis, showing an abnormal apical displacement of the tricuspid valve, particularly the septal leaflet. Treatment is supportive, including a prostaglandin infusion and administration of oxygen. With the postnatal fall in pulmonary vascular resistance, the pulmonary blood flow gradually improves and in many cases the hypoxia resolves. There are few surgical options for the neonate with Ebstein's malformation and intractable hypoxia.

Total anomalous pulmonary venous drainage

The non-obstructed type presents as heart failure in pink babies over 1 week of age, but the obstructed types cause early cyanosis and feeding difficulties. The clinical severity is determined by the degree of obstruction to the pulmonary venous return. Total anomalous pulmonary venous drainage mimics respiratory disease and can cause confusion with rising CO_2 and some response to an increase in F_iO_2.

The site of return of the anomalous veins may be supracardiac, cardiac or infracardiac; obstruction is particularly common and severe in the infracardiac group. Most commonly the pulmonary veins all enter a confluence behind, but separate from, the left atrium. Obstruction can occur at a number of sites, including the pulmonary vein orifices, the confluence, or on passage through the liver. In the last situation the cyanosis gets dramatically worse when the ductus venosus shuts.

There is a loud first heart sound and narrow fixed splitting of the second heart sound. A pulmonary ejection systolic murmur and a tricuspid flow murmur may be present, but with severe obstruction a loud pulmonary component of the second sound may be the only clue. Another clue may be the paradoxical finding of well-oxygenated blood from an umbilical venous catheter with deoxygenated blood from an umbilical artery catheter. The respiratory rate is increased, with dyspnoea proportional to the severity of obstruction. Hepatomegaly is present in most types of infracardiac drainage. A CXR shows a small heart with increased vascularity and venous congestion. With infracardiac drainage a total whiteout of the lung fields may be seen, and an erroneous diagnosis of lung disease is often made. Some babies present later on with chestiness and failure to thrive. In the first days of life the ECG is usually normal.

Cross-sectional echocardiography shows a small left atrium with no pulmonary veins entering it, and large right-sided chambers. The pulmonary venous confluence is seen behind the left atrium and often an ascending or descending vein can be demonstrated. Colour Doppler is of great value in tracing the flow of pulmonary venous blood. When there is infracardiac obstructed drainage, hugely dilated portal veins are seen within the liver.

Obstructed anomalous venous drainage is one of very few serious heart conditions presenting in the first few days of life that does not respond to a prostaglandin infusion. Urgent surgery to redirect the pulmonary veins to the left atrium is essential.

■ Arrhythmias in the neonatal period

Atrial ectopics

These are very common and they resolve within 3 months in 90% of cases. Atrial ectopics can be a marker for SVT, and may occasionally cause a ventricular bradycardia because they occur in a refractory period and conduction is blocked.

Paroxysmal supraventricular tachycardia

This occurs once in every 25 000 children. The heart rate during attacks ranges from 180 to over 300 beats/min, and the QRS complex is normal. Episodes usually begin and end abruptly. The child presents in heart failure with pallor, irritability and poor feeding. The diagnosis is made from the ECG. Look for an abnormal P wave axis or P wave morphology, or for a shortened PR interval and for the presence of delta waves (suggesting WPW syndrome) on the ECG during sinus rhythm. Death may occur if untreated for 48–72 hours. There is a 20% recurrence rate.

Treatment

The blood sugar level, electrolytes and acid–base status should be checked and corrected. Vagal stimulation, such as an ice bag to the face or immersion of the baby's face in cold water for a maximum of 10 seconds, is often successful. Attacks will usually respond to intravenous administration of adenosine, repeated after 20 minutes, if necessary (Fig. 22.5). In refractory cases an infusion of amiodarone over 20 minutes may be successful. If the baby is shocked, consider using synchronized DC cardioversion, starting with 1 J/kg. Flecainide can be considered but verapamil is contraindicated in the newborn.

Maintenance treatment may not be indicated if the attacks are rare, short and easily stopped; but if they are not, the baby should be treated with digoxin for 6–12 months. If the child has remained free from attacks at this age, an attempt should

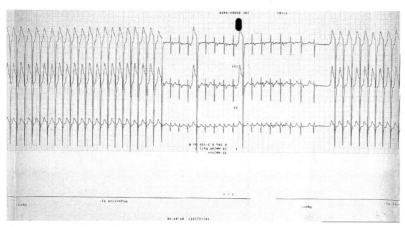

Fig. 22.5 Supraventricular tachycardia responding to an injection of adenosine and relapsing

be made to tail off drug treatment unless there is documented WPW syndrome. Oral maintenance treatment with other drugs in patients refractory to digoxin should be supervised by specialists.

Ventricular ectopics

Like atrial ectopics (see above), these are common and usually harmless. Review the baby in 6 weeks and check the QTc interval (p. 377). If this is prolonged, 24-hour monitoring is indicated to look for ventricular tachycardia.

Congenital heart block

Congenital heart block occurs once in 20,000 liveborn babies. Around 30% of cases of congenital atrioventricular block are associated with CHD, commonly atrioventricular septal defects and atrioventricular discordance (congenitally corrected transposition). Evidence of systemic lupus is commonly found in mothers of other cases. The babies present with bradycardia, often noted while still *in utero*, with Stokes–Adams attacks, or even with cardiac failure. There is usually an ejection murmur in the aortic area, and a mid-diastolic murmur at the apex, even without a structural heart abnormality.

Many babies are asymptomatic and do not require treatment. Mild congestive heart failure may respond to diuretics. Symptomatic cases require treatment with an isoprenaline infusion to raise the heart rate, followed by pacing. The indications for pacing in asymptomatic babies are controversial, but a mean heart rate below 50 beats/min or the presence of runs of ventricular tachycardia on a 24-hour ECG recording have been cited.

■ References

Ainsworth, S, Wyllie, JP, Wren, C (1999) Prevalence and clinical significance of cardiac murmurs in neonates. *Archives of Disease in Childhood*, **80**: F43–5.

Arlettaz, R, Archer, N, Wilkinson, AR (1998) Natural history of innocent murmurs in newborn babies: controlled echocardiographic study. *Archives of Disease in Childhood*, **78**: F166–70.

Benitz, WE (2010) Treatment of the persistent ductus arteriosus in preterm infants – time to accept the null hypothesis? *Journal of Perinatology*, **30**: 241–52.

Braudo, M, Rowe, RD (1961) Auscultation of the heart – early neonatal period. *American Journal of Disease in Children*, **101**: 67–78.

Ewer, AK, Furmston, AT, Bhoyar, A, *et al.* (2011) Pulse oximetry screening for congenital heart defects in newborn infants (PulseOx): a test accuracy study. *Lancet*, **378**: 785–94.

Franklin, RCG, Maccartney, FJ, Bull, K, Speigelhalter, DJ (1991) Evaluation of a diagnostic algorithm for heart disease in neonates. *British Medical Journal*, **302**: 935–9.

Fugelseth, D, Lindemann, R, Liestol, K, *et al.* (1997) Ultrasonographic study of ductus venosus in healthy neonates. *Archives of Disease in Childhood*, **77**: F131–4.

Wernovsky, G, Newburger, JW (2003) Neurological and developmental morbidity in children with complex congenital heart disease. *Journal of Pediatrics*, **142**: 6–8.

■ Further reading

Bernardini, S, Semama, DS, Huet, F, *et al.* (1997) Effects of cisapride in QTc interval in neonates. *Archives of Disease in Childhood*, **77**: F241–3.

Yates, R (2012) Cardiovascular disease. In Rennie, JM (ed.) *Rennie & Roberton's Textbook of Neonatology*, 5th edition. Edinburgh: Elsevier pp. 617–69.

23

Neonatal haematology

◼ Anaemia in the neonate

Key points

◼ Most anaemia in the non-jaundiced full-term baby is due to perinatal blood loss.

◼ Perinatal blood loss may cause nothing more than mild pallor requiring treatment with iron and folate, but is occasionally responsible for a pale shocked baby with a haemoglobin of <5g%.

◼ Anaemia of prematurity can be reduced by minimizing blood lost into the laboratory. Routine use of haematinics is of no value and we do not currently use erythropoietin.

◼ Consider haemolytic disease in all jaundiced babies in the first 24 hours.

◼ Most cases of haemolytic disease of the newborn are now due to ABO incompatibility, but other incompatibilities and red cell disorders such as spherocytosis present in a similar way.

Definition

Anaemia is defined as a haemoglobin less than 12g/dL in the first week or less than 10g/dL later in infancy.

Anaemia present at birth

This may be due to haemorrhage, haemolysis or rarely to impaired red cell production.

Haemorrhage

◼ Twin-to-twin transfusion.
◼ Fetal haemorrhage from normal or abnormal placental vessels, or from placental separation or injury (e.g. abruptio, placenta praevia, placental incision at caesarean section, ruptured velamentous insertion of the cord (vasa praevia)).
◼ Fetal or neonatal internal haemorrhage (ruptured liver or spleen, subgaleal haemorrhage p. 224).
◼ Feto-maternal haemorrhage.

Haemolysis

◼ Rhesus haemolytic disease (pp. 311–313).
◼ Other immune haemolytic processes, e.g. anti-Kell antibody, ABO incompatibility.
◼ Congenital infection (e.g. parvovirus B19, cytomegalovirus).

Impaired red cell production

■ Blackfan–Diamond syndrome and other disorders.
■ Rarities such as α-thalassaemia (baby often hydropic) (see Orkin *et al.* 2009).

Marked pallor in the neonate may also be due to severe asphyxia. A very tight nuchal cord can be associated with anaemia because of lack of placental transfusion.

Assessment of early anaemia

History and physical examination

■ Was there unusual blood loss in labour? Examine the placenta for abnormal vessels, especially vasa praevia (more common in twins or in low-lying or 'battledore' placenta).
■ Are there any findings in the baby to suggest bleeding (e.g. cephalhaematoma, boggy scalp swelling, rigid abdomen)? Or haemolysis (hepatosplenomegaly, jaundice)?
■ Was there a twin-to-twin transfusion? Compare haematocrits, discuss obstetric history.
■ Check the pulse and respiration. A steadily rising pulse rate, tachypnoea or air hunger are signs of massive haemorrhage.
■ *Always* measure the baby's blood pressure.

Investigation

■ Haemoglobin and packed cell volume (PCV) measurement. Remember, it takes 2–3 hours for these to fall after major acute haemorrhage.
■ Reticulocyte count.
■ Serum bilirubin.
■ Blood group and direct antiglobulin test (DAT) (Coombs' test).
■ pH. This is a good emergency test, since, when the cardiac output falls, tissue perfusion deteriorates and an acidaemia develops. Check lactate if available.
■ Check the mother's blood for feto-maternal haemorrhage using the Kleihauer test. It is possible to make an estimate of the quantity of blood from the Kleihauer test, although some laboratories are reluctant to attempt this estimation.

A diagnostic algorithm for neonatal anaemia is shown in Fig. 23.1.

Treatment

In an emergency the baby will be pale and showing signs of shock with weak pulses, often a tachycardia, shallow rapid respiration, hypotension and acidosis. In this life-threatening situation give an immediate transfusion (most easily through a umbilical venous catheter (UVC)) of 15–20 mL/kg over 5–10 minutes using uncrossmatched O-negative blood. Give oxygen if necessary, then insert an umbilical artery catheter for regular monitoring of PaO_2, blood gases and haematocrit. Correct any acid–base abnormalities. Check that vitamin K was given.

If the baby is still pale and hypotensive, repeat the transfusion over 15–20 minutes and if possible check the central venous pressure (CVP) through the UVC. Aim to achieve a normal blood pressure, normal pH and a haemoglobin above 12 g/dL.

If the baby with a haemoglobin of 8–10 g/dL is stable with no hypotension, tachycardia, acidaemia or respiratory distress, and in particular if no cause of acute blood loss can be found, he may be suffering from chronic, or acute on chronic, haemorrhage such as a feto-maternal or twin-to-twin haemorrhage during late pregnancy. In such babies haemodilution is likely to have occurred and they are

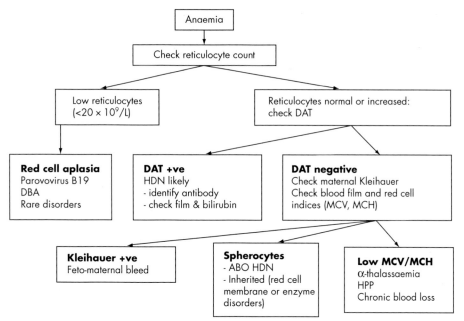

Fig 23.1 Diagnostic algorithm for neonatal anaemia. DBA, Diamond–Blackfan anaemia; DAT, direct antiglobulin test; HDN, haemolytic disease of the newborn; HPP, hereditary pyropoikilocytosis; MCH, mean corpuscular haemoglobin; MCV, mean cell volume

unlikely to be hypotensive: if the anaemia is even more severe it may have caused fetal heart failure, or even hydrops. In these situations, a single-volume (80 mL/kg) exchange transfusion using packed cells is the safest way of raising the haemoglobin without exacerbating the heart failure.

With anaemia of 10–12 g/dL in an asymptomatic baby, a top-up transfusion of 20–30 mL/kg can be given over 2 hours with furosemide cover, and the need for further transfusions reassessed afterwards.

Late-onset neonatal anaemia (2–28 days of age)

The conditions listed in Table 23.1 may be responsible for anaemia of below 10 g/dL occurring later in the neonatal period in otherwise well babies. The conditions fall into the same categories as before.

Table 23.1 Causes of chronic neonatal anaemia

Cause	Diagnosis
Haemorrhage	
Haemorrhage into the laboratory	Examine records of number of laboratory tests
Perinatal haemorrhage not recognized at the time of delivery	Check the history in more detail for such a problem
Chronic blood loss, especially from the gastrointestinal tract	Clinical examination, stool, urine analysis, iron-deficient picture on blood film

Cause	Diagnosis
Haemolysis	
Mild haemolytic disease of the newborn – insufficient to cause jaundice	Maternal history, direct antiglobulin (Coombs') test, antibody studies on the mother
Fragile red cells, e.g. spherocytosis	Blood film, family history
Enzyme deficiency (e.g. G6PD)	Enzyme assay, reticulocyte count
Chronic infection, especially urinary tract infection and occasionally congenital infections	Clinical examination, stool, urine analysis, iron-deficient picture on blood film
Impaired red cell/haemoglobin production	
Anaemia of prematurity	
Haemoglobinopathies	Hb electrophoresis, reticulocyte count, family studies
Drugs	History
Rare congenital bone marrow aplasias or congenital leukaemia	Physical examination for hepatosplenomegaly or skin infiltration; blood count, bone marrow

G6PD, glucose-6-phosphate dehydrogenase; Hb, haemoglobin.

Investigation and treatment

In most cases, if no diagnosis is obvious, it is reasonable to assume that the baby received no placental transfusion, or had a small unrecognized perinatal bleed. Helpful guidelines regarding transfusion can be found via the British Committee for Standards in Haematology (www.bschguidelines.com) and those at the time of writing are as shown in Table 23.2.

Anaemia of prematurity

The nadir in haemoglobin concentration in very low birth weight (VLBW) babies is around 8 g/dL at the age of 4–8 weeks and this section refers to babies presenting at this time. The nadir in preterm babies occurs earlier, and is lower, than that for term babies, which is around 11.4 g/dL at 8–12 weeks.

■ *Erythropoietin (EPO) deficiency* is almost certainly the single major cause of this disorder. EPO production switches off after birth in VLBW babies and rises only very slowly thereafter. There is a blunted EPO response to decreasing haemoglobin levels in preterm babies. In addition to EPO deficiency the *red cell survival* of premature babies is known to be short.

Table 23.2 Suggested transfusion thresholds for red blood cells in infants under 4 months of age (British Committee for Standards in Haematology)

Anaemia in the first 24 hours	Hb 12 g/dL (Hct 36%)
Cumulative blood loss in the first week	10% of blood volume
Neonate receiving intensive care	Hb 12 g/dL
Acute blood loss	10%
Chronic oxygen dependency	Hb 11 g/dL
Late anaemia, stable baby	Hb 7 g/dL

Hb, haemoglobin; Hct, haematocrit.

Table 23.3 Transfusion thresholds for preterm babies

Assisted ventilation			
	<28 days		≥28 days
	FiO₂ ≥0.3	FiO₂ <0.3	
Haemoglobin	<12 g/dL	<11 g/dL	<10 g/dL
PCV	<0.40	<0.35	0.30

Continuous positive airways pressure		
	<28 days	≥28 days
Haemoglobin	<10 g/dL	<8 g/dL
PCV	<0.30	<0.25

Breathing spontaneously (also consider reticulocyte count)		
	FiO₂ >0.21	Well in air
Haemoglobin	<8 g/dL	<7 g/dL
PCV	<0.25	<0.20

PCV, packed cell volume.

- *Folic acid deficiency.* Despite the fact that most premature babies, particularly those below 1.50 kg at birth, have low levels of serum folate by 6–8 weeks of age, megaloblastic change in the marrow is rare. However, we give babies below 2 kg, and those with rhesus haemolytic disease of the newborn (HDN), 0.1 mg of folic acid daily from 2 weeks of age while they are in the neonatal unit (NNU).
- *Vitamin E deficiency.* We no longer give vitamin E supplements routinely. Vitamin E deficiency was a feature of feeding babies with the older milk formulas which were high in polyunsaturated fats.
- *Iron deficiency.* This is not important in the anaemia of prematurity. Premature babies do eventually become iron deficient, so start iron supplements when they weigh 2 kg and are ready for discharge. For the first 6 months we give 2.5 mL Sytron (≅13.75 mg Fe, 95 mg iron edetate) as a single daily dose.

Management

Check the haemoglobin and reticulocyte count on all the asymptomatic growing premature babies in the NNU every week. Our current transfusion thresholds are shown in Table 23.3. Red blood cell (RBC) transfusion may be considered at higher thresholds than the above for neonates with hypovolaemia (unresponsive to crystalloid infusion), septic shock, necrotizing enterocolitis, undergoing/recovering from surgery. Transfusion should be with cytomegalovirus-negative, crossmatched blood from a 'pedi–pack' to minimize donor exposure. Irradiation (to reduce the risk of graft–versus–host disease) is a matter for local discussion.

Haemolytic disease of the newborn

Pathophysiology

Throughout all pregnancies, very small amounts of blood leak from the fetal circulation into the mother. If it is rhesus-positive blood, about 5% of rhesus-negative primiparae will develop a mild antibody response. However, in most women, major feto-maternal bleeding occurs only during labour, antepartum haemorrhage or spontaneous or therapeutic abortion. Although over 100 mL of blood may enter the mother's circulation in exceptional circumstances around the time of delivery, the usual volume is in the 0.5–5.0 mL range. This is, however, enough to evoke a major antibody response, which will be most marked against the D antigen of the rhesus group. The antibodies formed will be of the immunoglobulin (Ig)G class, which will cross the placenta and haemolyse fetal rhesus-positive red cells.

In the 5% of first pregnancies in rhesus-negative women where antibody is formed before delivery, the infant usually suffers only from mild rhesus HDN. In most first rhesus-incompatible pregnancies, no antibody is formed until after the feto-maternal bleed at delivery and so the infant has no neonatal problems. However, in subsequent pregnancies, if the fetus is again rhesus positive, the very small feto-maternal bleeds of 0.1–0.2 mL early in gestation will now evoke a major secondary antibody response in a sensitized woman. With each successive rhesus-positive fetus, larger amounts of anti-D will be made and the disease in the fetus will become more severe.

Not all rhesus-positive babies inside rhesus-negative women provoke an antibody response. The presence of ABO incompatibility between the mother and her fetus protects against rhesus HDN, since if A-positive fetal cells cross into an O-negative woman, her natural isoimmune anti-A will destroy the fetal RBCs before they evoke an antibody response to the rhesus antigen.

Antenatal care

There are three stages in the antenatal care:

1. Detect all rhesus-negative women and screen them for the presence of antibody by appropriate blood tests in the booking antenatal clinics. Many areas now offer anti-D prophylaxis during the first pregnancy. Anti-D should be given to cover events in pregnancy that might be associated with a feto-maternal haemorrhage, such as amniocentesis (see list below)(p. 22).
2. Assess how severely affected the baby is.
3. Plan the optimal time to deliver the baby.

Assessing severity

Management of rhesus-sensitized women is an area for highly specialized fetal medicine and is now concentrated in only a few centres since the welcome decline in the incidence of the condition. Management involves sampling fetal blood via the umbilical cord and intra-uterine transfusion where necessary. This treatment has revolutionized the outcome for affected babies, who are often maintained until after 34 weeks in good condition by repeated transfusions. Hydrops fetalis is now rarely seen as a consequence of haemolytic disease and is usually due to other causes (such as viral infection or heart disease).

Timing of delivery

Whenever possible the baby should be delivered at a time convenient for both the paediatrician and the transfusion service. Always ensure that at least two units of suitable fresh whole blood are available before delivery.

Postnatal care

- *Resuscitation*: in severely affected infants efficient resuscitation is paramount. If the infant is very anaemic it is easy to underestimate the severity of co-existing respiratory distress syndrome, since an anaemic baby cannot become cyanosed. Therefore, in severe rhesus HDN insert an arterial catheter as quickly as possible for assessment and control of PaO_2 and pH. All the tenets in Chapter 6 on first-hour care are particularly important to this group of infants.
- In low-risk infants, particularly where the infant is more than 36 weeks' gestation, difficulties at resuscitation are rare. Nevertheless, a paediatrician must attend all such deliveries in case the baby is unexpectedly severely affected, and also to get the initial investigations under way.
  - *Laboratory investigation*: the cord blood of babies born to all affected mothers must be analysed for blood group, DAT (Coombs' test), serum bilirubin and haemoglobin. The first two confirm the diagnosis, the second two give an indication of the severity of the disease. Haemoglobin values taken later in the first 4–6 hours of life are often 10–25% higher than the cord blood values.
  - *Anaemia*: the timing of the first exchange transfusion is decided on the basis of the *cord* haemoglobin results. Levels less than 10 g/dL are an indication for an immediate exchange transfusion; the further below 10 g/dL, the greater the urgency. With haemoglobin values between 10 and 12 g/dL an exchange will be needed within the next few hours. With cord haemoglobin values above 12 g/dL it is safe to wait and base the decision to do an exchange transfusion on the serum bilirubin values. Rate of rise of bilirubin is crucial information.
  - *Jaundice*: in all affected infants, estimate the bilirubin on capillary blood at least 6 hourly and record the results graphically (see Chapter 20). Start phototherapy immediately. Infants with cord bilirubin values exceeding 100–135 µmol (6–8 mg%), or who have a bilirubin rising faster than 8.5 µmol/L/h, will need an exchange transfusion. In premature infants who often have other problems increasing the risk of kernicterus, exchange transfusion should be carried out at lower bilirubin levels (Chapter 20).
- Always do a bilirubin estimation at the beginning and the end of an exchange transfusion, which should lower the plasma bilirubin by 50–60%. Immediately following the exchange there is a rapid rise in bilirubin as the tissue levels equilibrate with the plasma levels. Bilirubin levels should continue to be measured 4–6 hourly as before and repeated until the levels fall consistently or a further exchange is needed.
- Use intravenous immunoglobulin (500 mg/kg over 4 hours) as an adjunct to continuous multiple phototherapy in cases of rhesus haemolytic disease or ABO haemolytic disease when the serum bilirubin continues to rise by more than 8.5 µmol/L/h.
  - *Other haematological problems*: the infants may have a low platelet count, but bleeding problems are rare unless disseminated intravascular coagulation (DIC) develops in a severely affected infant. If DIC does develop, its treatment is that outlined on p. 318, and platelet transfusion should be given if the infant is bleeding and has a platelet count below $10 \times 10^9/L$ (10,000/mm³).
- Infants with severe rhesus HDN have many circulating nucleated red cells. These nucleated cells may cause confusion in white cell counts and in the examination of blood-stained cerebrospinal fluid.
  - *Cardiovascular status*: hepatosplenomegaly in the presence of extramedullary haemopoiesis, cardiomegaly in the presence of anaemia, and hydrops in the

presence of anaemia and hypoalbuminaemia are poor indicators of whether or not severely affected babies are in heart failure. On the contrary, many are markedly hypovolaemic and hypotensive. Blood pressure must therefore always be measured, and CVP as well, if possible, though it is often difficult to get a UVC through the ductus venosus, and the value of CVP measurements from a UVC wedged in the liver is uncertain. Hypotension should be treated vigorously: 20–30 mL/kg of saline may need to be given combined with dopamine or dobutamine.

- *Hypoglycaemia*: rhesus babies are prone to hypoglycaemia, especially after exchange transfusion. In infants with cord haemoglobin values below 10 g/dL, hypoglycaemia may arise at any time, and such babies should have regular glucose estimations for at least 48–72 hours after delivery. All babies need glucose measurements 1, 2 and 4 hours after exchange transfusions.
- *Late anaemia*: in DAT-positive infants who do not require exchange transfusion, anaemia of less than 6 g/dL may develop by 2–3 weeks of age. Similar but milder degrees of anaemia may also be seen in infants who have had an exchange transfusion. All survivors of HDN should be checked regularly during the first month of life and top-up transfusions given if the haemoglobin falls to less than 7 g/dL, particularly if the reticulocyte count remains low.
- *Folate deficiency*: survivors of HDN have low serum folate levels, and, although they rarely develop megaloblastic anaemia, their growth during the first year may be improved by giving them supplementary oral folate.

Treatment following intra-uterine transfusion

Irrespective of whether transfusions were given intraperitoneally or intravenously at cordocentesis, since rhesus-negative blood is given, the cord blood results will be peculiar – even suggesting that the baby is not affected because his haemoglobin will be normal and the DAT (Coombs' test) negative. Management of such babies is, however, no different to that outlined above. Not infrequently though, because most of their circulating red cells are rhesus negative, they do not require exchange transfusion.

Prevention of rhesus haemolytic disease

The antibody response following feto-maternal haemorrhage can be prevented by giving the mother 500 IU of anti-D immunoglobulin. This is routinely given intramuscularly to all rhesus-negative women who deliver rhesus-positive babies within 72 hours (ideally within 24 hours) of delivery. A maternal Kleihauer test (for fetal RBCs) should always be done and a further 125 units (1 mL) of anti-D immunoglobulin given for each 4 mL by which the feto-maternal transfusion is calculated to exceed 4 mL.

Anti-D immunoglobulin should always be given to all rhesus-negative women in pregnancy after any of the following complications:

1. spontaneous miscarriage;
2. ectopic pregnancy;
3. chorionic villus sampling;
4. amniocentesis;
5. termination of pregnancy;
6. antepartum haemorrhage;
7. road traffic accidents, falls and abdominal trauma;

8. external cephalic version;

The dose is 250 units at less than 20 weeks of pregnancy and 500 units thereafter.

These routines will prevent rhesus sensitization in 95% of women. As discussed above, it is now almost universal practice to try to protect the 5% of women who develop rhesus antibodies in response to the small feto-maternal haemorrhages which occur throughout pregnancy by offering primagravida 'prophylaxis'. This has led to some difficulty interpreting cord blood DAT results in babies of rhesus-negative mothers because the passive transfer of antibody can lead to a weakly positive DAT.

Our current guidelines regarding DAT-positive babies are as follows.

■ Guidelines for direct antiglobulin test-positive babies

DAT 1+ and DAT 2+

Routine follow-up and blood sampling NOT required UNLESS there is any one of the following:

1. jaundice identified <24 hours;
2. requirement for exchange transfusion;
3. jaundice requiring prolonged phototherapy.

THEN follow the guidelines for infants with DAT 3 + and 4 + including discharge on folic acid.

DAT 3+ and DAT 4+

1. Discharge on folic acid
2. 2/52 general review + Full blood count (FBC) + reticulocytes + prolonged jaundice screen if required.
3. 6/52 general review + FBC + reticulocytes. If normal FBC then discharge from follow-up.
4. Continue folic acid until fully weaned

ABO incompatibility (ABO haemolytic disease of the newborn)

Group A, B and most group O women have IgM isoagglutinins which do not cross the placenta, but about 10% of these women have an IgG anti-A haemolysin in their plasma (and rarely anti-B) which can cross the placenta and haemolyse the RBCs of a group A (or group B) infant.

The antibody is present before pregnancy and so first babies may be affected. Furthermore, it is unusual for the titres of these antibodies to rise as a result of feto-maternal bleeding at any stage of pregnancy, and successive pregnancies are therefore rarely more severely affected than the first one.

In absolute numbers ABO HDN is 5–10 times more common than rhesus HDN. Fortunately, since much of the antibody which crosses the placenta is absorbed by A and B antigens in body tissues other than the RBCs, and there are relatively few A and B antigenic sites on the fetal RBCs, ABO HDN rarely causes severe problems.

ABO HDN usually presents in the first 24 hours of life in an otherwise healthy full-term infant who rapidly becomes jaundiced. Jaundice recognized on the third or fourth day of life may also occasionally be due to ABO HDN. The haemoglobin is usually normal, and the DAT (Coombs' test) is either negative or weakly positive. The mother and baby are ABO incompatible. Proof of the diagnosis depends on identifying the haemolytic anti-A in maternal plasma or in the infant's plasma, after eluting it from his RBCs.

Treatment

If phototherapy is given from the time of diagnosis, the bilirubin rarely rises to dangerous levels. However, if it does exceed 350–400 µmol/L, an exchange transfusion is required in term babies, starting at lower levels in babies <37/40 (Chapter 20).

The other problems of rhesus HDN, such as hypoglycaemia, heart failure or chronic liver disease, are rarely seen, but babies who do not require exchange transfusion should be followed up carefully to ensure that anaemia does not develop.

Other blood group incompatibilities

The other rhesus groups C, E, c, e, and other groups such as Kell and Duffy, have all been responsible for HDN of varying severity, including rare cases of hydrops. The management is no different from that already described for rhesus disease. Anti-Kell may cause severe neonatal anaemia without jaundice.

Congenital spherocytosis

This can present within the first 48–72 hours with jaundice which may become severe enough to require exchange transfusion. The diagnosis can be made from the family history and the infant's blood film which shows many spherocytes, although less than in later life. The infant usually has a normal haemoglobin; but once spherocytosis is diagnosed, whether or not exchange transfusion is carried out, he should receive 1 mg of folic acid per day.

Non-spherocytic haemolytic anaemias

These are due to inherited red cell metabolic defects. Although they usually present later in life with a haemolytic anaemia, they occasionally present neonatally with severe jaundice requiring phototherapy or exchange transfusion.

■ Bleeding and bruising

Key points
- All babies should receive vitamin K to prevent haemorrhagic disease of the newborn. The most effective prophylaxis is obtained with 1 mg given intramuscularly shortly after birth.
- Late haemorrhagic disease of the newborn is virtually confined to breast-fed infants and those with liver disease, and is not reliably prevented by oral vitamin K prophylaxis.

- Thrombocytopenia and disseminated intravascular coagulation (DIC) are common in sick babies with many diagnoses.
- Platelet transfusion in the absence of overt bleeding is indicated if the platelet count is below $30 \times 10^9/L$: if bleeding is a clinical problem, give platelets if there is any thrombocytopenia.
- With DIC, treating the precipitating cause is the priority. Use fresh frozen plasma, cryoprecipitate, fibrinogen concentrate and platelets to control bleeding in severe cases.

The neonate, particularly if born prematurely, is deficient in all the factors involved in the intrinsic clotting mechanism with the exception of fibrinogen and factors V and VIII. The levels rise to adult values within a few weeks.

The levels of the natural anticoagulants antithrombin III and proteins C and S are low in neonatal plasma, as are levels of plasminogen. Although, in theory, this might make neonates hypercoagulable, this has not been found to be the case in practice.

Coagulation in the neonate is usually evaluated by a platelet count plus the prothrombin time (PT), thrombin time, fibrin degradation products (FDPs) and activated partial thromboplastin time (APTT) (Fig. 23.2). Beware of heparin in the sample, which can give rise to a prolonged APTT and a minor prolongation of the PT. The D-dimer test is the most sensitive indicator of intravascular formation of fibrin and the presence of D-dimers usually indicates DIC in the newborn. The PT in the normal term newborn is 13–16 seconds, being prolonged to about 13–20 seconds in preterms. This is often reported as an international normalized ratio which takes account of laboratory variation; this result centres around 1.0 with a range of 0.5–1.5 in term babies. The APTT also varies between laboratories, but is prolonged in babies compared with adults. Absolute values of 40–70 seconds at term and 40–100 seconds in preterms are usually reported. Interpretation of common patterns of abnormal test results is given in Table 23.4.

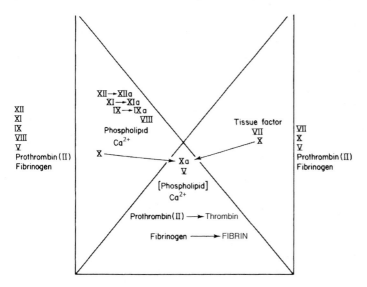

Fig. 23.2 Activated partial thromboplastin time (APTT) and prothrombin time (PT). Those portions of the coagulation mechanism measured by the APTT are in the triangle on the left; those measured by the PT are in the triangle on the right. Listed on the left are those factors which influence the APTT and on the right those which influence the PT. a, activated

Table 23.4 Interpretation of coagulation tests in neonatal bleeding

	Haemorrhagic disease of the newborn	DIC	Liver disease
PT	Very prolonged	Prolonged	Prolonged
APTT	Prolonged	Prolonged	Prolonged
TT	Normal	Prolonged	Prolonged
FDPs	Normal	Increased	Normal or ↑
Fibrinogen	Normal	Reduced	Reduced
Platelet count	Normal	Reduced	Normal or ↓
Response to vitamin K	Dramatic	No response	Diminished response

APPT, activated partial thromboplastin time; DIC, disseminated intravascular coagulation; FDP, fibrin degradation product; PT, prothrombin time; TT, thrombin time.

Haemorrhagic disease of the newborn (vitamin K deficiency bleeding)

This is due to a deficiency of the vitamin K-dependent clotting factors II, VII, IX and X and can be prevented by routine administration of 1 mg of the natural analogues of vitamin K (e.g. Konakion) intramuscularly at birth. This preventive treatment is recommended for all newborn babies. The incidence of the disorder if vitamin K prophylaxis is not used at all is about 1 in 10,000, whereas a single intramuscular dose of vitamin K prevents virtually all cases. Oral vitamin K regimens are not totally effective but are popular with some. There are three forms of the disorder: early, classical and late. The early form is limited to babies of mothers who have taken drugs such as anticonvulsants during pregnancy.

The classical form of vitamin K deficiency bleeding (VKDB) presents on the second to fourth day of life with umbilical stump haemorrhage, haematemesis and/or melaena, ecchymoses, epistaxis or scalp haemorrhage. The baby may also bleed from puncture sites and circumcision. The PT and APTT are very prolonged, but the thrombin time and fibrinogen level are normal (Table 23.4).

Once haemorrhage has occurred, the baby should be managed as on p. 311. An immediate replacement transfusion is indicated if the baby is shocked, but more gradual correction by exchange transfusion should be used if the baby has had time to haemodilute. Always give 1 mg vitamin K intravenously (to avoid a haematoma) irrespective of what was thought to have been given at delivery. Fresh frozen plasma (FFP) should be given at the same time because vitamin K takes several hours to correct the coagulation deficit.

Late VKDB is largely a disease of breast-fed babies. Intracranial haemorrhage is a devastating complication, which is seen in about a third of cases. There are often small warning bleeds from the gum or rectum. The time of onset has moved later (30–60 days) now that almost all babies receive at least a single oral dose of vitamin K as prophylaxis; it is now clear that more than one oral dose is required to prevent this disorder. The optimal oral regimen has not yet been devised; the manufacturers of Konakion MM recommend 2 mg orally on days 0, 28 and 56. Remember that VKDB is often the presenting condition in babies with liver disease.

Disseminated intravascular coagulation

This is seen in neonates with severe birth asphyxia, septicaemia, intracranial haemorrhage, hypothermia, hypotension, hypoxia and acidaemia. It usually presents as petechial bleeding into the skin, or oozing from skin puncture sites and the umbilicus, but haemorrhage may occur anywhere.

Neonatal haematology

Thrombin formation, triggered in vivo by microbial endotoxin or by thromboplastin released from damaged tissues and endothelial cells, results in intravascular coagulation which consumes platelets, factors II, VIII, XIII and fibrinogen, and leaves the baby with a bleeding diathesis. The fibrinolytic system is activated, and the FDPs so produced further aggravate the bleeding tendency by interfering with fibrin polymerization.

Diagnosis

The PT, APTT and thrombin time are all prolonged, confirming consumption of intrinsic coagulation factors and fibrinogen. FDPs will be increased in the blood. The platelet count is usually below 100×10^9/L (<100,000/mm³) and blood films show distorted RBCs. The D-dimer test may be available and levels are raised. The minimum criteria for the diagnosis of DIC are:

- compatible clinical signs;
- abnormal clotting studies, including a prolonged PT and APTT;
- some other laboratory evidence (e.g. fibrinogen consumption, low platelets, elevated FDP, elevated D-dimers).

Treatment

1. Remedy the underlying disease (e.g. correct hypotension or acidaemia).
2. Replace clotting factors by transfusing FFP (10–15 mL/kg). If the underlying condition is being adequately treated, FFP transfusion should not provide the fuel for further DIC.
3. In severely affected babies, or those with continuing DIC despite intravenous FFP, cryoprecipitate (which provides fibrinogen, factor VIII and von Willebrand factor) and fibrinogen concentrate (helpful especially in fluid restriction, e.g. hypoxic ischaemic encephalopathy (HIE)) can be used.
4. Give an extra dose of intravenous vitamin K.

Congenital deficiencies of coagulation factors

These may all present in the neonatal period, usually with bleeding from surgical incisions such as circumcision, but rarely from other sites. If bleeding in a neonate does not respond to vitamin K, and DIC is not present, specific assays for these conditions should be done. Haemophilia (factor VIII deficiency) is present in 90% of such cases. In the face of marked bleeding from the umbilical stump with normal coagulation times babies should be screened for factor XIII deficiency, which requires a special additional test. This very rare disease is more common in babies of consanguineous Pakistani or Bangladeshi parents.

Neonatal thrombocytopenia

The normal neonatal platelet count is the same as in the adult, 150×10^9/L. Thrombocytopenia is a common finding in the NNU, occurring in 20–30% of all admissions. The condition is rare (about 1%) in the general neonatal population, and in a well term baby the most likely cause is neonatal alloimmune thrombocytopenia or maternal idiopathic thrombocytopenic purpura. Thrombocytopenia usually presents with purpura, ecchymoses or large cephalhaematomata. Bleeding at other sites, including the gut, umbilicus, skin and central nervous system, can occur but is comparatively rare. Differential diagnosis is usually possible on the basis of a history, clinical examination, coagulation studies, platelet count (mother and baby), platelet antibody studies and occasionally bone marrow examination.

Causes include the following:

1. DIC, and hence all the conditions that may cause DIC, especially sepsis, HIE, necrotizing enterocolitis.
2. Neonatal alloimmune thrombocytopenia – usually a mother who is human platelet antigen (HPA)-1a negative with a HPA-1a-positive fetus.
3. Giant haemangiomas (Kasabach–Merritt syndrome).
4. Congenital infection including HIV and CMV.
5. Maternal idiopathic thrombocytopenia or systemic lupus erythematosus with transplacental passage of antiplatelet IgG.
6. In association with Rh HDN.
7. Marrow abnormalities (leukaemia, hypoplasia).
8. Drugs (administered to mother or baby – quinidine, thiazides).
9. Inherited abnormalities (e.g. Wiskott–Aldrich, thrombocytopenia – absent radius syndrome).
10. Maternal disease such as pre-eclampsia (PET).
11. Organic acidaemias (p. 247).

Treatment

One major anxiety is always whether the thrombocytopenia will lead to an intracranial haemorrhage, although for all the conditions listed above this seems to be exceptionally rare except in babies with alloimmune thrombocytopenia. In these groups neonatal treatment is always justified, and in neonatal alloimmune thrombocytopenia the risk of *in-utero* haemorrhage justifies the risk of antenatal platelet transfusion. In the other conditions specific therapy for thrombocytopenia is not indicated unless platelet counts are $<30 \times 10^9/L$ ($<50 \times 10^9/L$ if sick or very preterm in the first few days of life) *or* there are clinical problems with haemorrhage and any degree of thrombocytopenia.

Treatment of alloimmune thrombocytopenic purpura should be with transfusion of platelets from donors who are cytomegalovirus-negative and HPA-1a negative. In the UK this product has replaced washed maternal platelets, which carry a risk of graft-versus-host disease. Steroids and immunoglobulin (1 g/kg daily for 3 days) may prolong survival of the transfused platelets. In the non-immune thrombocytopenias such as DIC, platelet transfusion will usually control the bleeding.

Most cases of neonatal thrombocytopenia resolve quickly, either because underlying infection is treated or because the antibody responsible for the thrombocytopenia disappears. Only if thrombocytopenia is persistent should some of the rarer conditions listed above be sought. Persisting thrombocytopenia can be the only clue to congenital HIV infection.

Neonatal polycythaemia

The viscosity of blood increases linearly up to a PCV of 65%. Above this there is a progressively larger increase in viscosity for unit change in PCV. Furthermore, at a given PCV and shear rate in vitro, neonatal blood is more viscous than adult blood. Newborn babies become polycythaemic in the following situations:

1. recipients in twin-to-twin transfusion;
2. recipients of large placental transfusions;
3. small-for-dates babies;
4. babies of diabetic mothers;
5. rarities (e.g. neonatal thyrotoxicosis, Beckwith–Wiedemann syndrome).

Diagnosis

Polycythaemia should be diagnosed only if the venous haematocrit is greater than 65–70% since capillary haematocrits are inaccurate and may be 15% greater than the true central haematocrit. The symptoms which are attributed to hyperviscosity and polycythaemia are:

1. CNS depression, fits and cortical venous thrombosis;
2. heart failure;
3. respiratory distress, cyanosis and persistent fetal circulation;
4. jaundice;
5. hypoglycaemia;
6. hypocalcaemia;
7. renal vein thrombosis;
8. NEC.

Treatment

Some authorities recommend therapy for all babies with a venous haematocrit of 65–70%. However, we believe that therapy is needed for polycythaemia only when the central haematocrit exceeds 75%, or 70% in a baby with significant symptoms. The PCV can be lowered by carrying out an exchange transfusion using saline and exchanging 20 mL/kg depending on the degree of the polycythaemia. The full calculation is: volume in mL =

$$\frac{(\text{actual PCV} - \text{desired PCV})}{\text{actual PCV}} \times \text{weight (kg)} \times 80 \text{ (blood volume in mL/kg)}$$

■ Neonatal thrombosis

Increasing use of central lines and arterial catheters, sometimes combined with a genetic predisposition to thrombosis, has resulted in increasing problems with thrombotic disease in the newborn. It is important to make the diagnosis, as timely action can save a limb or minimize brain injury (from cerebral sinovenous thrombosis (CSVT)). Prevention should be attempted and all infusions into an arterial catheter should be heparinized.

Inherited disorders which increase thrombotic risk include:

■ factor V Leiden deficiency (activated protein C resistance);
■ protein C deficiency;
■ protein S deficiency;
■ prothrombin G20210A mutation;
■ homocystinuria due to cystathionine β-synthase deficiency;
■ antithrombin III deficiency;
■ increased lipoprotein A.

Diagnosis

Family history can be important: antithrombin deficiency is inherited in an autosomal dominant fashion. Healthy newborns have about half the adult levels of antithrombin III, and levels rise to the adult levels by about 6 months of age. As yet there is no suggestion that the management of newborns with a family history of thrombophilia should be any different from usual.

Clinical signs of venous obstruction include oedema and cyanosis of a limb, head and neck, or chest with increased collateral vessel circulation. There may be an abdominal mass and haematuria if the renal vein is thrombosed. Seizures may be the clue to CSVT.

Clinical signs of arterial thrombosis include a pale, cold limb with absent pulses which may be obviously painful, seizures, or increased ventilatory requirements owing to pulmonary emboli. Hypertension can be a clue to renal artery obstruction. Damping of a transduced arterial trace may be an early sign of thrombus formation.

The diagnosis can be confirmed with real-time and Doppler ultrasound or venography but may have to rest on clinical suspicion. MR angiography is available in a few centres.

Protein C deficiency may present as purpura fulminans, haemorrhagic necrosis of the skin with DIC.

Treatment

For arterial obstruction which is threatening a limb, surgical embolectomy should be seriously considered. If an arterial catheter is in situ, consider infusing tissue plasminogen activator down the catheter onto the clot before removing it. Anticoagulation therapy is emerging as possible treatment for babies with serious CSVT.

References

Orkin, SH, Nathan, DG, Ginsburg, D, et al. (2009) *Nathan and Oski's Hematology of Infancy and Childhood*, 7th edition. Philadelphia: Elsevier.

Further reading

Roberts, I, Murray, N (2012) Neonatal haematology. In Rennie, JM (ed.) *Rennie & Roberton's Textbook of Neonatology*, 5th edition. Edinburgh: Elsevier, pp. 755–90.

Web links

www.bcshguidelines.com
www.vasapraevia.co.uk

24

Genitourinary problems

Key points
- Renal failure in the neonate is diagnosed when the urinary output is <0.5 mL/kg/h in the first day and <1.0 mL/kg/h thereafter with a rising serum creatinine.
- Differentiating pre-renal from intrinsic renal failure can usually be done on the basis of the clinical findings and plasma and urine biochemistry.
- Conservative treatment with control of fluid balance and hyperkalaemia is sufficient in most cases as the oliguria is usually short-lived.
- Babies with renal malformations detected prenatally or in the neonatal period require assessment and follow-up in all cases.
- Male babies with bilateral ureteric dilatation and a thick-walled bladder on ultrasound have urethral valves until proved otherwise and must be investigated urgently.

Urine

Most babies pass urine at or immediately after birth; 97% have done so within 24 hours and all normal babies have passed urine within 48 hours. Breast-fed infants, who have a relatively low intake for the first 24–48 hours, pass little urine during this period. Following this, 40–60 mL/kg/24 h is produced. Passing less than 12 mL/kg/24 h (0.5 mL/kg/h) on day 1 and less than 24 mL/kg/24 h (1 mL/kg/h) thereafter is certainly abnormal and requires investigation. The most common cause of oliguria is pre-renal failure (Table 24.1). Polyuria is defined as more than 7 mL/kg/h of urine flow. Polyuria can be caused by a reduced antidiuretic hormone (ADH) concentration (diabetes insipidus) or resistance to ADH in the renal tubules (nephrogenic diabetes insipidus) but is more commonly seen in the polyuric phase of renal failure or in the diuretic phase of respiratory distress syndrome (RDS). Babies can concentrate their urine to about 500 mosmol/L (preterm) and 700 mosmol/L (term), but this is much less than the adult value of 1400 mosmol/L. The reasons are a shorter loop of Henle, reduced tonicity of the medullary interstitium, and reduced expression of aquaporins. Providing there is no glycosuria, proteinuria or haematuria, this corresponds to a specific gravity of 1002–1030. The pH of neonatal urine is usually between 5 and 8. For more information on neonatal renal function see p. 80.

Haematuria

This is comparatively common in very sick infants as a result of one of the conditions listed below. Haematuria is often misdiagnosed when a female infant has had a small

323

vaginal haemorrhage, and occasionally haematuria is diagnosed incorrectly when there are pink urate crystals on the nappy.

1. Bleeding tendency, particularly disseminated intravascular coagulation (DIC) (pp. 318–319). This is probably the most common cause of haematuria in very sick infants with RDS, septicaemia or necrotizing enterocolitis receiving intensive care.
2. Emboli from umbilical artery catheters (UACs), or with coagulase-negative staphylococci sepsis (endocarditis) in association with long lines.
3. Trauma, particularly after suprapubic bladder aspiration.
4. Hypoxic ischaemic encephalopathy (HIE) with associated tubular or cortical necrosis.
5. Renal artery or vein thrombosis (see below).
6. Urinary infection (p. 204).
7. Malformation, particularly from the wall of a trabeculated bladder in the presence of urethral valves (p. 328), or with hydronephrosis.
8. Other very rare causes of neonatal haematuria include drugs, tumours or polycystic kidney disease (the kidneys are often palpable and uraemia may be present).

Haemoglobinuria is very rare in the newborn except in the presence of DIC with intravascular haemolysis. In most of the conditions listed above the differential diagnosis is comparatively straightforward on clinical grounds, but, if any doubts remain, renal ultrasound is the investigation of choice.

Proteinuria

The normal newborn infant may excrete up to 1 g albumin/L during the first 24–48 hours of life, but the level falls rapidly after that period. Proteinuria in the neonatal period is rare as a primary finding. It is common in association with any of the severe illnesses such as septicaemia, HIE, hypotension and DIC, which compromise renal perfusion and in some cases also cause haematuria. Massive proteinuria occurs in congenital nephrotic syndrome.

Renal failure

Acute renal failure (ARF) can be defined biochemically or in terms of urine flow. Blood urea levels are unhelpful, but a creatinine above the normal range for gestation and postnatal age (100–130 µmol/L) (Appendix 5) and/or a rising creatinine during the first few days suggests renal failure. Creatinine usually falls steadily after birth. Any infant passing less than 0.5 mL/kg/h of urine with a rising serum creatinine is in renal failure. Most cases of ARF occur in neonates who have HIE, or are ventilated because of sepsis or RDS. In some of these babies renal failure is pre-renal due to over enthusiastic fluid restriction, but, in others, acute tubular necrosis or renal cortical necrosis may have occurred. Causes of ARF in the neonate are shown in Table 24.1.

Diagnosis

Most of these conditions can be established by taking the history, examining the baby (including catherization of the bladder if necessary) and doing a renal and bladder ultrasound scan. The important differential diagnosis then lies between pre-renal uraemia or renal failure. This differentiation can usually be made clinically

Table 24.1 Causes of renal failure in the neonate

Pre-renal	Intrinsic renal	Post-renal (obstructive)
Systemic hypovolaemia Any severe illness with shock Fetal or neonatal haemorrhage Operative fluid loss	Malformation (e.g. polycystic kidney disease)	Malformation (valves, pelvi-ureteric junction obstruction, recessive polycystic disease)
Renal hypoperfusion Severe illness, e.g. respiratory distress syndrome, asphyxia Drugs (e.g. indometacin) Coarctation of the aorta	Maternal drugs (captopril, indometacin)	Extrinsic compression (tumour)
	Acute tubular necrosis, acute cortical necrosis in severe illness	
	Renal vein/artery thrombosis	
	Pyelonephritis	
	Disseminated intravascular coagulation	

and confirmed by simultaneous measurements of serum and urinary sodium and osmolarity (Table 24.2). However, the biochemical discrimination is not so good in very low birth weight (VLBW) babies who have poor kidney function to start with and in whom sodium excretion may have been increased by furosemide.

If uncertainty persists, the 'fluid challenge' test beloved of nephrologists involves volume expansion with 10–15 mL/kg of normal saline. This test can be useful but is clearly ill advised in a hypotensive, oedematous ventilated 1 kg baby who is already requiring inotropic support. Such infants cope badly with a fluid load.

Treatment

If ARF is pre-renal, the correct treatment is volume expansion with blood or electrolyte solutions, maintaining a urine output of above 1 mL/kg/h and giving furosemide 2–4 mg/kg (which can be repeated daily if effective).

If there is intrinsic renal failure, the following regimen should be instituted:

1. Weigh the baby regularly (up to twice daily may be helpful).
2. Restrict fluid administration to insensible loss (20–30 mL/kg in a term baby) plus urine output. If the neonate is oedematous, replace insensible loss only. Flush arterial lines with the smallest possible volume of solution and remember to add this to the daily intake. Do not give potassium-containing solutions; add calcium to the intravenous fluid only if necessary; give enough sodium to keep at the plasma level at 135–145 mmol/L.

Table 24.2 Biochemical indices to differentiate pre-renal from intrinsic renal failure

	Pre-renal	Renal
Urinary Na (mmol/L)	<10	>40
Urine/plasma osmolarity	>2	<1.1

3. Measure plasma electrolytes and acid–base status at least twice a day.
4. Measure blood glucose every 12 hours and correct hypoglycaemia.
5. Correct metabolic acidaemia with bicarbonate if the Na^+ is less than 130 mmol/L.
6. Treat hyperkalaemia as appropriate. At levels above 8–9 mmol/L hyperkalaemia can cause severe cardiac disturbance and death. Emergency treatments include:
   - giving intravenous salbutamol 0.4 mg/kg over 20 minutes;
   - giving intravenous 10% calcium gluconate (2 mL/kg over 5–10 minutes) with electrocardiogram monitoring;
   - giving sodium bicarbonate (2 mEq/kg) over 5–10 minutes;
   - setting up a glucose/insulin infusion.
7. Treat *hypo*tension with dopamine; treat *hyper*tension with hydralazine.
8. Consider dialysis in appropriate cases (see below).

Most infants remain stable on this regimen and start to pass urine within 48–72 hours.

◼ Urinary tract infection

See p. 204.

◼ Congenital nephrotic syndrome

This is extremely rare but may present with hydrops or the clinical stigmata of nephrotic syndrome. The causes are:

1. 'Finnish' congenital nephrotic syndrome.
2. Congenital syphilis, or cytomegalovirus (that due to syphilis is treatable).
3. Renal vein thrombosis (RVT).

The treatment is to maintain serum albumin and try diuretics. The prognosis for babies with congenital nephrotic syndrome is poor and the condition is autosomal recessive.

◼ Renal malformations

Prenatally diagnosed renal malformations

Renal malformations are identified by antenatal ultrasound in about 1:800 pregnancies; about a fifth of childhood renal malformations are now detected this way. The most common problem identified antenatally is dilatation of the renal tract, but renal agenesis, malpositioned or multicystic kidneys are also found. All babies with an antenatally diagnosed problem should have a renal ultrasound scan within a week, and if the antenatal dilatation of the renal pelvis (pyelectasis) was 15 mm or more this scan should be done urgently, before the baby goes home from the maternity unit. This serves to identify those babies with problems who require early intervention, for example those with urethral valves. The yield of investigating babies with prenatal dilatation of the renal tract (pyelectasis) is as follows:

5–10 mm	approx 3% with abnormality;
10–15 mm	approx 50% with abnormality;
>15 mm	approx 94% with abnormality.

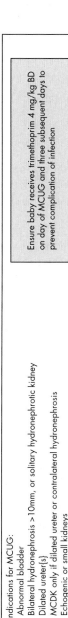

Antenatal hydronephrosis
(≥7mm 2nd trimester, ≥10mm 3rd trimester)

Copy details of antenatal imaging for the infant's notes
(if possible)

Antenatal history of:
- Abnormal bladder
- Oligo-or anhydramnios
- Bilateral hydronephrosis >20mm
- Unilateral hydronephrosis >20mm in a solitary kidney
- Bilateral echogenic and/or small kidneys

Prophylactic trimethoprim 2 mg/kg OD

Early ultrasound (ideally after 72 h) before discharge from hospital

Liaise with paediatric urology +/− nephrology

Many will require admission, serum electrolytes, MCUG and intervention

Indications for MCUG:
- Abnormal bladder
- Bilateral hydronephrosis >10mm, or solitary hydronephrotic kidney
- Dilated ureter(s)
- MCDK only if dilated ureter or contralateral hydronephrosis
- Echogenic or small kidneys
- Hydronephrotic duplex kidney

Antenatal history of:
- Bilateral hydronephrosis >15mm
- Unilateral hydronephrosis >15mm +/− ureteric dilatation
- Duplex kidney with ureterocele
- Large multicystic dysplastic kidney
- Incomplete history or lack of a reliable third trimester scan

Prophylactic trimethoprim 2 mg/kg OD

Ultrasound in the first 7–10 days

Liaise with paediatric urology +/− nephrology

Antenatal history of:
- Bilateral hydronephrosis 10–15mm
- Unilateral hydronephrosis 10–15mm with ureteric dilatation

Advise parents on signs of UTI and how to seek early help

Ultrasound in the first 2–3 weeks

Antenatal history of:
- Unilateral hydronephrosis 10–15mm no ureteric dilatation

When in doubt liaise with paediatric urology

Ensure baby receives trimethoprim 4 mg/kg BD on day of MCUG and three subsequent days to prevent complication of infection

Fig. 24.1 Flow chart detailing the initial steps in the investigation of the neonate with antenatally diagnosed hydronephrosis. From Smeulders and Wilcox (2012), with permission. BD, twice daily; MCDK, multicystic dysplastic kidney; MCUG, micturating cystourogram; OD, once daily; UTI, urinary tract in infection.

There is relative oliguria in the first days of life, so it is best to perform an ultrasound scan after day 2–3 of life. Formerly, all babies with renal 'pyelectasis' were discharged on trimethoprim prophylaxis, but recently we and many other units have restricted this treatment to those with an antenatal scan showing hydronephrosis of more than 15 mm, a duplex system, or a large multicystic dysplastic kidney. Our current protocol is shown in Fig. 24.1. The most common causes are pelvi-ureteric junction (PUJ) obstruction, vesico-ureteric junction (VUJ) obstruction, or reflux.

Pelvi-ureteric junction obstruction

This is diagnosed with MAG-3 renography, which confirms 'hold-up' at the PUJ level and provides information about renal function; this latter is the key to management. Minimal dilatation is usually defined as 7–12 mm, moderate as 12–20 mm and severe as >20 mm. Most cases of PUJ obstruction with mild to moderate dilatation of the renal tract and normal renal function will not deteriorate and can be watched safely. Those with severe dilatation are at risk of deteriorating renal function, and these children should be watched carefully with repeat isotope renograms and referred for consideration of pyeloplasty. Antibiotic prophylaxis should be continued.

Vesico-ureteric junction obstruction

This condition is also a common cause of antenatal pyelectasis. These babies have a megaureter. Management is similar to that of PUJ obstruction and the two can co-exist. Again, conservative management is indicated when the renal function is stable and the child is asymptomatic because the problem can resolve spontaneously. Antibiotic prophylaxis is recommended. Ureteroceles are more common in girls, and a prolapsed ureterocele can cause obstruction of a (commonly associated) duplex system upper pole and cause VUJ obstruction. Most ureteroceles respond to simple puncture carried out in the neonatal period.

Urethral valves

A posterior urethral valve (PUV) is a congenital membrane obstructing or partially obstructing the posterior urethra. PUV should be suspected in a male fetus with a thick-walled bladder and bilateral dilatation of the upper urinary tract. In the newborn, there can be symptoms of severe metabolic disorders related to renal failure, respiratory problems (spontaneous pneumothorax or pneumomediastinum) and urinary tract infections (UTIs). Ultrasound scan of the urinary tract is the first-line investigation. If confirmed it is essential to adequately drain the bladder by inserting either a transurethral or a suprapubic catheter. Surgical incision of the valve is performed endoscopically within the first week of life.

Vesico-ureteric reflux

This is diagnosed with micturating cystourogram (MCUG) done either because of follow-up of an abnormal antenatal renal scan or because of a diagnosis of UTI. Unfortunately no other test is available to make this diagnosis in infancy, although progress can be followed with isotope studies once the child is continent. These babies must remain on trimethoprim prophylaxis against infection. A DMSA scan should be done to look for renal scars. Most cases do not require re-implantation of the ureters, but those with breakthrough infections or deteriorating renal function should be considered for surgery. The natural history of reflux diagnosed in the neonatal period is that it will resolve, but prophylaxis needs to be continued until it does.

Potter's syndrome (renal agenesis plus pulmonary hypoplasia)

There is oligohydramnios during pregnancy and the fetal membranes show amnion nodosum. The baby has a squashed face, hypertelorism, epicanthic folds, micrognathia, low-set ears and large, floppy hands and feet. This condition presents at birth with severe dyspnoea due to pulmonary hypoplasia and the infants usually die within 2–3 hours. In those in whom the pulmonary abnormality is less severe, survival for 24–48 hours may occur. At postmortem the infants are anephric or have grossly abnormal, vestigial or multicystic kidneys, and the lung volume is usually less than 25% of normal.

Renal vascular thrombosis

Renal arterial thrombosis is rare except as a complication of UACs. RVT classically presents with haematuria, loin mass and thrombocytopenia, sometimes in association with maternal diabetes, dehydration, asphyxia or congenital heart disease. In about 50% of cases the thrombus extends into the inferior vena cava. Cases with inherited disorders resulting in a thrombotic tendency are being increasingly recognized, for example factor V Leiden deficiency (Lau *et al.* 2007). RVT is the most common non-catheter-related thrombosis in infancy. There is no evidence that anything other than conventional intensive care has any influence on outcome; treatment with low molecular weight heparin can be considered and may prevent spread of the thrombus to the other renal vein. The affected kidney usually becomes atrophic. The outcome in unilateral disease is good, but up to half of the babies with bilateral renal vein thrombi die. Hypertension occurs in 20% (Lau *et al.* 2007) and permanent renal failure is rare (3% according to Lau *et al.*), hence babies who have experienced RVT must be followed up.

Renal masses

Loin masses in the neonate due to kidney enlargement are usually caused by:

1. hydronephrosis ± outflow obstruction of any type;
2. cystic dysplasia/multicystic disease;
3. polycystic disease – infant or adult variety;
4. RVT (see above);
5. tumours;
6. adrenal haemorrhage or tumour.

Investigations should include:

1. electrolytes, urea and creatinine, urinary electrolytes;
2. blood pressure;
3. urine for chemistry, cytology, culture;
4. renal ultrasound;
5. DTPA, MAG-3, isotope scans;
6. intravenous urogram (IVU);
7. micturating cystogram;
8. renal arteriography and aortography.

According to the diagnosis, appropriate therapy can be instituted. Hydronephrosis will usually require surgical correction. With cystic dysplasia, prognosis depends on the amount of normal renal tissue present. Unilateral disease or local cysts may be surgically treatable.

Polycystic disease

The classification of polycystic disease is complex (Hildebrandt 1999). Both autosomal dominant and autosomal recessive forms may present in the neonatal period with marked kidney enlargement. The prognosis for the autosomal recessive form is poor. The autosomal dominant form, often associated with hepatic cysts and congenital hepatic fibrosis, has a reasonably good prognosis. Ultrasound cannot distinguish between the two.

Multicystic dysplastic kidneys

These are quite commonly detected antenatally. Postnatal management should include MCUG because 20% have reflux into the other kidney, which becomes a single kidney once the multicystic one shrivels up (half have involuted by 5 and two-thirds by 10 years of age). There is controversy about whether or not they should be surgically removed: our current practice is to remove those multicystic kidneys which fail to involute.

Nephrocalcinosis

Nephrocalcinosis is commonly diagnosed in VLBW babies on diuretics, particularly those who have received total parenteral nutrition. The crystals are calcium oxalate or calcium urate and eventually resolve. In term babies nephrocalcinosis can occur secondary to renal tubular acidosis or primary oxalosis.

Renal tubular acidosis

This is defined as a metabolic acidosis resulting from the inability of the kidney to excrete hydrogen ions or to reabsorb bicarbonate. There is an inappropriately high urinary pH given the systemic acidosis. Renal tubular acidosis can occur as a genetic defect, secondary to nephrocalcinosis, or be due to drugs. Treatment is with sodium bicarbonate orally.

■ Genitourinary tract anomalies

Hypospadias

Hypospadias is common, affecting 1:300 male births. It consists of an abnormally placed urethral meatus, chordee of the penis, and a foreskin which, instead of being wrapped around the penis, is present only on the dorsal side. In the majority, the hypospadias is an isolated problem that necessitates appropriate referral and requires surgical reconstruction between 1 and 2 years of age. It is essential to advise parents not to circumcise the baby as the foreskin tissue may be required for the surgical correction.

Undescended testicle

Testicular descent typically occurs from the fifth to the seventh months of gestation. In term boys, both testicles are usually descended at birth, but the incidence of undescended testis is about 1:50 to 1:100 births. Postnatally, descent can occur spontaneously but is rare after the first few months of life. Undescended testicles can be of two types: true undescended testicles, which lie along the original line of descent but which have not reached the scrotum, and ectopic testes, which have deviated from the normal line of descent. A retractile testis (which is normal) is often incorrectly diagnosed as an undescended testis. In most cases of true undescended testicle, a definitive operation to bring the testicle down into the scrotum is performed around 1 year of age.

Hydroceles

Congenital hydrocele results from an incomplete obliteration of the patent processus vaginalis. Fluid can enter and stay in the processus vaginalis, forming a hydrocele. Hydroceles usually present with a scrotal swelling which transilluminates. It is also possible to 'get above' a hydrocele – both features distinguishing it from a hernia. Surgical ligation of the processus vaginalis should be carried out if the hydrocele remains after 3 years, becomes symptomatic (very rare), or cannot be differentiated from a hernia.

Neonatal testicular torsion

Neonatal or intra-uterine torsion of the testicle usually presents as a swollen testicle. The scrotum is often red, oedematous, and may be tender on examination. The established treatment is early surgical exploration and fixation of the contralateral testis. However, if the scrotum has been red and oedematous from birth, the testicle is always necrotic and it is now common practice to treat the boy with analgesia and antibiotics alone in the immediate neonatal period. However, we believe it is prudent to perform surgical fixation of the contralateral testis before discharge.

Epispadias and bladder exstrophy

These are a spectrum of congenital malformations in which there is an abnormal development of the cloacal membrane and consequently incomplete midline fusion of the cloacal structures.

- In epispadias the bladder is covered and the urethra opens onto the dorsal surface of the penis. In girls the urethra is patulous and the clitoris has not fused in the midline. Surgical reconstruction is required.
- In bladder exstrophy, the bladder opens onto the abdominal wall, there is marked separation of the pubic bones and epispadias of the genitalia. Treatment requires closure of the bladder and pubic ring within the first few days of life, followed by a staged approach to correct the epispadias and reconstruct the bladder neck.
- Cloacal exstrophy is the most severe form – the bowel opens in the midline with two hemibladders lateral to it. There is also epispadias of the genitalia and pubic bone separation.

■ References

Hildebrandt, F (1999) Renal cystic disease. *Current Opinion in Pediatrics*, **11**: 141–51.

Lau, KK, Stoffman, JM, Williams, S, *et al.* (2007) Neonatal renal vein thrombosis: review of the English Language literature between 1992–2006. *Pediatrics*, **120**: e1278–84.

Smeulders, N, Wilcox, D (2012) Urology. In Rennie, JM (ed.) *Rennie & Roberton's Textbook of Neonatology*, 5th edition. Edinburgh: Elsevier, pp. 939–52.

■ Further reading

Dhillon, HK (1999) Antenatally diagnosed hydronephrosis. In Stringer, MD, Oldham, KT, Mouriquand, PDE (eds) *Pediatric Surgery and Urology: Long-Term Outcomes.* London: Saunders, pp. 479–86.

Modi, N (2012) Renal function, fluid and electrolyte balance and neonatal renal disease. In Rennie, JM (ed.) *Rennie & Roberton's Textbook of Neonatology*, 5th edition. Edinburgh: Elsevier, pp. 927–38.

25
Eye disorders

- The incidence of retinopathy of prematurity (ROP) can be minimized by meticulous attention to oxygen therapy, always keeping the PaO_2 less than 10 kPa and avoiding wide swings.
- ROP develops over a relatively narrow range of maturity, with 75% of the cases developing between 30 and 36 weeks of gestation.
- ROP developing after 36 weeks of gestation is unlikely to need treatment.
- All babies <32 weeks' gestation and <1.5 kg must have regular (1–2 weekly) ophthalmological assessment beginning at 32 weeks postconceptional age or 6 weeks actual age (whichever is the sooner), in order to identify those with threshold ROP who require treatment.
- Vision is impaired in 30% of babies who require treatment for ROP.
- Not all visual loss in ex-preterm survivors is due to ROP; some is due to cortical damage.

Retinopathy of prematurity

This disorder, formerly called retrolental fibroplasia, unique to the neonate, makes oxygen therapy difficult in babies with lung disease. It is a disease of prematurity with a very low incidence in babies over 32 weeks' gestation and 1500 g birth weight. Many regions have reported a reduction in incidence, for example in the Lothian region of Scotland the percentage of babies requiring treatment fell between 1990 and 2004 in spite of increased survival (Dhaliwal *et al.* 2008) (Table 25.1). The mildest stages of ROP, which do not progress to permanent damage, are best regarded as a normal variant in babies <28 weeks' gestation. As more extremely low birth weight babies survive, this type of ROP is more commonly seen.

A baby is at risk from ROP until he passes the postmenstrual age of about 32–34 weeks. Thus a 24-week gestation baby is at risk for 8–10 weeks after birth, whereas a 32-week baby is probably at risk for only a few days.

Classification of retinopathy of prematurity

This is done in three ways (CCRP 1987):

1. A classification of the acute stage. This is based on the fact that ROP is a disease of abnormal vascularization of the retina (Table 25.2). The eye is said to show plus disease if there is dilatation and/or tortuosity of the retinal vessels.
2. A description of the region of the retina affected (Fig. 25.1). Zone 1 is twice the distance from the disc to the macula. Zone 2 extends beyond this to the equator

Table 25.1 Incidence of retinopathy of prematurity (ROP) in Lothian 2000–2004

Birth weight (g)	Number screened	No ROP (%)	Stage 1, 2 ROP (%)	Stage 3 Untreated (%)	Stage 3 treated (%)
<750	48	18 (38)	7 (15)	11 (23)	12 (25)
750–999	82	51 (61)	16 (19)	6 (7)	10 (12)
1000–1249	118	106 (90)	7 (6)	3 (3)	2 (2)
1250–1499	117	116 (99)	0 (0)	1 (1)	0 (0)

Source: Dhaliwal et al. (2008)

Table 25.2 Classification of acute retinopathy of prematurity

Stage	Description
Stage 1	Demarcation line: a simple border or line seen at the edge of vessels dividing vascular from avascular retina
Stage 2	Ridge: the line structure of the previous stage has now acquired a volume and risen above the surface of the retina to become a ridge
Stage 3	Ridge with extraretinal fibrovascular proliferation: from the surface of the ridge, this extraretinal tissue may extend into the vitreous
Stage 4	Subtotal retinal detachment: forces developed from proliferating tissue in the vitreous or retina result in a traction type of retinal detachment. This is subdivided into: (a) detachment not involving the macula (b) subtotal retinal detachment involving the macula – resulting in poor vision
Stage 5	Total retinal detachment: a total funnel-shaped retinal detachment with very poor visual prognosis

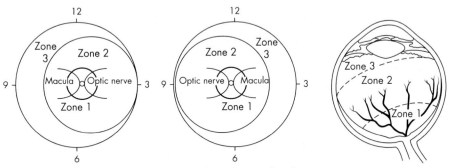

Fig. 25.1 Zones of the retina used for classifying retinopathy of prematurity in neonates
Source: CCRP 1987; Phelps 1998

of the eye, and zone 3 beyond the equator on the temporal side of the disc. The area involved can then be described by zone and by 'clock hour'.

3. A description of the regressed or cicatricial stage of the disease.

Documentation of the zone reached by the normal wave of vascularization – stage 0 – is useful to avoid stopping screening too soon.

More severe forms of ROP are associated with abnormalities of the posterior retinal and iris blood vessels termed plus disease. The posterior retinal blood vessels become dilated and tortuous, due to high levels of vascular endothelial growth factor (VEGF) in the vitreous. The presence of plus disease is very significant in the classification and treatment of ROP.

Aetiology and pathogenesis

Early gestation and low birth weight remain the strongest risk factors for the development of ROP. Of note, reduced postnatal growth velocity is an independent risk factor for the development of ROP. While it is well established that unrestricted oxygen greatly increases the risk of ROP, optimal oxygen levels have not been defined. In general, lower and more stable oxygen levels are thought to protect from ROP; however, this may be detrimental to other tissues and organs.

Premature birth interrupts normal retinal blood vessel development, with the physiological environment of the retina of a premature infant very different from that found *in utero*. Normal early retinal vessel development is driven by a 'physiological hypoxia', which is suppressed by oxygen therapy through reduced hypoxia-induced factor and VEGF. The overall result is reduced endothelial cell proliferation and migration and an inadequately vascularized retina at 6–10 weeks after birth. The peripheral, avascular retina continues to mature, becomes ischaemic and secretes high levels of tissue VEGF. This in turn results in abnormal angiogenesis.

Prevention

By far the most important component of this is strict monitoring of PaO_2. Transcutaneous PO_2 monitoring and oximetry are not adequate unless backed up by intermittent arterial sampling.

Diagnosis and screening

Guidelines for screening have been published and should be adhered to (RCPCH/RCOpth/BAPM 2008). All babies delivered at 32 weeks or less and/or <1501 g birth weight should be screened. The timing of first screen is dependent on gestational age (Table 25.3).

Table 25.3 Timing of first retinopathy of prematurity screen according to gestational age at birth

Gestational age	Age at first screen	
	Corrected gestational age	Postnatal age
22	30	8
23	30	7
24	30	6
25	30	5
26	30	4
27	31	4
28	32	4
29	33	4
30	34	4
31	35	4

Babies who are ≥32 weeks' gestational age at birth but <1501 g should be screened at 4–5 weeks postnatal age (day 28–35). Babies who qualify for screening must be re-examined by weekly screening if the vessels end in zone 1 or posterior zone 2, there is any plus or pre-plus disease, or there is any stage 3 disease in any zone. Other babies should be examined fortnightly until the criteria for termination have been reached. The eyes should be examined by an experienced ophthalmologist using indirect opthalmoscopy and after dilating the pupils with 0.5% cyclopentolate and 2.5% phenylephrine eye drops. An alternative combination is a preparation of tropicamide 0.2% and phenylephrine 1%.

Management

Timely treatment for ROP is effective at preventing severe visual impairment. Recent evidence has suggested that earlier treatment is more beneficial. The majority of treatment that is carried out now is laser coagulation. Treatment for ROP should be undertaken if any of the following indications are reached:

- zone 1, any ROP with plus disease;
- zone 1, stage 3 without plus disease;
- zone 2, stage 3 with plus disease.

Treatment for ROP should seriously be considered if the following indication is reached:

- zone 2, stage 2 with plus disease.

There is no specific evidence to guide the timing between reaching a grade of ROP that requires intervention and treatment for this; however, there are encouraging results of early treatment that takes place within 48 hours. Therefore babies with aggressive ROP should be treated as soon as possible and within 48 hours. ROP requiring treatment should normally be treated within 48–72 hours. Transpupillary diode laser therapy is recommended as the first-line treatment for ROP. Treatment with near-confluent (0.5–1 burn width) laser burn spacing should be administered to the entire avascular retina. The unavailability of diode laser equipment or the inability to transfer to another centre should not prevent or delay the treatment of ROP. In these situations, treatment with cryotherapy or argon laser may be completed by an ophthalmologist experienced in these techniques.

Prognosis

With meticulous control of oxygen therapy, effective screening and treatment, blindness from ROP should now steadily decline in incidence. However, survivors of both regressed and treated ROP have an increased incidence of myopia and squint and should be carefully followed up. Not all visual problems at follow-up are due to ophthalmic problems; there is a significant incidence of cortical visual problems, too. In the original EPIcure study of all births less than 26 weeks' gestation in the UK in 1995, 17% of survivors had visual impairment at 2.5 years, with 1.8% blind (Wood and Marlow 1999). Almost 20% of the whole cohort had required treatment for ROP.

▓ Buphthalmos (neonatal glaucoma)

The baby presents with irritability (due to pain), photophobia and tearing from the eye which has an acute increase in intraocular pressure. The eye has an enlarged corneal diameter (>11 mm) and is injected. This is an ophthalmic emergency if blindness is to be avoided.

■ Cataract

If a cataract is seen in the neonatal period, urgent ophthalmic referral is indicated, particularly for bilateral disease, to prevent amblyopia developing. Cataract is the most common cause of preventable childhood blindness. Many cases are genetic and further investigation is indicated.

■ Conjunctivitis

See pp. 189–190.

■ Strabismus

All babies have a tendency to transient alternating convergent strabismus. This is of no significance and the eyes gradually straighten by 3–6 months of age. Unless the eye position is constantly abnormal, observation is appropriate until the baby is 4 months old. A fixed strabismus may occur following birth trauma (usually a transient VIth nerve paralysis), or may be associated with retinoblastoma. In the latter case early diagnosis can be life-saving.

■ References

CCRP (Committee for the Classification of Retinopathy of Prematurity) (1987) The classification of retinal detachment. *Archives of Ophthalmology*, **105**: 906–16.

Dhaliwal, C, Fleck, B, Wright, E, *et al.* (2008) Incidence of retinopathy of prematurity in Lothian, Scotland, from 1990–2004. *Archives of Disease in Childhood*, **93**: F422–6.

Phelps, D (1998) Using new information in retinopathy of prematurity. In Hansen, TN, McIntosh, N (eds) *Current Topics in Neonatology 3*. London: WB Saunders, pp. 174–90.

RCPCH/RCOpth/BAPM (2008) Guideline for the Screening and Treatment of Retinopathy of Prematurity (ROP). Available from www.rcpch. ac.uk/.

Wood, N, Marlow, N (1999) Developmental and neurological disability in extremely preterm children at two and a half years. Proceedings of the Royal College of Paediatrics and Child Health Spring Meeting, *Archives of Disease in Childhood*, Suppl 1. V.

■ Further reading

American Academy of Pediatrics and American College of Obstetrics and Gynaecology (1997) *Guidelines for Perinatal Care*, 4th edition. Washington, DC: Library of Congress, pp. 188–92.

Fleck, B (2012) Neonatal ophthalmology. In Rennie, JM (ed.) *Rennie & Roberton's Textbook of Neonatology*, 5th edition. Edinburgh: Elsevier, pp. 837–48.

Phelps, D (1981) Vision loss due to retinopathy of prematurity. *Lancet*, **i**: 606.

26

Skin disorders

Key points

- Rashes and spots are common in the newborn period. Most of these are benign, requiring only parental reassurance.
- Early diagnosis of more severe and significant lesions is essential and requires experience as most diagnoses are made clinically.
- Birth marks are common, and many do not need intervention, but an understanding of possible underlying and associated conditions is essential.
- Vascular lesions are divided into haemangiomas, which are self-limiting and rarely need intervention, and vascular malformations, which may be capillary, venous, arterial or mixed.

One of the numerous roles of the neonatal resident is to identify the myriad skin presentations in the newborn period and, crucially, to differentiate the many benign skin conditions from more significant pathology, particularly infections which often require prompt identification and treatment (Table 26.1). This skill can only be acquired by exposure to hundreds of normal babies and the opportunity to learn from the experience of more senior clinicians. This chapter aims to be a guide to some of the more common and more significant skin presentations and pathologies.

Table 26.1 Infectious causes of skin lesions

Infection	Presentation	Treatment
Varicella (see p. 211)	Widespread vesicular or pustular disorder	Aciclovir IV
Herpes simplex (see p. 207)	Groups of blisters initially localized to the presenting part (often at site of scalp electrode), onset typically 4–8 days	Aciclovir IV
Superficial bacterial infections (see pp. 189–190) (Staphylococcus/ Escherichia coli)	Often originates in umbilical stump, lesions first appear as vesicles or pustules which rupture to form fast-spreading erosions	Flucloxacillin and an aminoglycoside IV
Localized Candida (see pp. 188–189)	Presents as napkin dermatitis with characteristic satellite lesions. Oral Candida presents as white plaques on the buccal mucosa and tongue	Topical antifungals, e.g. nystatin orally and cream to nappy area
Scabies	Presents from second week with widespread papules, nodules, vesicles and pustules, ofte n with facial and scalp involvement	Permethrin cream

IV, intravenous.

■ Common benign neonatal skin disorders

Erythema toxicum

This is a common self-limiting, benign, idiopathic condition which affects about two-thirds of term neonates. It appears as poorly demarcated erythematous macules, often with a raised central pale papule or less commonly pustule (an appearance originally described as a 'dewdrop on a rose petal'). Lesions can occur anywhere except the palms and soles. Most babies have a few spots, although it can be very florid in some cases. It normally appears between 24 and 48 hours, but may occur at any time from birth to 14 days. The cause is unknown, but pustular fluid contains high numbers of eosinophils and there is often a peripheral eosinophilia. Parental reassurance is the only management required.

Benign pustular dermatosis

This condition, formerly termed pustular melanosis, is often mistaken for infective pustules. In contrast to erythema toxicum, the rash is often present at birth, or in the first few hours after birth. The rash consists of pustules or blisters predominantly on the trunk and buttocks which burst, leaving an area of scaly skin which in dark skinned individuals has a transient post-inflammatory hyperpigmentation. The term dermatosis is better, because the depth of pigmentation (melanosis) varies according to skin colour. The pustules last for a day or two, but the pigmented freckle-like spots may persist longer, and there can be lesions of different ages, including established areas of flaky hyperpigmentation at birth.

The aetiology is unknown; pustular fluid contains neutrophils but fluid culture is sterile. If a confident diagnosis can be made – and this is easy if the typical hyperpigmented and scaly areas co-exist with pustules – parents should be reassured. Only if there are genuine concerns that pustules may be infective in origin should they be managed accordingly.

Milia

Milia, or miliaria, is a common skin condition affecting up to 50% of babies. Babies present with firm pearly-white 1–2 mm papules, particularly on the face. They usually disappear by 4 weeks of age. They are retention cysts of the pilosebaceous follicles.

Neonatal erythematous and scaly disorders

Seborrhoeic dermatitis (cradle cap)

This presents as a red erythema with a greasy yellow scale particularly affecting the scalp but sometimes more widespread. It is usually asymptomatic and self-limiting after the early months of life. Although the cause is unknown, it usually responds to weak steroids and anti-fungal agents.

Psoriasis

Napkin psoriasis is a severe form of the disorder which presents in the neonatal period with a well-demarcated, bright-red napkin rash with small scaly patches beyond the margins. This then disseminates with extensive psoriatic lesions to the scalp and face and trunk. The condition is usually self-limiting, resolving within a few weeks.

Disorders of keratin (ichthyoses)

The severe conditions collodion baby harlequin ichthyosis present at birth with generalized erythroderma and a shiny tight membrane with or without deep fissuring. The membrane peels off in days or weeks to leave various forms of ichthyosis, although occasionally the membrane peels off to leave normal skin. Neonatal problems include temperature instability, excessive fluid loss and secondary infection. The child should be barrier nursed in high humidity with intensive, supportive management.

Neonatal bullous skin disorders

Epidermolysis bullosa

This disorder, characterized by traumatic blistering of the skin, can be subdivided into multiple types dependent on the inheritance and cleavage plane of the blister. Severe forms present with extensive neonatal blistering, which may be first noticed when drying the baby after birth. In such cases immediate advice on skin management should be sought from the regional specialist centre. Pain control with Oramorph is generally required and vitamin K should be given orally (not intramuscularly); intravenous lines should be avoided if possible. Specialist dressings should be applied as advised by the regional specialist team.

Neonatal pemphigus

Mothers with pemphigus vulgaris or pemphigus foliaceus may transfer immunoglobulin G antibodies transplacentally, resulting in lesions which range from tense or flaccid bullae to large erosions. The condition is self-limiting and resolves with clearance of maternal antibodies.

■ Other miscellaneous neonatal skin conditions

Subcutaneous fat necrosis

Necrosis of subcutaneous fat is probably induced by ischaemia. It occurs only in full-term infants either with a history of a difficult labour and delivery or more recently as a complication of therapeutic hypothermia. The lesions appear 2–3 weeks after birth as tender, firm nodules, particularly on the buttocks, shoulders, upper back, proximal limbs and cheeks. They are usually self-limiting, resolving within a few months. Occasionally they become fluctuant, ulcerate or calcify. Calcified lesions may be associated with hypercalcaemia and occasionally nephrocalcinosis.

Neonatal lupus erythematosus

This results from transplacental passage of maternal anti-Ro or anti-La antibodies, which may also result in congenital heart block. The condition results in a photosensitive rash presenting as mauve erythema on the face, with a clear lower border on the cheeks, extending up around the eyes into the hairline. The condition is self-limiting, resolving after a few months, when the antibodies disappear.

Aplasia cutis

Aplasia cutis is a congenital absence of skin, usually localized but sometimes occurring as multiple lesions in a widespread distribution. The most common form presents as single or multiple round or oval lesions, with an intact but atrophic surface on the scalp or side of the face. Surgical repair is not usually indicated if the defect is small; the lesions resolve with gradual epithelialization and scar formation over a few weeks. Specialist advice should be sought, however, because of the risk of infection and bleeding, particularly if the lesion overlies a major cerebral venous sinus. In all scalp lesions, imaging of the skull should be performed, as there is often an underlying skull defect. Scalp aplasia cutis congenita is associated with a number of syndromes including trisomy 13, Adams–Oliver and Johanson–Blizzard syndrome.

Dermoid cysts

These are congenital cysts occurring along embryonic fusion lines as asymptomatic, non-compressible nodules. They occur most commonly over the anterior fontanelle, in the midline of the upper nose or at the lateral end of the eyebrow. Careful examination may reveal a punctum on the surface due to a dermal sinus. Prior to consideration of surgical excision for cosmetic reasons, imaging is required as many have underlying connections to the central nervous system (CNS).

■ Birthmarks and vascular disorders

Pigmented birthmarks

- Congenital melanocytic naevi are present at birth, appearing as raised verrucous or lobulated brown/black lesions with an irregular border and often with dark hairs. They vary in size from small to giant lesions (which carry approximately a 5% lifetime risk of malignancy). Lesions occurring over the spine may be associated with meningeal melanocytosis (especially if affecting the upper part of the spine), or with spinal dysraphism and tethered cord.
- Mongolian spots are flat, blue/grey lesions with poorly defined margins that occur predominantly on the lumbosacral area. They are common in Asian and black infants but may also occur in white infants, particularly those of Mediterranean origin. They usually fade considerably by puberty.
- Other important abnormalities of pigmentation include café au lait spots and hypopigmented macules, which may be part of a neurocutaneous disorder such as neurofibromatosis or tuberose sclerosis.

Vascular birthmarks

These can be divided into haemangiomas (proliferative vascular overgrowth) and vascular malformations (fixed collections of dilated abnormal vessels).

Haemangiomas

Infantile haemangiomas usually present in the first weeks of life and grow gradually into a typical lobulated 'strawberry naevus'. They are the most common vascular tumour encountered in infants, and may continue to grow for up to a year. They are more common in premature infants, and in girls. Deeper haemangiomas may occur alone or beneath a superficial lesion. The overlying skin is normal or bluish in colour. Resolution occurs by softening and shrinkage. Failure of complete resolution suggests the lesion to be a vascular malformation rather than a haemangioma. Most infantile haemangiomas do not require intervention and parents should be reassured. Complications of haemangiomas that may require treatment include:

- ulceration, which can be associated with significant bleeding and secondary infection;
- encroachment on vital structures such as closing an eye (risking ambylopia), the mouth (interfering with feeding) or the nose or airway (leading to respiratory difficulties).

Propranolol is now the drug of choice when treatment is required. The effect was a serendipitous discovery but the result is dramatic, although treatment may need to be continued for a year. Side effects are few. Failure to respond to propranolol, if started early, suggests an alternative diagnosis. In diffuse infantile haemangiomatosis there are multiple widespread small haemangiomas. In the systemic form, lesions may occur in many organs, particularly the liver, gastrointestinal tract, lungs and CNS. Patients with multiple cutaneous haemangiomas should have an ultrasound to exclude hepatic involvement, and be referred for specialist investigation and management.

Haemangiomas, particularly segmental haemangiomas, can be a clue to an underlying diagnosis. Segmental facial haemangiomas occur in PHACE (posterior fossa brain malformation, haemangioma, arterial abnormality, coarctation of the aorta and eye abnormality) syndrome.

Vascular malformations

Vascular malformations are structural abnormalities present at birth which grow in proportion to the patient and do not spontaneously resolve. They can be divided into capillary, arterial, venous, lymphatic and mixed. Broadly speaking, vascular malformations can be divided into slow flow (capillary, venous or lymphatic) and fast flow (arteriovenous malformations and fistulae). Ultrasound is the most useful non-invasive investigation and, along with history and clinical examination, can identify the elements of most vascular malformations and separate them from haemangiomas. Large vascular malformations can be troublesome to treat and require specialist advice.

- Capillary malformation (port-wine stain or naevus flammeus). This cutaneous vascular malformation is usually unilateral and occurs most commonly on the face. Treatment is with pulsed dye laser, best if started in the early months of life. Patients presenting with a capillary malformation in the ophthalmic (V1) and maxillary (V2) distributions of the trigeminal nerve should have early neurological and ophthalmological assessment to exclude Sturge–Weber syndrome, in which there is an associated vascular malformation of the ipsilateral meninges and cerebral cortex. An MRI scan may demonstrate the intracranial malformations in the first few months of life.
- Venous malformations usually have a bluish hue, and empty with pressure or when elevated.
- Lymphatic malformations (formerly called 'cystic hygromas' or 'lymphangiomas') are most common in the neck and axilla, where they can become huge and may be associated with hydrops fetalis during intra-uterine life.

▌ Further reading

Eichenfield, LF, Frieden, IJ, Esterly, NB (2008) *Neonatal Dermatology*, 2nd edition. Philadelphia: Elsevier Saunders.

Rogers, M (2012) Neonatal dermatology. In Rennie, JM (ed.) *Rennie & Roberton's Textbook of Neonatology*, 5th edition. Edinburgh: Elsevier, pp. 819–36.

27

Orthopaedic and bone disorders

Key points
- Neonatal fractures heal quickly and without residual deformity.
- Clinical screening for developmental dysplasia of the hip (DDH) misses many cases.
- Babies at risk for DDH (breech after 36 weeks' gestation or at delivery if earlier, positive family history, any abnormal clinical finding on examination of the hip) should have an ultrasound scan of the hips.
- All clinically abnormal hips should be referred for specialist orthopaedic opinion in the neonatal period.

Fractures

Skull

With modern standards of obstetric care, fractures of the skull are rarely seen. No treatment is required for a non-displaced linear fracture. Occasionally a depressed 'ping-pong' fracture may occur, especially if the baby for some reason has a thin skull vault – craniotabes. Although some surgeons recommend that all such fractures should be elevated, if the baby is neurologically normal, and there are no fragments of bone which could damage the cortex, no treatment is required and the vault bones should be allowed to grow and remodel.

Clavicle

This is commonly diagnosed when evaluating a baby with Erb's palsy. It may also present with a 'crack' heard during delivery, with limitation of arm movement from pain, or with swelling from angulation of the clavicle and callus formation. No treatment is usually needed; occasionally if the baby is in pain a figure-of-eight bandage can be applied. Healing is always rapid, without long-term deformity.

Humerus

This may be broken during extraction of the arm of a breech. It usually presents either with a 'crack' heard at delivery or with pseudoparalysis due to pain. The fracture is either a proximal epiphyseal fracture or is in the mid-shaft of the bone, where it may damage the radial nerve. Simple splinting, with either a large crepe bandage on the upper arm or firm but not tight bandaging of the arm to the baby's thorax, is all that is required. The fracture needs to be maintained in this way for only 2–3 weeks.

More commonly, fractures of the long bones and ribs are found in very low birth weight (VLBW) babies with osteopenia of prematurity. The fracture may result from handling, or from the baby trapping his arm between the tray and the wall of his incubator. The treatment is the same, plus aggressive management of osteopenia with appropriate nutritional support.

Femur

Delivery of the extended legs of a breech may be accompanied by a femur fracture, usually in the mid-shaft. If the diagnosis is not made then, the fracture usually presents with pseudoparalysis. Despite marked displacement and angulation on X-ray, reduction is not required and simple splinting with a bulky crepe/cotton wool bandage for 2–3 weeks is the only treatment needed. As with the humerus, a fracture of the femur should lead one to consider osteopenia, and at birth a fractured femur can be the first clue to bone disease or a myopathy – the baby's bones are thin because he has not moved very much *in utero*.

Cervical spine

A fracture dislocation of the cervical spine may occur during vaginal delivery of a breech with an extended head or during a difficult rotational forceps delivery. This usually results in severe damage to the cervical cord and produces a baby with a flaccid quadriplegia. If the cord is injured above the phrenic nerve, apnoea will result. Early exploration of the cervical spine is of no value. The long-term prognosis for such babies is very poor.

■ Dislocations

Apart from dislocation of the hip (see below), which is better termed developmental dysplasia of the hip (DDH), dislocations are rare. Congenital dislocation of the knee can occur and this is an orthopaedic emergency. The knee should be reduced and strapped.

■ Skeletal malformations

Limb malformations

Major reduction deformities of the limbs are rare. All such children should be referred early to an artificial limb centre with special interest and experience in the problems of limbless children.

Talipes calcaneovalgus

This usually requires no treatment other than gentle manipulations by the mother putting her baby's foot into the plantigrade position.

Talipes equinovarus

This needs treatment if the foot cannot be moved into the plantigrade position. Combined physiotherapy and orthopaedic assessment and appropriate management should be arranged. The best results are obtained with the Ponseti regimen. Furthermore, as some cases may be associated with a syndrome or neuromuscular problem, these should be examined for, and a hip ultrasound should be organized to exclude associated DDH.

Developmental dysplasia of the hip

This malformation may either be isolated or present in a child with other abnormalities. The incidence is 1:600 for females and 1:2500 for males. All neonatal residents must become skilled in the examination techniques used to exclude DDH in the neonatal period (Fig. 27.1).

Irrespective of the clinical findings, an ultrasound examination of the hips should be performed if the following are present:

1. A history of a first-degree family relative with hip problems that started when they were a baby or young child and needed treatment with a splint, harness or operation.
2. Breech presentation at or after 36 completed weeks of pregnancy (irrespective of presentation at delivery or mode of delivery), or at delivery if this is earlier than 36 weeks.

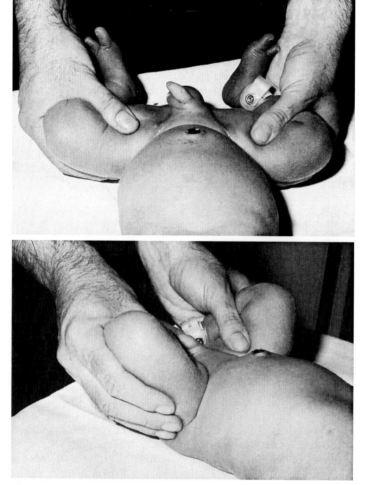

Fig. 27.1 Ortolani and Barlow manoeuvre

In the case of a multiple birth, if any of the babies falls into either of these categories, all babies in this pregnancy should have an ultrasound examination. There is some evidence of correlation with DDH with other conditions, including congenital talipes calcaneovalgus, metatarsus adductus, torticollis, oligohydramnios and a high female birth weight, but the NHS Newborn and Infant Physical Examination Programme (see Web link) does not mandate ultrasound examination of the hips in these groups. Once an abnormal hip has been identified, the baby should be referred for specialist orthopaedic opinion.

Short-limbed dwarfism

A large number of syndromes with short-limbed dwarfism are now recognized. In many of these the rib growth is also compromised, resulting in pulmonary hypoplasia, severe early respiratory distress and often death. The features of some of these conditions are given in Table 27.1.

Osteopenia of prematurity (neonatal rickets)

This condition occurs in VLBW survivors of neonatal intensive care. It is primarily a marker of the fact that it is difficult to get enough calcium and phosphorus into the diet of rapidly growing babies who weigh less than 1.5 kg at birth. It is not due to vitamin D deficiency, so the original name of rickets of prematurity is, strictly speaking, inappropriate.

Clinical features are rare. The disease usually presents radiologically with rachitic cupping visible in the ribs or at the wrists and knees, and is not usually found until 5–6 weeks of age. In severe cases there may be pathological fractures of the ribs, particularly in babies with severe persisting chronic lung disease. The calcium is usually normal, but may occasionally be raised; the phosphorus is low at 1 mmol/L or less, and the alkaline phosphatase markedly raised, often to values >1000 U/L.

Table 27.1 Features of some skeletal dysplasias presenting at birth

Syndrome	Bony features	Outcome
Asphyxiating thoracic dystrophy (AR)	Short ribs +++	Usually lethal but can survive
Achondroplasia (AD)	Narrow chest	Good
Diastrophic dwarfism (AR)	Short tubular bones, head large	Good
Camptomelic dwarfism (AR)	Thick, short tubular bones especially first metacarpal	Good
Rhizomelic chondroplasia punctata (AR)	Short femora and humeri Epiphyseal punctate calcification. Large head	Usually lethal. Low IQ
Osteogenesis imperfecta (AR)	Multiple fractures, poorly mineralized bones	Usually lethal; survivors have multiple fractures
Osteogenesis imperfecta (AD)	Thin, fractures in early life	Multiple fractures in early life – usually wheelchair bound
Hypophosphatasia (AR)	Marked bony underossification	Severe form lethal
Thanatotrophic dwarfism (sporadic)	Large head. Very small chest	Lethal

AD, autosomal dominant; AR, autosomal recessive.

The disease is largely preventable if preterm formula is used, or neonates taking expressed breast milk are given 1 mmol/kg/24 h of phosphate and vitamin D 400 U/day. If osteopenia does develop, the baby should receive 2 mmol/kg/24 h of phosphate and a total of 1000 U of vitamin D/day. Full recovery always occurs. If hypocalcaemia develops at any stage it should be treated with oral supplements of calcium gluconate.

▪ Further reading

Bishop, N (2012) Metabolic bone disease. In Rennie, JM (ed.) *Rennie & Roberton's Textbook of Neonatology*, 5th edition. Edinburgh: Elsevier, pp. 920–6.

Dare, CJ, Clarke, NMP (2012) Orthopaedic problems in the neonate. In Rennie, JM (ed.) *Rennie & Roberton's Textbook of Neonatology*, 5th edition. Edinburgh: Elsevier, pp. 967–88.

Faix, RG, Donn, SM (1983) Immediate management of the traumatised infant. *Clinics in Perinatology*, **10**: 487–506.

Graf, R (1984) Classification of hip joint dysplasias by means of ultrasonography. *Archives of Orthopaedic and Trauma Surgery*, **102**: 248–55.

Jones, DA (1998) *Hip Screening in the Newborn: A Practical Guide*. Oxford: Butterworth-Heinemann.

▪ Web link

www.newbornphysical.screening.nhs.uk

28

Neonatal abstinence syndrome

Maternal illicit drug use remains common – around 14% of women aged 16–34 years in England and Wales have used cannabis in a year, 4.5% cocaine, 3% ecstasy and 2% amphetamines. Substance abuse during pregnancy has effects on the health of the mother, the pregnancy, the fetus and the newborn infant. In addition there are associations between drug addiction, alcohol misuse, HIV, hepatitis B/C infection, unemployment/poverty, squalid accommodation, parental imprisonment and social isolation, all of which present a threat to babies cared for by these chaotic families.

A wide spectrum of drugs taken by women can induce abstinence syndrome in their babies (Table 28.1).

■ Maternal opiate abuse

Of babies born to opiate-using mothers, 60–90% develop withdrawal, usually in the first 24 hours. During pregnancy the aim is to reduce fetal exposure to fluctuating levels, and in general this means replacing heroin with methadone. Babies born to drug-abusing mothers are often preterm and small-for-dates, but are protected against respiratory distress syndrome (RDS) because many of these drugs mature

Table 28.1 Drugs associated with a neonatal withdrawal syndrome

Drug		Time of onset of withdrawal
Opiates	Heroin	0–96 h (peak 12–24 h)
	Methadone	12 to >72 h (peak 24–48 h); can be up to 2 weeks
	Codeine	<24 h
	Dihydrocodeine	<48 h
	Pentazocine	<24 h
Barbiturates	Short acting	<24 h
	Longer acting	>7 days
Benzodiazepines	Diazepam	2–6 h
	Chlordiazepoxide	3 weeks
Antidepressants	Tricyclics	0–72 h
	SSRI/SNRI	0–72 h
Alcohol		<24 h

SNRI, Serotonin–norepinephrine reuptake inhibitor; SSRI, Selective serotonin reuptake inhibitor.

Table 28.2 Signs of opiate withdrawal

Jitteriness, irritability, shrill cry
Hyperactivity, poor sleeping, wakefulness
Excessive sucking, hyperphagia
Seizures
Diarrhoea, vomiting, reflux
Snuffles, sneezing, salivation
Tachypnoea
Yawning, hiccoughs
Sweating, fever

the surfactant synthesizing enzymes. The clinical features of those who do develop symptoms are summarized in Table 28.2. The typical baby is intensely irritable and miserable with jitteriness, poor sleeping, crying, snuffles and feeding problems. These babies frantically suck at their hands, and are excessively alert and agitated. If their milk intake is not controlled they will exhibit hyperphagia, often taking in large volumes of more than 300 mL/kg/day. In spite of all the sucking they are not good at coordinating swallowing, and vomiting and diarrhoea are frequent. If the drug use is concealed, urine or hair can be analysed to make the diagnosis.

An important part of the management of these babies is good nursing care, swaddling, a quiet environment and small, frequent feeds. Several scoring systems have been devised, and one such chart is reproduced as Fig. 28.1. At any time the baby may score 0 or 1 for each item, with a maximum total score of 10. Babies who score more than 6 on two occasions more than 2–4 hours apart should be treated. We use oral morphine, which prevents seizures. The dose of oral morphine is 0.5 mg/kg/dose given four times a day, and it can be increased to 0.75 mg/kg/dose. Wean by 0.05 mg/dose every 2–3 days.

Cocaine

Maternal abuse of this drug causes major problems to the fetus, largely because of its vasocontrictor and hypertensive effects. These damage tissues by ischaemia and vascular disruption, and include fetal cerebral infarction or haemorrhage, bowel atresia, limb reduction defects and renal tract dilatation. In addition, as with opiates, these babies may be born prematurely and small for gestational age, and have a reduced incidence of RDS. More specifically, abruptio placenta occurs in a high proportion of pregnancies (Jones 1991). Exposure *in utero* to cocaine may lead to fetal cerebral infarction or intracranial haemorrhage (McGlone *et al.* 2009) and it is our practice to undertake a cranial ultrasound in these babies.

Cannabis/marijuana

The extensive literature on this subject has been reviewed by Day and Richardson (1991). If maternal cannabis use has any deleterious effects on the fetus or on the neonate, they are small.

Alcohol

Although binge drinkers are likely to produce babies with fetal alcohol syndrome or abstinence syndrome, a study from Scotland among women without associated

DRUG WITHDRAWAL CHART

Score 1 if item present, 0 if absent

NAME

HOSPITAL NUMBER

DATE OF BIRTH

1	Irritability with scratching or excessive wakefulness							
2	High-pitched cry							
3	Tremors							
4	Hypertonicity							
5	Convulsions							
6	Hyperthermia >38°C or tachypnoea >60							
7	Vomiting or diarrhoea							
8	Yawning or hiccoughs							
9	Salivation or stuffy nose or sneezing							
10	Sweating or dehydration							
	TOTAL SCORE							
	Time							
	Date							

Fig. 28.1 Drug withdrawal chart. After Rivers (1999)

problems such as malnutrition and drug abuse showed no ill effects from social alcohol consumption during pregnancy (Forrest *et al.* 1991).

Selective serotonin reuptake inhibitors/serotonin–norepinephrine reuptake inhibitors

Selective serotonin reuptake inhibitors (SSRIs) and serotonin–norepinephrine reuptake inhibitors (SNRIs) are widely used antidepressants known to cause symptoms in the newborn. Infants exposed to third-trimester SSRIs or SNRIs may suffer withdrawal, with predominantly central nervous system symptoms within 24 hours of birth which usually resolve spontaneously within a few days and are rarely serious. There is, however, an increased risk of developing persistent pulmonary hypertension of the newborn with paroxetine, sertraline or fluoxetine (Chambers *et al.* 2006).

■ References

Chambers, CD, Hernandez-Diaz, S, Van Marter, LJ, *et al.* (2006) Selective serotonin-reuptake inhibitors and risk of persistent pulmonary hypertension of the newborn. *New England Journal of Medicine*, **354**(6): 579–87.

Day, NL, Richardson, GA (1991) Perinatal marijuana use: epidemiology, methodologic issues and infant outcome. *Clinics in Perinatology*, **18**: 77–91.

Forrest, F, Florey, C du V, Taylor, D, *et al.* (1991) Reported social alcohol consumption during pregnancy and infants' development at 18 months. *British Medical Journal*, **303**: 22–6.

Jones, KL (1991) Developmental pathogenesis of defects associated with prenatal cocaine exposure: fetal vascular disruption. *Clinics in Perinatology*, **18**: 139–46.

McGlone, L, Mactier, H, Weaver, LT (2009) Drug misuse in pregnancy: losing sight of the baby? *Archives of Disease in Childhood*, **94**(9): 708–12.

Lawn, C, Aiton, N (2012) Infants of drug addicted mothers. In Rennie, JM (ed.) *Rennie & Roberton's Textbook of Neonatology*, 5th edition. Edinburgh: Elsevier, pp. 431–443.

■ Further reading

Bauer, CR (1999) Perinatal effects of drug exposure: neonatal effects. *Clinics in Perinatology*, **26**(1) 87–106.

Lawn, C, Aiton, N (2012) Infants of drug addicted mothers. In Rennie, JM (ed.) *Rennie & Roberton's Textbook of Neonatology*, 5th edition. Edinburgh: Elsevier, pp. 931–42.

United Kingdom New Developments, Trends and In-depth Information on Selected Issues: 2008 National Report (2007 data) to the EMCDDA. European Monitoring Centre for Drugs and Drug Addiction (2008), A

Neonatal abstinence syndrome

PART 5
Procedures and their complications

Procedures and iatrogenic complications

An iatrogenic disorder is any adverse condition that occurs as a result of a diagnostic procedure or therapeutic intervention that is not the natural consequence of the underlying disease. The most common iatrogenic events in neonates include nosocomial infections, catheter-related complications, unplanned extubations and intubation injury. To minimize the risk of nosocomial infections, good infection control and effective hand-washing policies are essential. Medication errors occur all too frequently in busy neonatal units (NNUs), but these can be minimized by safe drug prescribing and administration practices and the inclusion of an experienced neonatal clinical pharmacist in daily ward rounds to check drug and total parenteral nutrition prescription charts and to give advice about safe drug use. Other advances increasingly being used include electronic prescribing, smart infusion pumps and the use of standardized drug infusion concentrations.

■ Neonatal procedures

Implicit consent is considered acceptable for most routine, low-risk procedures performed in neonatology; however, explicit consent should be taken for complex or high-risk procedures. In an emergency, essential procedures should be performed, but clinical staff should inform parents as soon as possible after an emergency procedure has been performed.

■ Blood sampling and cannulation

Capillary heel pricks

Capillary blood samples from heel pricks are the most common performed procedure on the NNU. They have the advantage of conserving the veins in sick and preterm babies and can be used for most blood sampling requiring less than 1.5 mL with the exception of blood cultures. A specifically designed automated device should always be used.

1. Ensure that the foot is warm and well perfused.
2. Clean the heel with an antibacterial swab and allow to dry.
3. The preferred areas for capillary sampling are the outer aspects of the heel (Fig. 29.1). Do not sample from the end of the heel as there is an increased risk of osteomyelitis.

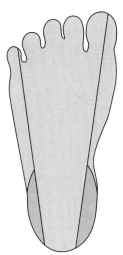

Fig. 29.1 The darker shaded areas indicate the lateral and medial aspects of the heel, which are suitable for heel pricks

4. Dorsiflex the foot, hold the automated device against the skin and activate. Apply gentle pressure and allow a drop of blood to form.
5. When samples have been collected, apply pressure with sterile cotton wool or gauze and dress with a plaster.

Venepuncture blood samples

For routine blood samples always use the smallest veins possible to preserve larger veins for cannulation or long-line insertion. If performing a venepuncture, always consider inserting a cannula if appropriate.

1. Clean skin with antiseptic or with an alcohol swab and allow to dry.
2. Occlude the vein proximally, using with gentle pressure
3. Insert the needle or butterfly, at an angle of 30–45° to the skin. Inserting the needle where the vein bifurcates prevents the vein from rolling away from the point of the needle.
4. Allow blood to drip into the specimen bottles from the needle.
5. After needle removal, apply gentle pressure with sterile gauze to prevent bruising/haematoma formation.

Peripheral venous cannulation

Veins in the back of the hand, forearm and foot should be used first. Confirm that the vessel empties following proximal occlusion and fills distally.

1. Flush the extension tubing with saline.
2. Clean skin with antiseptic and allow to dry.
3. Occlude the vessel proximally and apply gentle traction to the skin.
4. Insert the cannula, at an angle of 30–45° to the skin. As the needle pierces the vein, blood will appear in the hub of the cannula. Advance the cannula in a further 1–2 mm, partially withdraw the needle and advance the cannula forward into the vessel. Remove the needle. Collect blood samples if required by the drip method or by aspirating blood from the hub of the cannula with a needle and syringe.

5. Connect the extension tubing to the cannula and flush gently with saline.
6. Secure the cannula using Steri-strips and a transparent adhesive dressing to allow inspection of the cannula site (transparent dressings should be omitted in extremely preterm infants with gelatinous skin). Do not apply the dressing around the whole circumference of the limb.
7. Use a size-appropriate splint if the cannula is inserted over the elbow or ankle joint. Do not fix the limb too tightly to the splint.

Percutaneous central venous catheters

The veins most commonly used for peripheral inserted central venous catheters (CVCs) include those in the antecubital fossa, the axillary vein, the long and short saphenous veins and scalp veins.

1. Identify the vein. If an upper limb or scalp vein is being catheterized, measure the distance to the top of the sternum. If a lower limb vein is used, measure from the insertion up to the xiphisternum.
2. Scrub up and put on gown and sterile gloves. Using a full aseptic technique, clean the skin and drape.
3. Apply a sterile tourniquet (a piece of sterile gauze can be wrapped around the limb and secured tightly with artery forceps).
4. Flush the CVC and any extension with saline.
5. Insert the introducer needle into the vein. Release the tourniquet and thread the catheter into position with non-toothed fine forceps.
6. Remove the introducer needle. Secure the line with Steri-strips and apply pressure over the insertion site to secure haemostasis.
7. Neatly coil the external length catheter and fix to the skin with Steri-strips. Place a small square of gauze under the hub to protect the skin and apply a temporary sterile dressing to the insertion site.
8. Flush the line with 0.5 mL of contrast material and X-ray to confirm the position of the catheter tip.
   • For arm or scalp veins, the tip of the line should lie in the superior vena cava, outside of the cardiac silhouette.
   • For leg veins, the tip of the line should lie just below the diaphragm (T9–10).
9. Maintain a sterile field while the X-ray is taken.
10. Shorten the CVC if it is too long; never advance lines that are too short owing to the risk of infection. If the line has coiled back on itself or is kinked or misplaced, replace the line or pull it back to a short-line position (mid-humerus or femur) to use for a few days. However, CVCs inserted from the arm that are seen to go up into the jugular vein often 'flip' into the correct position if they are left with an infusion of 0.45 saline (0.5 mL/h) for a few hours. The line position must be reconfirmed before use with any other fluids.
11. Finally, apply a transparent adhesive dressing to cover the insertion site, catheter and hub of the extension set.

Complications of venous cannulation

1. Haematoma formation: apply gentle pressure to secure haemostasis before applying the dressing.
2. Thrombophlebitis may occur, resulting in redness and tenderness over the vein. It usually resolves with removal of the cannula.

3. Infection: *Staphylococcus epidermidis* (coagulase-negative *Staphylococcus*) is the most common cause of catheter-related infections. It is much more common with CVCs than with peripheral cannulae.
4. Extravasation injury is a common complication, presenting with pain and swelling that progresses to superficial blistering, ischaemia and tissue necrosis.

Management of extravasation injury

1. Extravasation injuries must be treated promptly in order to minimize tissue damage and subsequent scarring.
2. Stop the intravenous infusion immediately, but do not remove the cannula.
3. Remove the dressing and elevate the limb.
4. Try to aspirate fluid from the extravasated area via the cannula, using a 1mL syringe.
5. If there is blistering or discoloration of the skin or if the infusion contained astringents such as calcium, potassium, sodium bicarbonate, discuss with the plastic surgeons and consider using hyaluronidase.
   - After cleaning and infiltrating the area with 1% lidocaine, inject 500–1000 U of hyaluronidase subcutaneously (this can be done through the cannula if still in situ). Make two to four small stab incisions at the periphery of the injury.
   - Inject up to 500 mL of saline through a blunt cannula inserted through one of the puncture sites and flush the saline towards the other incisions to wash out the extravasated material.

Arterial puncture

The radial artery is most commonly used, providing the ulnar collateral circulation is intact. The posterior tibial and dorsalis pedis arteries can also be used. Avoid end arteries such as the brachial or femorals. If arterial blood is needed, e.g. for blood gas, consider whether an arterial line should be placed.

1. Before proceeding, perform the modified Allen's test: elevate the arm and occlude both the radial and ulnar arteries at the wrist. Release pressure on the ulnar artery and ensure colour returns to the hand in less than 10 seconds.
2. Identify the artery, using palpation and/or transillumination with a cold light.
3. Extend the wrist in a supine position, but do not overextend the wrist.
4. Clean skin with antiseptic and allow to dry.
5. Insert the needle at an angle of ~30°; blood should flow freely into the needle.
6. Blood can be collected with a syringe or by the drip method.
7. Remove the needle and apply compression with a sterile gauze swab for 5 minutes, or until haemostasis is achieved.

Peripheral arterial cannulation

Identify a suitable peripheral artery, usually the radial or posterior tibial arteries. Do not use the ulnar artery if the radial artery in that arm has been punctured or cannulated previously. Always perform the modified Allen's test before cannulating the radial artery (see above).

1. Clean the skin with antiseptic solution or alcohol. Using a no-touch technique, insert the cannula into the artery at an angle of 30–45°; as blood flushes into the chamber, advance the needle 1–2 mm and then slide the catheter forward into the artery.

2. Apply pressure proximal to the cannula and remove the needle. Attach a pre-flushed Luer-lock extension set and flush with saline.
3. Secure the cannula with Steri-strips or tape and dress with Tagaderm or similar transparent dressing.
4. Apply a splint to the limb and ensure that the tips of fingers or toes are easily visible and commence infusion with heparinized saline.
5. Remove the cannula without delay if it stops sampling or if there is loss of the arterial pressure wave-form. Do not flush the cannula to remove clots.

Complications of arterial puncture/cannulation

Major complications of peripheral arterial lines are reported to occur in less than 2% of babies. They include haemorrhage/haematoma formation, trauma to the vessel wall with aneurysm formation or to adjacent nerves, infection and thromboembolism/vasospasm and distal ischaemia.

Remove the arterial line immediately if distal perfusion is compromised, if the line stops sampling or fails to give a reliable blood pressure trace. Application of 1/4 of a cutaneous glyceryl trinitrate patch over the ipsilateral brachial or popliteal artery may improve the distal circulation.

■ Umbilical catheterization

Umbilical artery catheterization

An umbilical artery catheter (UAC) provides relatively long-term access to the circulation, but usually should not remain in place for longer than 10–14 days. Before you scrub up for the procedure, estimate how far to insert the line by one of the following methods:

- measuring the distance from the tip of the left shoulder to the base of the umbilicus + stump length (cm);
- using the following calculations to estimate insertion length:
  - infants >1500 g = (birth weight in kg × 3) + 9 cm + stump length (cm);
  - infants <1500 g = (birth weight in kg × 4) + 7 cm + stump length (cm).

Appropriate catheters are FG2.5 for babies <1000 g, FG3.5 for babies <1500 g and FG5.0 for those >1500 g.

1. Scrub up and put on gown and sterile gloves.
2. Using a full aseptic technique, clean the skin and drape.
3. Flush the catheter and three-way tap with saline.
4. Place a sterile cord tie loosely around the base of the stump. This can be tightened to control blood loss.
5. Use a scalpel to cut the umbilical cord horizontally, 1–2 cm above the skin margin.
6. Apply two artery forceps to the umbilical stump and roll the edges of the cord outwards.
7. Identify the two thick-walled arteries and a single thin-walled gaping umbilical vein.
8. One of the arteries should be gently dilated with a probe or an iris dilator and then introduce the catheter into the artery using non-toothed forceps to the calculated length. It should be easy to aspirate blood when the catheter is in the correct position.

9. The catheter should be secured using a suture that is carefully inserted into the umbilical stump. H-tape bridges or commercial devices can be attached to the abdominal wall to secure the line.
10. A chest and abdominal X-ray must be taken to confirm the position of the line. The tip of the UAC can be safely positioned above the diaphragm at a level between the sixth and ninth thoracic vertebrae. UACs can also be positioned between the third and fifth lumbar vertebrae but this is associated with more complications than the 'high' position.
11. If the line is too long it can be brought back to the correct position. Lines that are too short or misplaced should be removed and a new line inserted.
12. The UAC must be removed if perfusion problems persist or if it is no longer clinically required.

Umbilical venous catheterization

Before you scrub up for the procedure, estimate how far to insert the line by one of the following:

- measuring the distance from the base of the umbilicus to the xiphisternum plus the length of the umbilical stump;
- insertion length = (birth weight in kg × 2) + 5 cm + stump length (cm).

Use a larger catheter, e.g. FG 4.5–5.0. Double-lumen catheters are available and can be useful in babies likely to require multiple infusions.
1. Scrub up and put on gown and sterile gloves.
2. Using a full aseptic technique, clean the skin and drape.
3. Flush the catheter and three-way tap with saline.
4. Place the sterile cord tie loosely around the base of the stump. This can be tightened to control blood loss.
5. Use a scalpel to cut the umbilical cord horizontally, 1–2 cm above the skin margin.
6. Apply two artery forceps to the umbilical stum and roll the edges of the cord outwards.
7. Identify the two thick-walled arteries and a single thin-walled gaping umbilical vein.
8. The vein often does not require dilation. Insert the catheter the appropriate distance. Using a syringe, gently aspirate: blood will usually flow smoothly down the line if it is correctly sited.
9. Secure the umbilical vein catheter (UVC) with a suture and confirm the position of the UVC with a chest/abdominal X-ray with the tip of the umbilical catheter at the level of the ninth–tenth thoracic vertebra.
10. Remove the UVC if it is in the liver.

Complications of umbilical catheters

- Trauma during insertion creating a false passage, haematoma, peritoneal perforation, vessel perforation.
- Vasospasm is the most frequent complication seen with UACs, presenting with blanching or duskiness of the lower limbs or toes. The line should be removed if perfusion does not improve within 15 minutes.
- Air embolism.
- Arterial thromboembolism resulting in pallor or coldness of the lower limbs, gluteal skin necrosis, absent pulses, haematuria, systemic hypertension and renal failure. Low-dose heparin should be infused via the UAC to reduce the risk of catheter occlusion. For intravascular thrombosis, consider intravenous infusion of Alteplase (rt-PA).

- Misplacement of UVC and venous thromboembolism.
- Catheter breakage.

Intraosseous lines

These are in routine use in paediatric resuscitation and can be useful in neonates for emergency access to the circulation when other routes have failed. We now keep these as standard equipment on our resuscitation trolleys.

1. Scrub up and put on gown and sterile gloves.
2. Using a full aseptic technique, clean the skin and drape.
3. Insert the intraosseous needle into the anterior medial aspect of the tibia, 1–2 cm below the tuberosity, at an angle of 10–15° towards the foot. Using a twisting motion, insert the needle to a depth of ~1cm. You should feel a sudden give as the needle enters the marrow cavity.
4. Remove the trochar; the needle should stay in place without support.
5. Aspirate a sample of marrow for crossmatch and culture.
6. Attach a syringe and inject 2–3 mL of saline to ensure the needle has penetrated the bone correctly.
7. Start infusing drugs and fluids to restore circulation. Observe for signs of extravasation.

Complications of intraosseous lines include fractures and damage to the growth plate of the tibia. Angle the needle towards the foot to minimize the risk of extravasation and compartment syndrome. Infection is another risk.

Endotracheal intubation

This is one of the most commonly performed life-saving procedures. It is generally accepted that premedication drugs should be used for all elective or semi-elective intubations where intravenous access is established or can easily be obtained. Drugs that are commonly used include fentanyl (preferable to morphine as immediate onset), suxamethonium/atracurium and atropine (may be required only if the baby becomes bradycardic).

The orotracheal route is best for emergency intubations. To minimize hypoxia, each intubation attempt should last no more than 20–30 seconds.

1. Position the baby's head in the midline in a neutral position. Do not hyperextend the neck as this makes visualization of the cords more difficult.
2. Use gentle suctioning to clear the oropharynx.
3. Hold the laryngoscope in the left hand and introduce the blade into the right-hand side of the mouth, sweeping the tongue to the left as the blade is advanced.
4. The tip of the blade should be introduced into the vallecula. (In extremely preterm infants, the vallecula may be too small, in which case gently elevate the epiglottis with the laryngoscope blade.)
5. Apply gentle anterior traction to the laryngoscope, avoiding applying pressure to the upper gum. Applying cricoid pressure will help to bring the vocal cords into view.
6. Under direct vision, the endotracheal tube (ETT) tip should be inserted about 1 cm below the cords. Do not try to pass the ETT down the laryngoscope blade as this will obstruct your line of sight. Do not force the ETT through closed cords.
7. Confirm the position of the tube by looking for symmetrical chest wall movement and listening for equal breath sounds over both lung fields. Colorimetric end-tidal CO_2 detectors can be used to confirm that the tube is lying within the trachea.

Table 29.1 Estimated insertion lengths and endotracheal tube (ETT) sizes as given in the work of Kempley (2009)

Gestational age (weeks)	Weight (g)	ETT size (internal diameter mm)	Approx. length for orotracheal route (cm)
23–24	500–600	2–2.5	5.5
25–26	700–800	2.5	6.0
27–29	900–1000	2.5	6.5
30–34	1000–2000	3.0	7–7.5
34–38	2000–3500	3–3.5	7.5–8.0
>38	>3500	3.5–4.0	8.5–9.0

8. Secure the ETT using adhesive tape, or a purpose-made fixation device.
9. After fixation, listen to the breath sounds again and observe chest wall movement. Shorten the ETT to reduce dead space.
10. The ETT position must be confirmed with a chest X-ray. The tip of the ETT is best placed opposite the body of the first thoracic vertebra (T1). Estimated insertion lengths and ETT sizes are given in Table 29.1.

Nasotracheal tubes may be preferred in infants who are very active on the ventilator. Do not use an introducer.

1. Insert the laryngoscope to visualize the oropharynx. Avoid hyperextending the neck.
2. Insert a lubricated straight ETT through the nostril, following the curve of the nasopharynx, until the tip is in line with the glottis.
3. Apply gentle cricoid pressure and advance the tube through the cords under direct vision. Magill's forceps can be used in larger babies to thread the tip of the ETT through the cords.
4. Nasal ETTs are commonly secured with two half-split tapes. One half of each split tape is used to encircle the tube, while the remainder of the tape adheres to a hydrocolloid dressing on the upper lip and cheek.

Complications of intubation

Minor degrees of stridor secondary to laryngeal oedema are common in the first 24 hours following extubation. The risk of iatrogenic intubation injury increases with decreasing gestational age and birth weight. Complications include nasal damage, pharyngeal tear, laryngeal injury including trauma to vocal cords and arytenoids, subglottic stenosis, subglottic granuloma or cysts, tracheal tear, palatal grooves and defective dentition.

Needle thoracocentesis

For a pneumothorax:

1. Confirm the diagnosis: mediastinal shift, abdominal distension and increasing oxygen requirement, transilluminate the chest, chest X-ray if unsure (but do not delay treatment of tension pneumothorax).
2. Scrub up and put on gown and sterile gloves. Using a full aseptic technique, clean the skin and drape.

3. Attach a three-way tap, open to air, to the tubing of the butterfly needle and place under water. The weight of the three-way tap will keep the end of the tubing submerged.
4. Using a non-touch technique, insert the needle into the second intercostal space in the mid-clavicular line.
5. Air will bubble out, confirming the diagnosis of a pneumothorax. If the pneumothorax was under tension, leave the needle in situ, while preparing to insert a formal chest drain.
6. In the case of a simple pneumothorax, a syringe can be attached to the three-way tap to remove any residual air. When all the air has been aspirated, remove the needle and repeat a chest X-ray.

For a pleural tap of effusion:

1. Confirm the diagnosis: reduced/absent breath sounds, chest X-ray or ultrasound to assess size of effusion.
2. Scrub up and put on gown and sterile gloves.
3. Using a full aseptic technique, clean the skin and drape.
4. Using a non-touch technique, insert a cannula needle into the fourth–fifth intercostal space in the mid-axillary line, keeping the needle at right angles to the skin until the pleural space is penetrated. Advance the catheter over the needle and withdraw the needle. Attach a short extension to the catheter and aspirate the pleural fluid slowly with a syringe.
5. When enough fluid has been aspirated, remove the catheter and apply a sterile gauze dressing.

Chest drain insertion

Classic (blunt dissection) method

1. Ensure adequate analgesia with local anaesthetic infiltrated into the skin and opiate parenteral analgesia.
2. Position the infant with a towel under the back so the affected side is raised ~30° above the horizontal. Ask an assistant to hold, or secure, the arm above the infant's head.
3. Scrub up and put on gown and sterile gloves.
4. Using a full aseptic technique, clean the skin and drape.
5. Identify the fourth or fifth intercostal space, mid-axillary line.
6. Assemble the equipment and remove the trochar from the chest drain tube.
7. Using a no. 11 scalpel blade, make a 1 cm long incision in the skin, parallel to and just above the rib. Insert a pair of artery forceps into the incision and, keeping the forceps perpendicular to the chest wall, use blunt dissection to penetrate the muscle layer.
8. The pleura can be incised with the scalpel or opened by applying pressure with the closed tip of the forceps. A definite give will be felt as the tip of the forceps pierces the pleura. Use your index finger as a guard to prevent the forceps from penetrating too deeply.
9. Keep the forceps in place and thread the chest drain tube between the opened tips of the forceps and advance it 2–3 cm into the pleural space.
10. Direct the chest drain anteriorly and apically to drain a pneumothorax and posteriorly to drain a pleural effusion. Ensure that all of the side holes in the chest drain tube are contained within the pleural cavity.

11. Connect the tube to the drainage system with an underwater seal and look for bubbling and/or a swinging meniscus.
12. Secure the chest drain to the skin with a simple suture: the ends of the suture should be tied around the chest drain tube four or five times and knotted securely. An additional suture may be required to close the incision. Do not use a purse string suture as this leaves an unsightly scar.
13. Apply a small square of gauze to the insertion site and secure the chest drain tube at right angles to the skin with two transparent adhesive dressings, applied to the tube and chest wall in an 'inverted T'.
14. X-ray to confirm the position of the chest drain and that the pneumothorax has resolved.
15. A low-pressure vacuum (-5–$10\,cmH_2O$) can be applied to the drainage system to assist with drainage of a pneumothorax.
16. If a large pleural effusion is present, control the rate of drainage by intermittent clamping of the drain.

Seldinger technique

If appropriate equipment is available, this is a less traumatic procedure. Straight or pig-tail chest drain tubes are available for use in neonates.

1. Position the baby and clean and drape the skin as before.
2. Infiltrate the skin and subcutaneous tissues with local anaesthetic and make a 0.5 cm incision in the skin. Remember to aspirate on the needle before infiltrating the local anaesthetic. Attach a saline-filled syringe onto the introducer needle and insert the introducer needle into the pleural space, keeping the needle at right angles to the skin. Fluid or bubbles of air should be aspirated into the syringe to confirm that the needle lies in the pleural space.
3. Remove the syringe and pass the guide wire into the pleural space and remove the introducer needle.
4. Thread a dilator over the guide wire and gently dilate the tract, using a twisting motion.
5. Remove the dilator and thread the chest drain tube over the guide wire, angling the tube anteriorly for a pneumothorax and posteriorly for a pleural effusion.
6. Withdraw the guide wire, secure the chest drain in place, connect to the underwater drain and apply an adhesive dressing as described above.
7. Confirm the position of the tube with an X-ray.

Complications of chest drains

- Haemorrhage from intercostal arteries or veins.
- Trauma to the lung, pericardium including haemorrhagic pericardial effusion and tamponade, thoracic duct damage with resultant chylothorax and phrenic nerve injury.
- Infection.
- Failure to drain/re-accumulation of the pneumothorax.

Chest drain removal

Once the pneumothorax or pleural effusion has resolved, clamp the tube for several hours. Removal of the chest drain is also painful and requires systemic analgesia.

1. Remove dressings and clean the skin in the area of the chest drain with antiseptic solution.
2. Remove any suture(s).
3. Pull the chest drain out, keeping the edges of the wound approximated. Apply Steri-strips to close the wound. Use a simple suture if the wound is gaping or if the Steri-strips do not stick. Dress with sterile gauze and cover with a transparent dressing.
4. Perform a chest X-ray to exclude re-accumulation of the pneumothorax.

Needle pericardiocentesis

Consider a diagnosis of tamponade in any baby with a central venous or arterial access who presents with severe cardiorespiratory compromise. Confirm the diagnosis with ultrasound, but do not delay the procedure if the baby is in extremis.

1. Clean the skin. Assemble equipment (FG 21–25 venous cannula, extension set, three-way tap and syringe).
2. Using a non-touch technique, insert the cannula just below the xiphoid cartilage and 0.5 cm to the left of the midline, directing the needle towards the left shoulder while aspirating gently on the syringe.
3. Continue advancing the needle until air or fluid is obtained, usually at a depth of 1–2 cm. Slide the catheter over the needle and remove the needle to avoid traumatizing the heart as the fluid or air is removed.
4. Evacuate as much air or fluid as possible from the pericardial sac. Removal of 5–10 mL of fluid will effect a significant improvement in cardiac output within seconds.

Complications include cardiac puncture, pneumopericardium, pneumothorax and cardiac arrhythmas.

■ Urine collection

Suprapubic aspiration

1. An assistant should hold the baby in a supine, frog-leg position with a pot ready to perform a clean urine catch if the baby has other plans.
2. Using ultrasound, confirm that the bladder is full.
3. Clean the skin between the umbilicus and symphysis pubis with antiseptic solution.
4. Insert the needle through the anterior abdominal wall in the midline, 1 cm above the pubic symphysis. Apply gentle suction with the syringe and advance the needle to a depth of 1–2 cm until urine is obtained. Withdraw the needle and apply pressure over the puncture site with sterile gauze.

Transurethral catheterization

1. Clean the external genitalia with antiseptic solution and allow to dry.
2. Lubricate the outside of the catheter with sterile KY jelly.
3. Using a non-touch technique, insert the catheter through the urethral meatus into the bladder.
4. Urine should drain freely.

5. Fix the catheter to the thigh with adhesive tape and attach to the collecting system.
6. Remove the catheter as soon as possible to minimize the risk of infection.

Complications of urine collection include trauma, haemorrhage and infection.

■ Cerebrospinal fluid collection

Lumbar puncture

Lumbar puncture is performed to collect cerebrospinal fluid (CSF) for investigation of infection or neurometabolic disorders, or for the drainage of CSF in babies with post-haemorrhagic hydrocephalus.

1. The baby should be held by an experienced assistant on a firm surface, in a left-side-down position.
2. Scrub up and put on gown and sterile gloves.
3. Using a full aseptic technique, clean the skin and drape.
4. The assistant then should flex the spine to open the intervertebral spaces.
5. Identify the L4 spinous process, which lies on an imaginary line joining the top of the right and left iliac crests.
6. In a term infant, insert the needle through the midline of the intervertebral space at L3/4 or L4/5, aiming towards the umbilicus. A change in resistance can be felt as the ligamentum flavum and dura are penetrated.
7. Remove the stylet. If an opening pressure measurement is required, a three-way tap and manometer should be attached to the hub of the spinal needle.
8. Collect CSF into sterile universal containers. If there is no flow, carefully rotate the needle. A traumatic tap (with blood-stained CSF that clears as the samples are collected) occurs when the needle damages the epidural venous plexus on the posterior surface of the vertebral bodies. Uniformly blood-stained CSF is seen with intraventricular and, more rarely, subarachnoid haemorrhages.
9. At the end of the procedure, replace the stylet before removing the needle. Apply a sterile dressing.

Ventricular tap

Ventricular tap is performed to drain CSF in babies with obstructive (e.g. post-haemorrhagic) hydrocephalus where lumbar puncture has not been successful (i.e. non-communicative).

1. Confirm that there is progressive ventriculomegaly on cranial ultrasound examination and estimate the depth for needle insertion.
2. Use scissors to trim any hair that overlies the lateral angle of the fontanelle. Do not shave the scalp.
3. An assistant should hold the baby's head in the neutral position.
4. Scrub up and put on gown and sterile gloves.
5. Using a full aseptic technique, clean the skin and drape.
6. Insert the spinal needle at the lateral angle of the fontanelle and advance to the required depth, aiming towards the inner canthus of the eye.
7. Remove the stylet from the needle and attach a three-way tap and manometer to measure the opening pressure.

8. Allow the CSF to drain, or aspirate slowly at a rate of 1–2 mL/min. Remove a maximum of 10–15 mL/kg of CSF.
9. Remove the needle and apply pressure for 2–3 minutes until CSF stops leaking from the puncture site. Dress with sterile gauze.

Complications of cerebrospinal fluid drainage

1. Infection – there is a possibility of introducing micro-organisms during CSF sampling. This should be minimized by strict aseptic technique. Babies with suspected central nervous system infections will already be on antibiotics.
2. Haemorrhage – is usually local and settles spontaneously. To minimize the risk a normal clotting and platelet count should be confirmed in sick babies prior to CSF drainage.
3. Trauma to brain tissue will occur with repeated venticular taps – parenchymal cysts frequently develop along the needle track. The need for repeated ventricular taps is an indication to refer to a neurosurgeon for consideration of a ventriculoperitoneal shunt or reservoir.

■ Reference

Kempley, S (2009) Neonatal endotracheal intubation: the 7–8–9 rule. *Archives of Disease in Childhood. Education and Practice Edition*, **94**: 29.

■ Further reading

Harding, S (2012) Procedures. In Rennie, JM (ed.) *Rennie & Roberton's Textbook of Neonatology*, 5th edition. Edinburgh: Elsevier, pp. 126–91.

PART 6
Useful information

Appendix 1
Growth charts

All babies should be plotted on the age-appropriate growth chart after birth. From birth until 2 weeks after the expected date of delivery (EDD) the measurements should be plotted on the **23–42 weeks' gestation** chart. Gestational correction is always required when plotting babies born before 37 completed weeks of gestation.

In preterm infants, if the EDD is not known, plot birth weight at the exact gestational age and then calculate the date of the *next completed* week (e.g. for date of birth (DOB) 24/2/09 at 27 weeks + 3 days' gestation, date at 28 weeks' gestation will be 28/2/09). Then write in the date (day and month only) at each completed week of gestation until the EDD is reached. If the EDD is known, write into the date box marked EDD, then work backwards on the 23–42 weeks chart, writing in the date (day and month only) for each completed week of gestation until birth gestation is reached.

Weight and head circumference should be plotted weekly for all babies resident on the neonatal unit as part of their ongoing care. As good nutrition is the key to most neonatal care, this should be seen as an essential part of the care of the infant and not as a weekly chore.

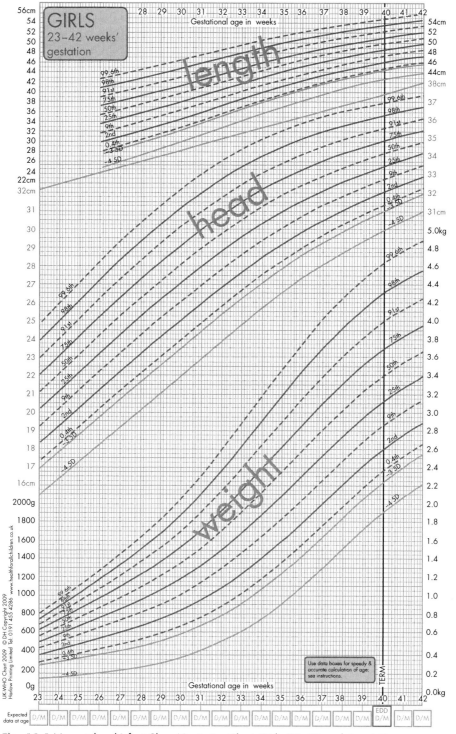

Fig. A1.1 Neonatal and Infant Close Monitoring Chart. Girls: 23–42 weeks' gestation. Reproduced with permission of the Royal College of Paediatrics and Child Health

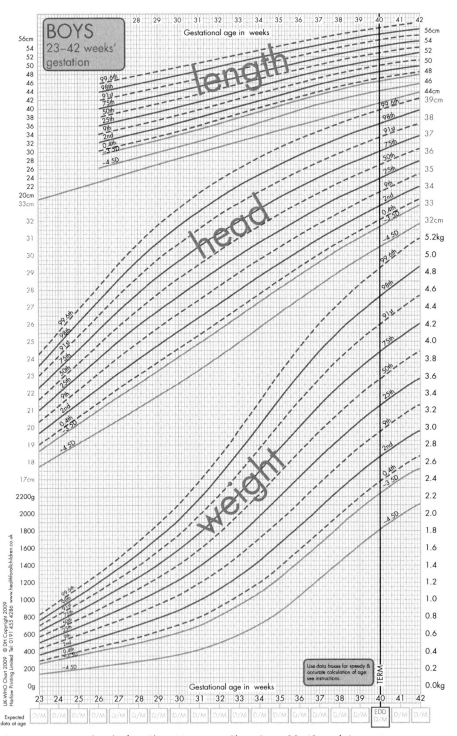

Fig. A1.2 Neonatal and Infant Close Monitoring Chart. Boys: 23–42 weeks' gestation. Reproduced with permission of the Royal College of Paediatrics and Child Health

Appendix 2
Assessing the ill neonate

Many attempts have been made to develop scoring systems which can be applied to neonates in the first few hours of life.

■ Respiratory severity scoring

1. Alveolar–arterial oxygen difference (A–aDO$_2$): this requires a calculation of the alveolar oxygen tension (PAO_2) using the alveolar air equation:

$$PAO_2 = PIO_2 - \frac{PACO_2}{R} + \{PACO_2 \times FIO_2 \times \frac{1 - R}{R}\}$$

where:

- PIO_2 is the partial pressure of inspired O$_2$ in mmHg and equals 160 mmHg when breathing air at sea level;
- FIO_2 [as a fraction] × 760 [atmospheric pressure] – 47 [water vapour pressure];
- $PACO_2$ is the alveolar CO$_2$ partial pressure – assumed to be the same as $PaCO_2$, in mmHg;
- R is the respiratory quotient – assumed to be 0.8.

The A–aDO$_2$ is then the arterial PaO_2 subtracted from the PAO_2. A normal adult breathing air with a PaO_2 of 100 mmHg has an A–aDO$_2$ of 8 mmHg, whereas a baby with a PaO_2 of 50 mmHg in 100% oxygen has an A–aDO$_2$ of 628 mmHg. Babies with an A–aDO$_2$ of more than 610 mmHg are in serious trouble.

2. a–AO$_2$ ratio (arterial–alveolar oxygen ratio).

This also requires a calculation of the PAO_2 as above. The ratio of PaO_2 and PAO_2 is then expressed numerically.

In general, babies with a–AO$_2$ ratios < 0.1 are seriously ill.

3. Oxygenation index OI.
4.

$$OI = \frac{\text{mean airways pressure (cm H}_2\text{O)} \times F_1O_2}{PaO_2 \text{ (post-ductal) mmHg}} \times 100$$

The units are the same as for calculating A–aDO$_2$.
An OI >40 identifies a baby with a severe oxygenation deficit

Birth weight (g) and gestation (weeks):

The maximum (worst) score for birth weight and gestation is 15, which is obtained for a 22-week male infant of less than 501 g birth weight

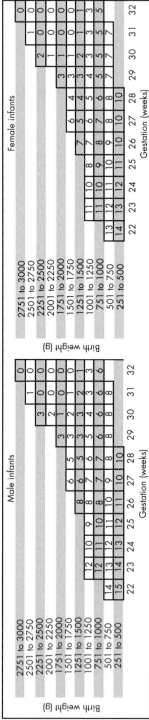

Male infants and **Female infants** — Birth weight (g) versus Gestation (weeks) score grids.

Temperature at admission (°C):

Temperature at admission (°C)	
≤29.6	5
29.7 to 31.2	4
31.3 to 32.8	3
32.9 to 34.4	2
34.5 to 36.0	1
36.1 to 37.5	0
37.6 to 39.1	1
39.2 to 40.7	2
≥40.8	3

Base excess (mmol/L):

Base excess (mmol/L)	
<−26	7
−26 to −23	6
−22 to −18	5
−17 to −13	4
−12 to −8	3
−7 to −3	2
−2 to 2	1
≥3	0

Sex, birth weight (g) and gestation (weeks):
Temperature at admission (°C):
Base excess (mmol/L):

The logistic regression equation relating CRIB II to mortality (CRIB II algorithm) is:

Log odds of mortality $= G = -6.476 + 0.450 \times$ CRIB II

Probability of mortality $= \exp(G)/[1 + \exp(G)]$

The range of possible CRIB II scores is 0 to 27

Total CRIB II score

Fig. A2.1 Clinical Risk Index for Babies (CRIB) II scoring

Clinical Risk Index for Babies – CRIB II score

This is a simple scoring system to estimate the mortality risk for neonates based on the following criteria:

- gender;
- gestation weeks;
- birth weight;
- admission temperature;
- base excess.

A number of other scoring systems are in use, including the Score for Neonatal Acute Physiology (SNAP II) and a simplified version (SNAPE II). Overall CRIB II appears to be one of the most discriminatory, although risk adjustment using all scores is imperfect. An online calculator for CRIB score is available at www.sfar.org/scores2/crib22.html.

Further reading

Gagliardi, L, Cavazza, A, Brunelli, A, *et al.* (2004) Assessing mortality risk in very low birthweight infants: a comparison of CRIB, CRIB-II, and SNAPPE-II. *Archives of Disease in Childhood. Fetal and Neonatal Edition* 89(5): F419–22.

Parry, G, Tucker J, Tarnow-Mordi, W (2003) UK Neonatal Staffing Study Collaborative Group. CRIB II: an update of the clinical risk index for babies score. *Lancet*, 361(9371): 1789–91.

Appendix 3
Normal blood pressure

Term neonates

Good normative data on blood pressure in healthy term newborns are surprisingly hard to find. Various techniques can be used to measure blood pressure, while indwelling arterial pressure measurements are the 'gold standard'. The technique is clearly invasive and study populations in which this technique has been used are, by definition, not 'normal' babies. Most studies in healthy term babies use non-invasive oscillometric techniques; overall an association is seen with postnatal age and possibly with birth weight. Table A3.1 shows that a normal term newborn baby has a blood pressure of around 65/45 mmHg (mean 50) in the first few days of life; a systolic blood pressure of over 90 mmHg is usually considered hypertensive.

Preterm infants

As with term neonates what constitutes a 'normal' blood pressure is difficult to define. Several studies have demonstrated that the blood pressure of preterm babies rises rapidly over the first few days of life and continues gradually to increase over the first 2 weeks. In assessing a preterm infant in the first few days a basic start point is that the mean blood pressure is approximately equal to the gestational age in weeks, for infants born between 24 and 32 weeks (Fig. A3.1). However, blood pressure is generally being used as a surrogate of tissue perfusion, and interpretation of blood pressure should also take into account other factors such as capillary refill, urine output and blood lactate measurements as proxy measures of end-organ perfusion. Also take care in infants with 'low blood pressure' resulting from a low diastolic pressure in the presence of a patent ductus arteriosus.

By 2 weeks of life blood pressure has normally stabilized. This has led Dionne *et al.* (2012) to devise a helpful table of values of normal blood pressure (Table A3.2).

Table A3.1 Normal blood pressure (BP) by day of life in 406 healthy term newborns (Kent *et al.* 2007)

BP in mmHg	Day 1 (range)	Day 2 (range)	Day 3 (range)	Day 4 (range)
Systolic	65 (46–94)	68 (46–91)	69.5 (51–93)	70 (60–88)
Mean	48 (31–63)	51 (37–68)	44.5 (26–61)	54 (41–65)
Diastolic	45 (24–57)	43 (27–58)	52 (36–70)	46 (34–57)

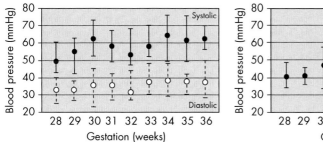 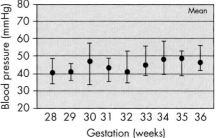

Fig. A3.1 Tenth, 50th and 90th percentiles of systolic, diastolic and mean blood pressure plotted for each week of gestation on day 2 of life. From Meskell *et al.* (2009) with permission

Table A3.2 Estimated blood pressure values after 2 weeks of age in infants from 26 to 44 weeks postconceptional age (from Dionne *et al.* 2012, with permission)

Postconceptional age		50th percentile	95th percentile	99th percentile
44 weeks	Systolic	88	105	110
	Diastolic	50	68	73
	Mean	63	80	85
42 weeks	Systolic	85	98	102
	Diastolic	50	65	70
	Mean	62	76	81
40 weeks	Systolic	80	95	100
	Diastolic	50	65	70
	Mean	60	76	80
38 weeks	Systolic	77	92	97
	Diastolic	50	65	70
	Mean	59	74	79
36 weeks	Systolic	72	87	92
	Diastolic	50	65	70
	Mean	57	72	77
34 weeks	Systolic	70	85	90
	Diastolic	40	55	60
	Mean	50	65	70
32 weeks	Systolic	68	83	88
	Diastolic	40	55	60
	Mean	49	64	69
30 weeks	Systolic	65	80	85
	Diastolic	40	55	60
	Mean	48	63	68

Postconceptional age		50th percentile	95th percentile	99th percentile
28 weeks	Systolic	60	75	80
	Diastolic	38	50	54
	Mean	45	58	63
26 weeks	Systolic	55	72	77
	Diastolic	30	50	56
	Mean	38	57	63

■ References

Dionne, JM, Abitbol, CL, Flynn, JT (2012) Hypertension in infancy: diagnosis, management and outcome. *Pediatric Nephrology*, **27**(1): 17–32. Erratum in *Pediatric Nephrology* (2012) **27**(1): 159–60.

Kent, AL, Kecskes, Z, Shadbolt, B, Falk, MC (2007) Normative blood pressure data in the early neonatal period. *Pediatric Nephrology*, **22**: 1335–41.

Kent, AL, Meskell, S, Falk, MC, Shadbolt, B (2009) Normative blood pressure data in non-ventilated premature neonates from 28–36 weeks gestation. *Pediatric Nephrology*, **24**: 141–6.

Appendix 4
The neonatal electrocardiogram

The electrocardiogram (ECG) remains essential in the study of cardiac arrhythmias and can help in assessing chamber enlargement, hypertrophy and strain. A systematic approach to the ECG enables the maximum information to be extracted from it and should include an assessment of rate, rhythm, axis, atrial and ventricular information.

■ Rate and rhythm

The normal heart rate for babies varies according to age. On the first day the range is 95–145 with a mean of 120 beats/min. By the end of the first month the mean heart rate is 150 beats/min with a range of 115–185. Extrasystoles of supraventricular or ventricular origin are not rare, but in the absence of congenital heart disease they usually subside spontaneously over the first week. In sinus rhythm every QRS complex is accompanied by a P wave; the distance between the two is the PR interval. The P waves should be upright in lead I and V_6. If they are not, either the atria are not normally sited or there is a supraventricular rhythm.

The PR interval

The PR interval is measured in lead II from the beginning of the P wave to the beginning of the QRS complex. It increases slightly with age and is normally of no more than 0.12 seconds' duration in neonates. The PR interval is reduced to less than 0.07 seconds in nodal rhythm and in Wolff–Parkinson–White syndrome. A long PR interval indicates first-degree block. This can be familial or due to structural disease, e.g. atrial septal defect.

■ The axis

The cardiac axis can be estimated by looking at which limb lead (I, II, III, aVR, aVL or aVF) the QRS complex has the greatest net positive deflection. This is done by counting the number of small squares of the positive R deflection and subtracting any downward Q or S deflections. The angle is then estimated from the chart in Fig. A4.1. An alternative method is to look at two perpendicular leads, e.g. leads I and aVF, and calculating the net positive or negative deflections for each lead. These are then used to create a two-dimensional vector from which the axis can be drawn. The mean neonatal frontal QRS axis is + 135° with a normal range between + 110° and + 180°. There is a rapid change to the left (i.e. a less positive or more negative axis) in the first month, to a mean axis of + 75°, and then a further, more gradual, change to the left until adult life is reached. Left axis deviation (sometimes called a superior axis) is seen in tricuspid atresia, atrioventricular septal defects and babies with pulmonary stenosis and Noonan syndrome.

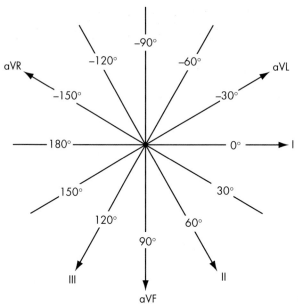

Fig. A4.1 Mean QRS axis

■ Information about the atria

The P wave

A peaked P wave more than 3 mm tall, best seen in lead II and V_1, indicates right atrial enlargement. This is seen in anomalies with a high right atrial pressure, tricuspid and pulmonary atresia, or a very dilated right atrium, Ebstein's anomaly. The normal P wave is not more than 2.5 mm high and lasts for less than 0.12 seconds. A bifid P wave lasting more than 0.12 seconds, or late inversion of the P wave greater than 1 mm in V_1, suggests left atrial enlargement.

■ Information about the ventricles

The QRS complex

QRS voltages may be very low in the first week, particularly in preterm babies. At birth the R wave should be dominant in V_1, and in V_6 the S wave is commonly, but not invariably, dominant. However, by 1 month the R wave should be dominant in V_6 too. The RS complex represents depolarization of the ventricles and rarely exceeds 0.08 seconds in duration. Complexes exceeding 0.08 seconds indicate prolongation of intraventricular conduction, but partial right bundle branch block is the normal pattern in 20% of neonates. The QRS complexes evolve across the chest leads from a dominant R in V_1 to more S in V_6.

The Q wave

The Q wave represents septal depolarization. Absent (40%) or small Q waves may be seen in the left chest leads in the perinatal period, but deflections of more than

The neonatal electrocardiogram

Table A4.1 Criteria for diagnosing ventricular hypertrophy on neonatal ECGs

Right ventricular hypertrophy
1. R in V$_1$ 20 mm or more
2. S in V$_6$ 0–7 days 14 mm or more, 8–30 days 10 mm or more
3. R/S ratio in V$_1$ 0–3 months 6.5:1 or more
4. T upright in V$_1$ after 4 days
5. Q wave in V$_1$
Left ventricular hypertrophy
1. S in V$_1$ more than 20 mm
2. R in V$_6$ more than 20 mm
3. Q in V$_5$, V$_6$ more than 4 mm

4 mm are abnormal and indicate septal hypertrophy. A Q wave in V$_1$ is abnormal and indicates right ventricular hypertrophy, or may be seen in congenitally corrected transposition. An rsR pattern is normal but may easily be confused with a qR pattern, if the primary r wave is very small.

The ST segment

Normally this begins from a point within 2 mm of the isoelectric line (TP segment). Elevation of the ST segment is seen with myocardial injury, in myocarditis or acute ischaemia. ST segment depression may occur with electrolyte disturbances, digoxin therapy, ischaemia, 'strain' – pressure overload of either ventricle – and endocardial fibroelastosis.

The QT interval

The QT interval is measured from the beginning of the QRS complex to the end of the T wave. It varies with heart rate and should not exceed 0.28 seconds at a heart rate of 160 beats/min, and 0.31 seconds at a heart rate of 120 beats/min. The QT interval corrected for heart rate, or QTc, is the QT interval divided by the square root of the RR interval. The RR interval measured is the one immediately preceding the QRS complex whose QT interval has been measured. There is disagreement about the upper limit of the normal QTc interval in neonates, with no published data on the values in preterm babies. Certainly a value of above 0.5 seconds is prolonged. A prolonged QTc is seen with hypocalcaemia, and marked prolongation is seen with the rare QT prolongation syndrome, which is associated with potentially lethal ventricular arrhythmias.

Table A4.2 ECG standards (neonatal period)

Age in days	Centile	Rate	QRS axis	PR (ms)	P II (mV)	R V$_1$ (mV)	R V$_5$ (mV)	R V$_6$ (mV)	S V$_1$ (mV)	S V$_6$ (mV)	R/S ratio V$_1$
0–1	95%	150	+185	140	0.25	2.35	1.8	1.0	1.8	0.8	7.0
	50%	120	+135	105	0.16	1.3	1.0	0.4	0.8	0.3	2.5
	5%	100	+90	82	0.07	0.7	0.3	0.1	0.1	0.0	0.4
1–3	95%	150	+185	132	0.25	2.4	1.9	1.0	1.8	0.75	6.0
	50%	120	+135	105	0.16	1.5	1.1	0.4	0.8	0.3	2.5
	5%	100	+90	85	0.05	0.7	0.4	0.1	0.1	0.0	0.4
3–7	95%	160	+180	130	0.27	2.1	1.9	1.1	1.5	0.8	7.0
	50%	125	+135	103	0.17	1.25	1.3	0.5	0.7	0.3	2.9
	5%	100	+90	80	0.08	0.5	0.5	0.15	0.1	0.0	0.5
7–30	95%	175	+150	128	0.28	1.7	2.1	1.3	1.0	0.8	6.3
	50%	145	+110	100	0.18	1.0	1.4	0.5	0..4	0.3	3.7
	5%	110	+75	75	0.08	0.4	0.6	0.25	0.1	0.0	1.0

Values relate to term neonates. From: Daignon *et al.* (1979/80) Normal ECG standards for infants and children. *Pediatric Cardiology*, **1**: 123–31 and 133–52.

At a paper speed of 25 mm/s, 1 mm = 0.04 s = a small square; 5 mm = 0.2 s = 1 large square: for the rate, count the number of divisions between two RR complexes and divide into 300.

Appendix 5

Normal biochemical values in the newborn

The values here have been derived from many sources in the literature and appendices to major textbooks of neonatology. For simplicity in many cases we have rounded up or down some numbers.

Table A5.1 Normal blood urea and electrolyte values

	Preterm	Full term	1 week	1 month	Child
Na (mmol/L)	130–145	130–145	–	–	136–145
K (mmol/L)	4.5–7.2	3.6–5.7	4.0–6.0	4.0–6.0	3.3–4.6
Cl (mmol/L)	95–117	92–109	92–109	92–109	95–108
Ca (mmol/L)	1.75–2.80	2.10–2.70	2.20–2.70	2.15–2.65	2.2–2.5
PO$_4$ (mmol/L)	1.00–2.60	1.8–3.0	1.4–3.0	1.7–3.0	–
Mg (mmol/L)	0.62–1.25	0.7–1.0	0.85–1.05	0.65–1.0	0.7–0.95
Urea (mmol/L)	0.5–6.7	1.6–10.0	1.6–5.0	1.9–5.2	3.3–6.6
Creatinine µmol/L	55–150	35–115	14–86	12–48	–

Other blood biochemical values

Albumin	19–44 g/L
Alkaline phosphatase	125–373 IU/L up to 500 IU/L in preterm babies
Alpha-1-antitrypsin	1.0–2.2 g/L (values <1.0 suggest deficiency)
Alpha-fetoprotein	<55,000 U/mL at term. Levels decline rapidly after birth, and are higher still in preterm babies
Ammonia	20–160 µmol/L
Aspartate aminotransferase	20–100 IU/L
Bicarbonate	18–22 mmol/L
Bilirubin	up to 200 µmol/L in the first 10 days
	Conjugated bilirubin <20 µmol/L
Cholesterol	1.5–4.0 mmol/L

Copper	1.4–11.0 μmol/L
Cortisol	330–1700 nmol/L (at birth), 1st week 200–770 nmol/L
Creatinine kinase	< 500 IU/L (may be higher <hours)
Ferritin	150–900 μg/L (preterm infants)
Folic acid	5–21 ng/mL
Red cell folate	>160 ng/mL
Gamma-glutamyl transpeptidase	<250 IU/L in the first 2 weeks <150 IU/L 2–4 weeks
Growth hormone (1st week)	15–404 ng/mL
17-hydroxyprogesterone	<30 nmol/L (2–7 days), <14 nmol/L (>6 days)
IgA	<0.1 g/L
IgG	5–17 g/L
IgM	<0.2 g/L
Immunoreactive trypsin	up to 120 μg/L
Insulin	Usually <20 mU/L; should suppress with hypoglycaemia
Iron	10–33 μmol/L (higher at birth)
Lactate	0.8–1.2 mmol/L after 24 hours
Lactate dehydrogenanse	325–1825 μ/L
Osmolality	275–300 mosmol/kg H_2O
Proteins: total	55–75 g/L (5.0–7.5 g%)
Proteins: albumin	25–45 g/L (2.5–4.5 g%)
Pyruvate	up to 120 μmol/L
Testosterone	<10 nmol/L (male) <2 nmol/L (female)
Thyroid-stimulating hormone	<10 mU/L after 3 days
Free thyroxine (T_4)	75–300 nmol/L (<200 in pre term infant >100 at term)
Triiodothyronine (T_3)	0.8–4.0 nmol/L
Triglycerides	0.06–1.60 mmol/L (5–140 mg%)
Uric acid	0.15–0.5 mmol/L
Vitamin A	15–50 μg/dL
Vitamin D	7–19 μg/dL
Vitamin E	1.0–3.5 μg/dL
Zinc	8–20 μmol/L

Normal urine biochemistry

Calcium	0.2–1.6 mmol/L	0.05–0.21 mmol/kg/24h
Phosphate	<10 mmol/L	5–25 μmol/kg/24h
Sodium	1–15 mmol/L	0.8–2.2 mmol/kg/24h (much higher in preterm infants)
Potassium	2–28 mmol/L	0.2–5.0 mmol/kg/24h
Chloride	5–30 mmol/L	1.3–3.3 mmol/kg/24h
Urea	1–9 mmol/L	1.3–5.9 mmol/kg/24h
Creatinine clearance	15–25 mL/min/1.73m^2 in preterm infants <1 week 20–45 mL/min/1.83m^2 in full-term infants	
7 Ketosteroids	<2.5 mg/24h	
Pregnanetriol	<0.2 mg/24h	

Appendix 6
Haematological
values in the newborn

The normal haemoglobin at birth is about 14 g/dL in babies at 28 weeks' gestation, and about 17.0 g/dL at term (Table A6.1). The haematocrit is about 55% at term; the capillary haematocrit is always about 15% higher than arterial or venous haematocrit. Up to $0.5 \times 10^9/L$ nucleated red cells may be present in the blood of the normal term neonate, and up to $1.5 \times 10^9/L$ in the premature baby. Very high levels of nucleated red cells have been recorded after fetal stress and haemorrhage. These usually disappear within 48 hours of delivery.

Following the rise in PaO_2 after delivery, the level of erythropoietin falls, and it is undetectable in the plasma for 1–2 months. This is associated with a dramatic decrease in red cell production, which is very high in fetal life. In both full-term and premature babies the haemoglobin falls as a consequence, and in premature babies it reaches a nadir of 7–8 g/dL by the end of the second month. After the first few days when the reticulocyte count is $150–200 \times 10^9/L$ (about 4–5%), it stays below $50 \times 10^9/L$ (about 1–2%) for most of the first 1–2 months in all babies (Table A6.1).

The white blood count varies considerably during the first month of life in term and premature babies. The normal values for neutrophils and lymphocytes are given in Table A6.2.

The platelet count in the neonate averages $150–450 \times 10^9/L$, but it may be up to $600 \times 10^9/L$ by 2–4 months. Platelet function is virtually normal in the neonatal period; although abnormalities of function can be demonstrated in a test tube, the bleeding time is normal.

The reference ranges for coagulation times are given in Table A6.3.

Table A6.1 Haematological values during the first weeks of life in term babies (95% intervals in brackets) (adapted from Brugnara and Platt 1998)

Value	Cord blood	Day 1	Day 3	Day 7	Day 14
Haemoglobin (g/dL)	16.8 (13.7–20.1)	18.4 (14–22)	17.8 (13.8–21.8)	17.0 (14–20)	16.8 (13.8–19.8)
Venous Hct (%)	53	58	55	54	52
Red cells ($10^3/$ mm^3)	5.25	5.8	5.6	5.2	5.1
MCV (FL)	107	108	99	98	96

Hct, haematocrit; MCV, mean cell volume.

Value	Cord blood	Day 1	Day 3	Day 7	Day 14
MCH (pg)	34	35	33	32.5	31.5
MCHC (%)	31.7	32.5	33	33	33
Reticulocytes (%)	3–7	3–7	1–3	0–1	0–1
Nucleated RBC/mm³	500	200	0–5	0	0

Hct, haematocrit; MCH, mean corpuscular haemoglobin; MCHC, mean corpuscular haemoglobin concentration; MCV, mean cell volume; RBC, red blood cell.

Table A6.2 Neutrophil and lymphocyte count $\times$ 10^9/L (mean and range) in full-term and premature babies (derived from various sources in the literature)

Age	Neutrophil		Lymphocyte	
	Full term	Premature	Full term	Premature
0	11 (5–26)	5 (2–9)	5.5 (2–11)	4 (2.5–6)
24 hours	11 (5–21)	7.5 (3–9)	5 (2–9)	3.5 (1.5–3)
72 hours	5.5 (2–7)	4.5 (3–7)	3.5 (2–5)	3 (1.5–4)
1 week	5 (2–8)	3.5 (2–7)	5 (3–6)	4.3 (2.5–7.5)
1 month	3.8 (1–9)	2.5 (1–9)	6 (3–15)	6.5 (2–15)

Table A6.3 Reference values for coagulation tests in healthy term infants (means and standard deviations) and preterm infants (means and 95% range)

Test	Term infant			Preterm infant		
	Day 1	Day 5	Day 30	Day 1	Day 5	Day 30
PT (s)	13 ± 1.43	12.4 ± 1.46	11.8 ± 1.25	13 (10.6–16.2)	12.5 (10.0–15.3)	11.8 (10.0–13.6)
APPT (s)	42.9 ± 5.8	42.6 ± 8.62	40.4 ± 7.42	53.6 (27.5–79.4)	50.5 (26.9–74.1)	44.7 (26.9–62.5)
TT (s)	23.5 ± 2.38	23.1 ± 3.07	24.3 ± 2.44	24.8 (19.2–30.4)	24.1 (18.8–29.4)	24.4 (18.8–29.9)
Fibrinogen (g/L)	2.83 ± 0.58	3.12 ± 0.75	2.7 ± 0.54	2.43 (1.5–3.73)	2.8 (1.6–4.2)	2.54 (1.5–4.14)

APPT, activated partial thromboplastin time; PT, prothrombin time; TT, thrombin time.

References

Brugnara, C, Platt, OS (1998) The neonatal erythrocyte and its disorders. In Nathan, DG, Orkin, SH (eds) *Nathan and Oski's Haematology of Infancy and Childhood*, 5th edition. Philadelphia: WB Saunders, pp. 19–52.

Appendix 7

Normal cerebrospinal fluid values in the newborn

Table A7.1 Normal values of neonatal cerebrospinal fluid. All values are given as mean and range

Type of infant	White cell count (count/mm³)	Protein (g/L)	Glucose (mmoL/L)
Preterm <28 days	9 (0–30)	1 (0.5–2.5)[a]	3 (1.5–5.5)
Term <28 days	6 (0–21)	0.6 (0.3–2.0)[a]	3 (1.5–5.5)

[a]Protein values are higher in the first week of life and depend on the red cell count.

- A white cell count of more than 21/mm³ with a protein value of more than 1 g/L with less than 1000 red cells is suspicious of meningitis.
- A high white cell count with a negative gram stain is highly suspicious of herpes simplex encephalopathy. These infants must be treated with aciclovir in addition to antibiotics.
- Cerebrospinal fluid (CSF) glucose is usually 70–80% of plasma glucose, and at least 50% of it. Take the plasma glucose sample before doing the lumbar puncture (LP) to avoid the effect of stress.

■ Traumatic lumbar puncture

Traumatic LP is common in the newborn (incidence varies depending on the definition). It has been suggested by various authors that it is possible to apply a formula to compare observed and predicted white cell counts in CSF samples with high red cell counts thought to be due to a 'traumatic tap'. None of the formulae can be used with confidence, and most recent reports doubt their value (Greenberg *et al.* 2008). In suspicious clinical cases the appropriate course is to repeat the LP after 24–48 hours and to treat for meningitis in the meanwhile. A normal CSF result obtained on the repeat specimen probably excludes meningitis.

■ Reference

Greenberg, RG, Smith, PB, Cotton, CM, *et al.* (2008) Adjustment of cerebrospinal fluid cell counts for a traumatic lumbar puncture does not aid diagnosis of meningitis in neonates. *Pediatric Infectious Disease Journal*, 27: 1047–51.

Index

Golden hour, 47
Graft versus host disease, 267
Graseby monitor, 55
Graves' disease, 25, 73
Group B beta-haemolytic *Streptococcus*, 11, 46, 127, 188
Growth charts, 366–368
Guedel airway, 42
Guthrie blood spots, 255
Guthrie card, 48

H

Index